Lecture Notes in Computer Science 5624

Commenced Publication in 1973
Founding and Former Series Editors:
Gerhard Goos, Juris Hartmanis, and Jan van Leeuwen

W0080509

Ben-Tzion Karsh (Ed.)

Ergonomics and Health Aspects of Work with Computers

International Conference, EHAWC 2009
Held as Part of HCI International 2009
San Diego, CA, USA, July 19-24, 2009
Proceedings

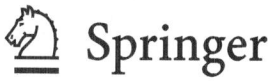 Springer

Volume Editor

Ben-Tzion Karsh
University of Wisconsin-Madison
Department of Industrial and Systems Engineering
Madison, WI 53706-15721513, USA
E-mail: bkarsh@engr.wisc.edu

Library of Congress Control Number: Applied for

CR Subject Classification (1998): H.5, H.4, C.3, I.5, K.6, H.5.2

LNCS Sublibrary: SL 3 – Information Systems and Application,
incl. Internet/Web and HCI

ISSN   0302-9743
ISBN-10   3-642-02730-X Springer Berlin Heidelberg New York
ISBN-13   978-3-642-02730-7 Springer Berlin Heidelberg New York

springer.com

© Springer-Verlag Berlin Heidelberg 2009
Printed in Germany

Typesetting: Camera-ready by author, data conversion by Scientific Publishing Services, Chennai, India
Printed on acid-free paper   SPIN: 12703876   06/3180   5 4 3 2 1 0

Foreword

The 13th International Conference on Human–Computer Interaction, HCI International 2009, was held in San Diego, California, USA, July 19–24, 2009, jointly with the Symposium on Human Interface (Japan) 2009, the 8th International Conference on Engineering Psychology and Cognitive Ergonomics, the 5th International Conference on Universal Access in Human–Computer Interaction, the Third International Conference on Virtual and Mixed Reality, the Third International Conference on Internationalization, Design and Global Development, the Third International Conference on Online Communities and Social Computing, the 5th International Conference on Augmented Cognition, the Second International Conference on Digital Human Modeling, and the First International Conference on Human Centered Design.

A total of 4,348 individuals from academia, research institutes, industry and governmental agencies from 73 countries submitted contributions, and 1,397 papers that were judged to be of high scientific quality were included in the program. These papers address the latest research and development efforts and highlight the human aspects of the design and use of computing systems. The papers accepted for presentation thoroughly cover the entire field of human–computer interaction, addressing major advances in knowledge and effective use of computers in a variety of application areas.

This volume, edited by Ben-Tzion Karsh, contains papers in the thematic area of Ergonomics and Health Aspects of Work with Computers, addressing the following major topics:

- Ergonomics and Health in the Workplace
- New Trends in Ergonomics
- Interaction Devices and Environments

The remaining volumes of the HCI International 2009 Proceedings are:

- Volume 1, LNCS 5610, Human–Computer Interaction—New Trends (Part I), edited by Julie A. Jacko
- Volume 2, LNCS 5611, Human–Computer Interaction—Novel Interaction Methods and Techniques (Part II), edited by Julie A. Jacko
- Volume 3, LNCS 5612, Human–Computer Interaction—Ambient, Ubiquitous and Intelligent Interaction (Part III), edited by Julie A. Jacko
- Volume 4, LNCS 5613, Human–Computer Interaction—Interacting in Various Application Domains (Part IV), edited by Julie A. Jacko
- Volume 5, LNCS 5614, Universal Access in Human–Computer Interaction—Addressing Diversity (Part I), edited by Constantine Stephanidis
- Volume 6, LNCS 5615, Universal Access in Human–Computer Interaction—Intelligent and Ubiquitous Interaction Environments (Part II), edited by Constantine Stephanidis

- Volume 7, LNCS 5616, Universal Access in Human–Computer Interaction—Applications and Services (Part III), edited by Constantine Stephanidis
- Volume 8, LNCS 5617, Human Interface and the Management of Information—Designing Information Environments (Part I), edited by Michael J. Smith and Gavriel Salvendy
- Volume 9, LNCS 5618, Human Interface and the Management of Information—Information and Interaction (Part II), edited by Gavriel Salvendy and Michael J. Smith
- Volume 10, LNCS 5619, Human Centered Design, edited by Masaaki Kurosu
- Volume 11, LNCS 5620, Digital Human Modeling, edited by Vincent G. Duffy
- Volume 12, LNCS 5621, Online Communities and Social Computing, edited by A. Ant Ozok and Panayiotis Zaphiris
- Volume 13, LNCS 5622, Virtual and Mixed Reality, edited by Randall Shumaker
- Volume 14, LNCS 5623, Internationalization, Design and Global Development, edited by Nuray Aykin
- Volume 16, LNAI 5638, The Foundations of Augmented Cognition: Neuroergonomics and Operational Neuroscience, edited by Dylan Schmorrow, Ivy Estabrooke and Marc Grootjen
- Volume 17, LNAI 5639, Engineering Psychology and Cognitive Ergonomics, edited by Don Harris

I would like to thank the Program Chairs and the members of the Program Boards of all thematic areas, listed below, for their contribution to the highest scientific quality and the overall success of HCI International 2009.

Ergonomics and Health Aspects of Work with Computers

Program Chair: Ben-Tzion Karsh

Arne Aarås, Norway
Pascale Carayon, USA
Barbara G.F. Cohen, USA
Wolfgang Friesdorf, Germany
John Gosbee, USA
Martin Helander, Singapore
Ed Israelski, USA
Waldemar Karwowski, USA
Peter Kern, Germany
Danuta Koradecka, Poland
Kari Lindström, Finland

Holger Luczak, Germany
Aura C. Matias, Philippines
Kyung (Ken) Park, Korea
Michelle M. Robertson, USA
Michelle L. Rogers, USA
Steven L. Sauter, USA
Dominique L. Scapin, France
Naomi Swanson, USA
Peter Vink, The Netherlands
John Wilson, UK
Teresa Zayas-Cabán, USA

Human Interface and the Management of Information

Program Chair: Michael J. Smith

Gunilla Bradley, Sweden
Hans-Jörg Bullinger, Germany
Alan Chan, Hong Kong
Klaus-Peter Fähnrich, Germany
Michitaka Hirose, Japan
Jhilmil Jain, USA
Yasufumi Kume, Japan
Mark Lehto, USA
Fiona Fui-Hoon Nah, USA
Shogo Nishida, Japan
Robert Proctor, USA
Youngho Rhee, Korea

Anxo Cereijo Roibás, UK
Katsunori Shimohara, Japan
Dieter Spath, Germany
Tsutomu Tabe, Japan
Alvaro D. Taveira, USA
Kim-Phuong L. Vu, USA
Tomio Watanabe, Japan
Sakae Yamamoto, Japan
Hidekazu Yoshikawa, Japan
Li Zheng, P.R. China
Bernhard Zimolong, Germany

Human–Computer Interaction

Program Chair: Julie A. Jacko

Sebastiano Bagnara, Italy
Sherry Y. Chen, UK
Marvin J. Dainoff, USA
Jianming Dong, USA
John Eklund, Australia
Xiaowen Fang, USA
Ayse Gurses, USA
Vicki L. Hanson, UK
Sheue-Ling Hwang, Taiwan
Wonil Hwang, Korea
Yong Gu Ji, Korea
Steven Landry, USA

Gitte Lindgaard, Canada
Chen Ling, USA
Yan Liu, USA
Chang S. Nam, USA
Celestine A. Ntuen, USA
Philippe Palanque, France
P.L. Patrick Rau, P.R. China
Ling Rothrock, USA
Guangfeng Song, USA
Steffen Staab, Germany
Wan Chul Yoon, Korea
Wenli Zhu, P.R. China

Engineering Psychology and Cognitive Ergonomics

Program Chair: Don Harris

Guy A. Boy, USA
John Huddlestone, UK
Kenji Itoh, Japan
Hung-Sying Jing, Taiwan
Ron Laughery, USA
Wen-Chin Li, Taiwan
James T. Luxhøj, USA

Nicolas Marmaras, Greece
Sundaram Narayanan, USA
Mark A. Neerincx, The Netherlands
Jan M. Noyes, UK
Kjell Ohlsson, Sweden
Axel Schulte, Germany
Sarah C. Sharples, UK

Neville A. Stanton, UK

Xianghong Sun, P.R. China

Andrew Thatcher, South Africa

Matthew J.W. Thomas, Australia

Mark Young, UK

Universal Access in Human–Computer Interaction

Program Chair: Constantine Stephanidis

Julio Abascal, Spain

Ray Adams, UK

Elisabeth André, Germany

Margherita Antona, Greece

Chieko Asakawa, Japan

Christian Bühler, Germany

Noelle Carbonell, France

Jerzy Charytonowicz, Poland

Pier Luigi Emiliani, Italy

Michael Fairhurst, UK

Dimitris Grammenos, Greece

Andreas Holzinger, Austria

Arthur I. Karshmer, USA

Simeon Keates, Denmark

Georgios Kouroupetroglou, Greece

Sri Kurniawan, USA

Patrick M. Langdon, UK

Seongil Lee, Korea

Zhengjie Liu, P.R. China

Klaus Miesenberger, Austria

Helen Petrie, UK

Michael Pieper, Germany

Anthony Savidis, Greece

Andrew Sears, USA

Christian Stary, Austria

Hirotada Ueda, Japan

Jean Vanderdonckt, Belgium

Gregg C. Vanderheiden, USA

Gerhard Weber, Germany

Harald Weber, Germany

Toshiki Yamaoka, Japan

Panayiotis Zaphiris, UK

Virtual and Mixed Reality

Program Chair: Randall Shumaker

Pat Banerjee, USA

Mark Billinghurst, New Zealand

Charles E. Hughes, USA

David Kaber, USA

Hirokazu Kato, Japan

Robert S. Kennedy, USA

Young J. Kim, Korea

Ben Lawson, USA

Gordon M. Mair, UK

Miguel A. Otaduy, Switzerland

David Pratt, UK

Albert "Skip" Rizzo, USA

Lawrence Rosenblum, USA

Dieter Schmalstieg, Austria

Dylan Schmorrow, USA

Mark Wiederhold, USA

Internationalization, Design and Global Development

Program Chair: Nuray Aykin

Michael L. Best, USA

Ram Bishu, USA

Alan Chan, Hong Kong

Andy M. Dearden, UK

Susan M. Dray, USA

Vanessa Evers, The Netherlands

Paul Fu, USA

Emilie Gould, USA

Sung H. Han, Korea
Veikko Ikonen, Finland
Esin Kiris, USA
Masaaki Kurosu, Japan
Apala Lahiri Chavan, USA
James R. Lewis, USA
Ann Light, UK
James J.W. Lin, USA
Rungtai Lin, Taiwan
Zhengjie Liu, P.R. China
Aaron Marcus, USA
Allen E. Milewski, USA

Elizabeth D. Mynatt, USA
Oguzhan Ozcan, Turkey
Girish Prabhu, India
Kerstin Röse, Germany
Eunice Ratna Sari, Indonesia
Supriya Singh, Australia
Christian Sturm, Spain
Adi Tedjasaputra, Singapore
Kentaro Toyama, India
Alvin W. Yeo, Malaysia
Chen Zhao, P.R. China
Wei Zhou, P.R. China

Online Communities and Social Computing

Program Chairs: A. Ant Ozok, Panayiotis Zaphiris

Chadia N. Abras, USA
Chee Siang Ang, UK
Amy Bruckman, USA
Peter Day, UK
Fiorella De Cindio, Italy
Michael Gurstein, Canada
Tom Horan, USA
Anita Komlodi, USA
Piet A.M. Kommers, The Netherlands
Jonathan Lazar, USA
Stefanie Lindstaedt, Austria

Gabriele Meiselwitz, USA
Hideyuki Nakanishi, Japan
Anthony F. Norcio, USA
Jennifer Preece, USA
Elaine M. Raybourn, USA
Douglas Schuler, USA
Gilson Schwartz, Brazil
Sergei Stafeev, Russia
Charalambos Vrasidas, Cyprus
Cheng-Yen Wang, Taiwan

Augmented Cognition

Program Chair: Dylan D. Schmorrow

Andy Bellenkes, USA
Andrew Belyavin, UK
Joseph Cohn, USA
Martha E. Crosby, USA
Tjerk de Greef, The Netherlands
Blair Dickson, UK
Traci Downs, USA
Julie Drexler, USA
Ivy Estabrooke, USA
Cali Fidopiastis, USA
Chris Forsythe, USA
Wai Tat Fu, USA
Henry Girolamo, USA

Marc Grootjen, The Netherlands
Taro Kanno, Japan
Wilhelm E. Kincses, Germany
David Kobus, USA
Santosh Mathan, USA
Rob Matthews, Australia
Dennis McBride, USA
Robert McCann, USA
Jeff Morrison, USA
Eric Muth, USA
Mark A. Neerincx, The Netherlands
Denise Nicholson, USA
Glenn Osga, USA

Dennis Proffitt, USA
Leah Reeves, USA
Mike Russo, USA
Kay Stanney, USA
Roy Stripling, USA
Mike Swetnam, USA
Rob Taylor, UK

Maria L.Thomas, USA
Peter-Paul van Maanen, The Netherlands
Karl van Orden, USA
Roman Vilimek, Germany
Glenn Wilson, USA
Thorsten Zander, Germany

Digital Human Modeling

Program Chair: Vincent G. Duffy

Karim Abdel-Malek, USA
Thomas J. Armstrong, USA
Norm Badler, USA
Kathryn Cormican, Ireland
Afzal Godil, USA
Ravindra Goonetilleke, Hong Kong
Anand Gramopadhye, USA
Sung H. Han, Korea
Lars Hanson, Sweden
Pheng Ann Heng, Hong Kong
Tianzi Jiang, P.R. China

Kang Li, USA
Zhizhong Li, P.R. China
Timo J. Määttä, Finland
Woojin Park, USA
Matthew Parkinson, USA
Jim Potvin, Canada
Rajesh Subramanian, USA
Xuguang Wang, France
John F. Wiechel, USA
Jingzhou (James) Yang, USA
Xiu-gan Yuan, P.R. China

Human Centered Design

Program Chair: Masaaki Kurosu

Gerhard Fischer, USA
Tom Gross, Germany
Naotake Hirasawa, Japan
Yasuhiro Horibe, Japan
Minna Isomursu, Finland
Mitsuhiko Karashima, Japan
Tadashi Kobayashi, Japan

Kun-Pyo Lee, Korea
Loïc Martínez-Normand, Spain
Dominique L. Scapin, France
Haruhiko Urokohara, Japan
Gerrit C. van der Veer, The Netherlands
Kazuhiko Yamazaki, Japan

In addition to the members of the Program Boards above, I also wish to thank the following volunteer external reviewers: Gavin Lew from the USA, Daniel Su from the UK, and Ilia Adami, Ioannis Basdekis, Yannis Georgalis, Panagiotis Karampelas, Iosif Klironomos, Alexandros Mourouzis, and Stavroula Ntoa from Greece.

This conference could not have been possible without the continuous support and advice of the Conference Scientific Advisor, Prof. Gavriel Salvendy, as well as the dedicated work and outstanding efforts of the Communications Chair and Editor of HCI International News, Abbas Moallem.

I would also like to thank for their contribution toward the organization of the HCI International 2009 conference the members of the Human–Computer Interaction Laboratory of ICS-FORTH, and in particular Margherita Antona, George Paparoulis, Maria Pitsoulaki, Stavroula Ntoa, and Maria Bouhli.

Constantine Stephanidis

HCI International 2011

The 14th International Conference on Human–Computer Interaction, HCI International 2011, will be held jointly with the affiliated conferences in the summer of 2011. It will cover a broad spectrum of themes related to human–computer interaction, including theoretical issues, methods, tools, processes and case studies in HCI design, as well as novel interaction techniques, interfaces and applications. The proceedings will be published by Springer. More information about the topics, as well as the venue and dates of the conference, will be announced through the HCI International Conference series website: http://www.hci-international.org/

General Chair
Professor Constantine Stephanidis
University of Crete and ICS-FORTH
Heraklion, Crete, Greece
Email: cs@ics.forth.gr

Table of Contents

Part I: Ergonomics and Health in the Workplace

Part II: New Trends in Ergonomics

Part III: Interaction Devices and Environments

Part I

Ergonomics and Health in the Workplace

Effects of the Workplace Game: A Case-Study into Anticipating Future Behavior of Office Workers

Annelise de Jong[1], Merlijn Kouprie[1], and Evi De Bruyne[2]

[1] Delft University of Technology, Faculty of Industrial Design Engineering
Landbergstraat 15, 2628 CE Delft, The Netherlands
[2] Center for People and Buildings,
Kluyverweg 6, 2629 HT Delft, The Netherlands
{A.M.deJong,E.deBruyne}@tudelft.nl, merlijnkouprie@gmail.com

Abstract. This paper describes the evaluation of the Workplace Game regarding the type of information that it provides. The Workplace Game is intended to make employees aware of the changes in the office and the implications thereof on their behaviour and way of working. The game might also be helpful for designers or architects of future flexible offices. To find out what type of information the game provides and if the information can be of use for designers the game was evaluated in an observational study of two playing sessions. The study showed that the Workplace Game stimulates employees to talk about their behaviour. The game makes players talk about their *future* work behaviour by eliciting information about their *present* work behaviour. However, the game needs adaptation to provide directions for designing future flexible offices. Recommendations how the game can be made helpful to designers of future flexible offices are discussed.

Keywords: flexible office, participatory design game, empathic design, user experience, office layout, innovative office design, office behaviour.

1 Introduction

In modern society the needs of organizations change, not only in terms of internal economic growth but also due to the dynamic environment that they are a part of. It is essential to be able to adapt the workspace to these changing needs to support people in carrying out their activities, for instance in a proper exchange of knowledge when workers are dislocated. This adaptation of workspace often does not only entail a physical change of the office environment, but involves also a social change in people's ways of working.

More and more Dutch companies change their existing office environment into an environment that is designed to stimulate flexibility, adaptation and social interaction. Office innovation often is a radical change and its success is largely dependent on the ways people are able to adapt to this new work environment, especially on the ways people are willing to adapt and committed to the change. Often, the failure of such a change is due to the fact that employees are not sufficiently involved in the creation of this new flexible office. They are not consulted on their present working behaviour or

B.-T. Karsh (Ed.): Ergonomics and Health Aspects, HCII 2009, LNCS 5624, pp. 3–12, 2009.

asked to elaborate on their views of this future office environment. This makes them feel disengaged, which strongly influences their willingness to adapt to the new work environment.

To engage people more into the process of changing the office environment, the Center for People and Building developed The Workplace Game. This game is in essence a communication tool that enables office workers to exchange ideas about their (future) office environment and clarifies future implications of the changes. It consists of a game board that is designed to resemble an office floor plan, and a set of playing cards with multiple-choice questions that are divided into three categories: workplaces, meeting places, and facilities. Since the Workplace Game is designed to make employees have an open discussion about their office environment, the information it generates could be helpful for office space designers or architects, in the way that it could provide them with (future) behavioural information about the office workers [4].

This paper evaluates the Workplace Game in terms of the information that it provides for office space designers. We evaluate what type of information about work behaviour (in future flexible offices) the Workplace Game elicits and draw conclusions for its potential use in designing future flexible office spaces.

2   The Workplace Game

In two previous articles the Workplace Game and its elements are explained in detail [3]. Here we will shortly summarise the goal of the game and introduce the case studies that were analysed in the present research.

2.1   Goal

The Workplace Game is a tool to facilitate user involvement in the implementation and management of innovative offices. It is developed as an evaluation tool to make employees aware of the changes in the office and the implications thereof on their way of working. When companies introduce a new office concept it is not enough to merely introduce the workers to this environment. Office users will need time to adapt to the new work situation, change and learn new behaviours that fit the new office situation. Simply telling the users what to do and how to react to the new situation often does not lead to the desired working behaviour. The Workplace Game facilitates broad user involvement in the process of change and helps people to prepare for and adapt to the future situation.

The game has five goals: (1) it stimulates awareness of employees about the changes (to come) in the work environment, (2) it stimulates discovering of and discussion on *new* desired behaviour, (3) it creates awareness of employees about their own points of view, (4) it stimulates the development of shared values and norms, and (5) it creates input for the development of rules of conduct for the new situation. Using the game to provide input for a design process was not a consideration when it was first developed.

The Workplace Game is aimed at the user (to be) of an innovative office environment and can be played before, during or after the implementation of the new context. One precondition is that the employees must have experience with, rather than knowledge of, flexible offices. The most important ingredients of the game are the questions, which state rather down-to-earth situations and workers' responses to it. Each question is assigned to one of the following themes: information & knowledge, attitude & behaviour, and values & norms, which reflects loosely the layer theory of organisational culture of Schein [3].

2.2 Case Studies

We analyzed two case studies in which the Workplace Game was played. Both were executed in one company that was about to change their existing office structure into a more dynamic structure, thus it was a scenario that was actually happening for the employees of the company and not just a simulation. The Workplace Game was played with the intention of introducing workers to their future working situation. We provided them with materials and guidelines to do so, and at the same time allow us to evaluate the game. Each study contained multiple groups, and each group consisted of several (3 to 5) employees. Before playing the game there was a short introduction, explaining the goal and the rules. The game ended after approximately one hour of playing, and afterwards there was a group discussion. We consider the discussion as part of the Workplace Game, because it forms a significant part of the game where shared values and norms can be created with the entire group. The two studies that we observed differed from each other: In the first session the choice of an innovative flexible office concept was presented without illustration of specific floor plan details, whereas in the second session the architect gave a detailed presentation of the future flexible office. In this paper we analyse both case studies, trying to discover the experiences of the players regarding future flexible offices.

3 People's Experiences

The experiences that people have are unique for each individual. If we can access those experiences we can use them as information and inspiration for designing new products and services. To study these experiences several methods can be applied [6].

Sanders and Dandavate [9] discussed the main issues designers have to deal with when trying to access these user experiences in terms of knowledge. People have *explicit* knowledge, which is knowledge on which they can inform us, because they are able to express this knowledge in words. Designers should listen to what users tell about their past experiences in interviews, however, they should be aware that the user could leave out significant details. Furthermore, designers can look at what people do, which provides them with *observable* information. Designers should look at how people behave and how they use products. Again, however they should be aware that significant information could be missing; one can only observe present behaviour, not future behaviour or needs. To truly understand people's experience a designer needs to gain a deep understanding of users and empathize with them [5]. Understanding how people feel provides the designer with *tacit* knowledge, knowledge that users cannot express in words, but that is of great importance to the designer. It reveals latent needs that can only be recognised in the future. Generative techniques enable us to reveal people's knowledge, feelings and dreams for the future. Figure 1 shows the relationships between the various techniques of gathering data described, and their ability to access these knowledge levels [10].

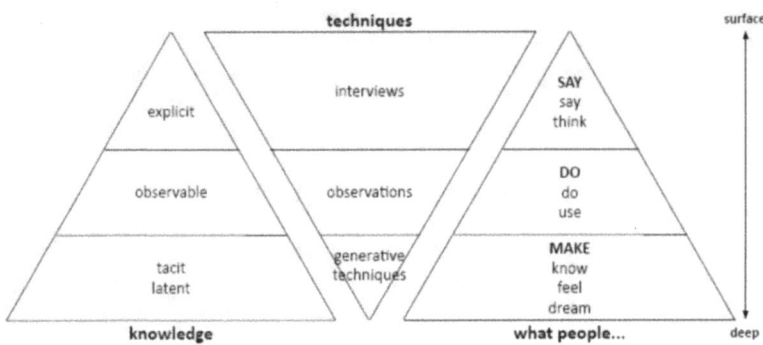

Fig. 1. Different levels of knowledge about experience are accessed by different techniques

3.1 Empathic Design Techniques

Truly understanding people's behaviour and intentions is difficult. Now that we are aware what layer of user knowledge we need to reach to get to know people's dreams for the future, the question is *how* we can reach this layer, and whether the Workplace Game could be used to obtain access to it.

Empathic design aims to *"provide designers access to how users experience their material surroundings and the people in it, including themselves as key characters of their everyday lives"* [7]. Techniques within the field of empathic design, such as generative techniques, often succeed in reaching the deeper levels of user experiences. What these techniques have in common is that they are primarily visual and focus on the creativity of a user, which serves as a common ground for connecting people from different disciplines. A designer can use empathic design techniques to explore the user's life and to gain a deeper understanding of this life. Next to this, the designer is also inspired to imagine new and better possibilities for people. This inspiration can be used to create more useful and enjoyable things for people [5].

According to this theory Sanders [8] developed the 'Make Tools', which facilitate exchange between people who experience products and the people who design for experiencing. The user is given a playful assignment around a certain theme and is asked to create something out if this, in a safe environment. By having users make artefacts and by asking them to tell stories about it they will be able to express their thoughts, feelings, and dreams for the future. The aim of the present study is to reveal whether the Workplace Game provides the designer with a deeper understanding of the user by accessing his or her latent needs, and if so, if the Workplace Game can be used as inspiration for designing *new* flexible offices.

4   Evaluating the Workplace Game

In the study presented here, we did a qualitative analysis of the game. We observed two sessions and compared the results in our analysis. Our aim was to gain an understanding of what type of information about working behaviour (in future flexible offices) the Workplace Game elicits. The main research questions were: do players talk about past, present, and/or future behaviour? And, do players talk about their preferences for their future flexible office? For the analysis we observed players and their utterances during the two sessions of the workplace game.

4.1   The Sessions

Session 1 – Results of the observations. The participants are very open when they start playing the game. It is explained that playing the game is about creating awareness about the workplace and their behaviour in it. One participant expresses her worries in advance that the management will only use the game for creating awareness. She emphasizes that if they would discover a real problem while playing, the management will need to take this problem into consideration. Awareness should not be the only outcome of the game, according to her, she also wants the management to use its output in the implementation of the future office environment.

– The game stimulates talking about behaviour.

Participants mainly talk about their behaviour in certain and specific situations, not about details regarding the layout of the new office. This could be explained by the fact that there already is a lot of clarity about the physical conditions of the new workplace. Questions about facts (*"Can you do office work, like phoning, in a concentration cell?"*) and about rules (*"Can your colleague leave his coat in the hallway, because he has no desk, however he has a locker?"*) are clear and do not need any discussion. Questions about personal feelings (*"Two colleagues are chatting in an open work space, what do you think about this?"*) makes them talk about their own situation (*"I would find it irritating, but I know I am a chatterbox too."*) and they open up to each other. Players conclude that the game made them think about their present behaviour.

– The game stimulates talking about *future* behaviour.

Most questions more or less steer the discussion towards a present or future situation (e.g. *"Imagine, the concentration-cell is always occupied by the time you arrive at the office, what do you do?"*). Sometimes the participants mention that it is difficult to imagine how it could be in the future, but they solve this by focusing on how they value their own and others behaviour at present. They say that whatever changes in the physical layout of the office, the present behaviour should be maintained or avoided. They conclude that it is important to make a list of rules about the most simple situations and behaviour in these situations.

– The game stimulates talking about preferences concerning the future flexible office.

When the question describes a problem that can occur in the workplace and asks for a solution the group discusses about what they would like themselves and what they find irritating. They think of physical solutions for this problem that can cause this negative behaviour to turn positive. For example: *"Meeting places for informal discussions are not used, how can you solve this problem?"* They point out that the rooms are situated too far away from the workplaces, and that the chairs in the rooms are not suitable for discussions, but more for studying individually. They state that if the location and the interior of the rooms were more inviting and attractive, they would go there more often.

Session 2 – Results of the observations. This session starts off a bit awkward, when one of the players does not seem to like to begin with the game, because the introduction of the workshop included a presentation of the design of the future office, which brought up many issues to deal with.

– The game stimulates talking about behaviour.

One participant wants to keep working the way he is working at present and he does not want to change his behaviour. After some questions he realizes that next to his own norms and values there are other people that you have to deal with in an open environment. He opens up a little, and says that he *might* has to adjust his behaviour in *some* situations, but he remains very sceptical about flexible offices.

– The game stimulates talking about *future* behaviour.

They discuss how situations are at present and project this to future situations. However, the employees have difficulties imagining how it would be like to work in an open office environment. The game made them realize that there obviously is a need for guidelines in the new environment. The current environment also has rules, but this behaviour seems more 'natural': no one ever thought about it. For the new environment different or additional rules must be developed to prevent workers from returning to their old habits and to stimulate them to make use of the new situation.

– The game stimulates talking about preferences for the future flexible office.

Players go into detailed descriptions of physical objects they want to have (e.g. *"I want to have a place where I can plug in my water cooker."*). They start fantasizing about how they want their new office to be, especially in the discussion afterwards, when they have warmed up, the players start dreaming. Their enthusiasm however is slightly tempered by the presence of the architect. He mentions that the goal of this afternoon is to get to know the wishes of the employees, but he rejects many of their ideas. The main reason for this is that the basic layout and floor plan are already de-signed. It is obvious that the employees are disappointed that their opinion is asked too late in the design process. They want to convey their preferences for the work en-vironment, but the things that are still to be decided and open for discussion are minimal (e.g. *"How many whiteboards does your department need?"*). The architect tries to convince the employees by talking about his own experiences, but he does not ask people *why* they want things or *why* they feel a certain way. For example, one person wants a cabinet of 1.80m high, but it is not allowed to have higher cabinets than 1.20m. The interesting question here is why this person wants a cabinet of 1.80m high: does he have prototype models of 1.80m high? Does he have many documents to store? Or does he want privacy?

To conclude we could say that the Workplace Game stimulates employees to talk about their behaviour. The game makes players talk about their *future* work behaviour by eliciting information about their *present* work behaviour. The players extrapolate this knowledge about their likes and dislikes to the future and imagine how they would behave. The playing cards with questions trigger them to talk about their pref-erences for the future. Thus, the Workplace Game provides us with feelings of office workers in present situations ánd with dreams for future situations.

5   Discussion

5.1   Conclusion

Looking back to Figure 1, one might say that the Workplace Game uses the interviewing technique to get information. Participants were asked questions, which they answered. To a certain extent this is true, however from the analysis we learned that people *do* talk about dreams and feelings about the new work situation, which is information from the deeper level of user knowledge. By playing the game the architect can reach a deeper understanding of the user, because tacit knowledge is brought up by revealing latent needs.

It can be concluded that the Workplace Game has elements of generative techniques. The questions themselves are an interviewing technique, but because of the way the questions are asked –by means of playing a game- they stimulate employees to dream about the future. Looking at literature about using games in design, games seem to be very useful in revealing unmet user needs. Games are helpful in creating a future vision, because they are structured, have explicit rules for participation and consist of carefully prepared activities. This makes the player feel engaged and the atmosphere informal, which allows players to communicate on the same level. Open-ended assignments, like the questions of the Workplace Game, give the participants opportunity to interpret and influence according to their own opinion; and game-boards and 3D pieces stimulate creativity [1], [2].

However, the Workplace Game does not provide directions for designing future flexible offices. This is mainly because the game is not aimed at generating ideas - it is designed as an evaluation and communication tool- so it does not stimulate creativity. But the main reason for the lack of creativity is that the game was played in a situation where the office design was almost completely determined. One participant mentioned that the game does not elicit what would be the most ideal workspace for herself, because it entailed the decision that was already taken of implementing flexible offices. Had the company not yet decided to take this direction, she might have expressed more latent needs and useful information for the architect. Other players wondered whether the moment the game was played is the right moment for playing, because it had already been decided that a flexible office would be their future. The architect who was present in the second session did not realize enough that he could still gain much inspiration from the employees, although he already designed much of the office; instead, he mainly defended his own design.

Looking at literature that integrates understanding user needs and creating new ideas, e.g. contextmapping, we can see that a specific structured process is followed. The aim of contextmapping is twofold: it is used to elicit user information and it is also concerned with bringing the information to the design team so that it can serve as inspiration for new design ideas [10]. The process that is followed stimulates this. First the user is warmed up by means of sensitizers (i.e. *"participants are triggered, encouraged and motivated to think, reflect, wonder and explore aspects of their personal context in their own time and environment."*) and after a week or so the individuals come together in a session in which the participants do generative exercises. The most useful information for the designer is a result of the sessions, since participants then start talking about the stories that are hidden behind the created artefacts. The generative exercises reveal people's knowledge, feelings, and dreams for the future.

In the sessions with the Workplace Game we can conclude that the game functioned as a sensitizing tool, it warmed up the people and made them aware. The discussion afterwards however, could have given much more useful information to the architect. To a certain extent the discussion revealed interesting information, but it did not provide a more profound understanding of the employees.

5.2 Recommendations

If the Workplace Game were ever to be used as a helpful tool for designing future office spaces, three important recommendations for adapting it are discussed: the moment in the design process to play the game, the people that are involved in playing the game, and the product (the game) itself.

First of all, deciding on the moment to play the game in the design process (before, during, or after the design is made) is important for the results. When you want to engage employees in the process of changing a traditional office into a flexible office, it is important to involve them as soon as possible. At this time employees can still have the feeling that nothing has been decided and that they can fully participate in developing the future office space. The information that results from playing can be used by an architect or designer as a source of inspiration to create innovative flexible offices. On the contrary if the game is played after the flexible office is introduced the focus will lie more on evaluating and discussing behaviour. This results mainly in creating awareness amongst the employees and providing information about details for the architect.

Secondly, the people that are involved in playing the game have a large influence on the end result. Players in the first session mention that they are already open for innovative offices, because they are members of a board that is concerned with these changes. They think that their less open minded colleagues might have a more difficult time playing this game, because they will more often be confronted with new situations. However, these employees should also be consulted in a session of the game, because they can provide insight into why there is resistance. Also, when the architect of the flexible office is present he should be aware of his position. He should solicit employees more for their opinion and should be open to all kinds of input from them. The employees are to be considered as experts of their own experiences, and the architect is the expert on the design. Not all experiences can be implemented in the design, but an attempt should be made by the architect to listen more attentively to discussion between the employees and be creative with their wishes.

Thirdly, the Workplace Game itself, the product, has two elements that steers the information that results from the game session in a certain direction. First there are the playing cards that contain questions regarding present or future situations that steer the answers of the employees in a certain direction. When the architect focuses on discovering dreams for the future, it is important to find a good balance between present and future behaviour. It might prove to be useful to make the employees more aware of their changing behaviour by clearly separating the present and future and then making of using that by letting people compare the two situations, as far as possible. A second element that predetermines the game results is the consensus coin. We noticed that people often try to reach consensus, even though this is not necessary and differences in opinion are always allowed. When they focus too much on reaching consensus they might not express their individual dreams, and thus not provide the architect with adequate information about their latent needs. In a situation where players instantly agree on an answer, there is no group discussion, which means that if this situation takes place, the architect is also left with very little information.

6 Future Research Focus

Although the Workplace Game does seem to provide interesting information for the architect, further research is recommended if it is to be used for designing future office spaces. It could be interesting to do a case study with a group of employees at the *start* of the office change process. The employees should have some knowledge about the change and be interested in thinking about it, but there should not be a already determined office design. An architect could take part in the session to receive information, but he or she should be instructed to not be too critical, or possibly a moderator should be used that leads the discussion. This can reveal what information the game actually provides for architects and what information is not provided.

Another interesting focus for future research could be to use the Workplace Game as a sensitizing tool and develop a second Workplace Game which focuses on eliciting useful information for the architect to serve as inspiration for a future flexible office. Two questions come to mind: Does an architect wants to involve users in his design process, and, is a game the right format to elicit user information?

Acknowledgements. Thanks to the employees of an internationally operating company that creates innovative products and services in Life Sciences and Materials Sciences for participating in the case studies, and to Sanne Valkenburg for her help and advice with the analysis of the Workplace Game.

References

1. Brandt, E.: Designing exploratory design games: a framework for participation in Participatory Design? In: 9th Conf. on Participatory Design: Expanding Boundaries in Design, Trento, Italy, August 01-05, 2006, pp. 57–66. ACM Press, New York (2006)
2. Brandt, E., Messeter, J.: Facilitating Collaboration through Design Games. In: 8th Conference on Participatory Design: Artful Integration: Interweaving Media, Materials and Practices, Toronto, Ontario, Canada, July 27-31, pp. 121–131. ACM Press, New York (2004)
3. De Bruyne, E., De Jong, A.: The Workplace Game: Exploring End Users' New Behaviour. In: Applied Human Factors and Ergonomics 2008 Int. Conf., Las Vegas (2008)
4. De Jong, A., De Bruyne, E.: Participatory design of office spaces by game playing? In: Applied Human Factors and Ergonomics 2008 Int. Conf., Las Vegas (2008)
5. Fulton Suri, J.: Empathic Design: Informed and Inspired by Other People's Experience. In: Koskinen, I., Battarbee, K., Mattelmäki, T. (eds.) Empathic Design, User Experience in Product Design, pp. 51–57. IT Press, Helsinki (2003)
6. Koskinen, I.: Empathic Design in Methodic Terms. In: Koskinen, I., Battarbee, K., Mattelmäki, T. (eds.) Empathic Design, User Experience in Product Design, pp. 59–65. IT Press, Helsinki (2003)

7. Koskinen, I., Battarbee, K.: Introduction to User Experience and Empathic Design. In: Koskinen, I., Battarbee, K., Mattelmäki, T. (eds.) Empathic Design, User Experience in Product Design, pp. 37–50. IT Press, Helsinki (2003)
8. Sanders, E.B.-N.: Postdesign and Participatory Culture. In: Useful and Critical: The Position of Research in Design, University of Art and Design, Tuusala, Finland, September 9-11, pp. 87–92 (1999)
9. Sanders, E.B.-N., Dandavate, U.: Design for Experiencing: New Tools. In: Proceedings of the 1st International Conference on Design and Emotion. University of Technology, Delft (1999)
10. Sleeswijk Visser, F., Stappers, P.J., Van der Lugt, R., Sanders, E.B.N.: Contextmapping: Experiences from Practice. CoDesign 1(2), 119–149 (2005)

Management Support and Worksite Health Promotion Program Effectiveness

David M. DeJoy, Heather M. Bowen[1], Kristin M. Baker[1], Bethany H. Bynum[2],
Mark G. Wilson[1], Ron Z. Goetzel[3], and Rod K. Dishman[4]

[1] The University of Georgia, College of Public Health, Department of Health Promotion and
Behavior, Athens, Georgia 30602
{dmdejoy,hmbowen,kmbaker,mwilson}@uga.edu
[2] The University of Georgia, Franklin College of Arts and Sciences, Department of
Psychology, Athens, Georgia 30602
bhhoff2@uga.edu
[3] Emory University, Rollins School of Public Health, Institute for Health and Productivity
Studies, 4301 Conneticut Avenue, NW, Suite 330, Washington, DC 20008
Ron.Goetzel@thomsonreuters.com
[4] The University of Georgia, College of Education, Department of Kinesiology, Athens,
Georgia 30602
rdishman@uga.edu

Abstract. The purpose of this paper is to describe the development and use of
management support measures in two worksite health promotion intervention
trials. Results from the two intervention trials suggest that management support
for health promotion can be assessed and tracked over time using both perceptual and observational measures. These results also provide initial evidence that
an increase in management support can contribute to positive changes in health
related behaviors and outcomes. Specifically, longitudinal results from the two
studies suggest that interventions designed to increase management support for
health promotion resulted in changes in perceptions of management support, actual changes in the work and organizational environment. Preliminary results in
these studies also suggest that increased management support is important in
weight loss.

Keywords: health promotion, management support, organizational climate,
workplace, worksite.

1 Introduction

Management support is typically viewed as a critical prerequisite to the success of
workplace health promotion programming [5,23]. In our review of the relevant workplace literatures, we found that management support is frequently mentioned and discussed but seldom operationalized or measured. Published reports of workplace health
promotion interventions often address the steps that were taken to gain or build management support, and such activities are sometimes viewed as key components of the
intervention. Occasionally, informant interviews or other qualitative data are presented
to gauge the extent to which management facilitated or impeded implementation, or the

B.-T. Karsh (Ed.): Ergonomics and Health Aspects, HCII 2009, LNCS 5624, pp. 13–22, 2009.
© Springer-Verlag Berlin Heidelberg 2009

general extent to which efforts to boost support were successful. Actual attempts to quantitatively assess or track management support across time or between treatment conditions are quite rare.

The basic idea of assessing management support intersects with the concept of organizational climate. Organizational climate has been defined as the shared perceptions held by members of an organization concerning the practices, procedures, and types of behaviors that get rewarded and supported in a particular setting [18]. In general, employee perceptions of management support play a key role in the formation of climate perceptions. Today, it is generally accepted that organizations have multiple climates rather than a single, all-inclusive climate. These so-called facet-specific climates may include climates for customer service, occupational safety, innovation, risk-taking, and so forth. The climate literature contains numerous studies and instruments assessing the climate for workplace safety, but very few assessing the climate for health promotion. Published reviews of safety climate research indicate that perceptions of management support/commitment are perhaps the single most dominant component of safety climate [9,12,15].

Ribisl and Reischl's [20] health climate questionnaire represents one of the few attempts to assess health-related climate factors within work organizations. Their instrument features 12 subscales. One of the subscales, "employer health orientation", provides a global assessment of management support for health promotion. More recently, Barrett and colleagues [1] developed an organizational leadership scale as part of the Alberta Health Project in Canada. This scale follows an organizational learning perspective, but is oriented more towards communities than workplaces.

The purpose of this paper is to describe the development and use of management support measures in two worksite health promotion intervention trials. Both of these trials included intervention components that were specifically directed at demonstrating management support. Both intervention packages were developed using social-ecological frameworks [4].

2 Worksite Physical Activity Trial

This study evaluated the efficacy of a social-ecological intervention delivered at the workplace to increase leisure-time physical activity. A group–randomized 12-week intervention consisting of organizational action and personal and team goal-setting was implemented with 1,442 employees at 16 worksites of a large national retailer [8]. Change in physical activity was analyzed using latent growth modeling (LGM) and latent transition analysis. Participants in the intervention had greater increases in moderate and vigorous physical activity and walking compared to participants in a health education control condition. The proportion of participants that met a public health recommendation for regular participation in either moderate or vigorous physical activity remained near 25% at control sites during the study but increased to 51% at intervention sites.

The organizational action component of the intervention consisted of ecologically-based environmental changes designed to integrate personal and environmental resources to promote physical activity. Specific components included: 1) senior management endorsement, 2) joint worker-management participation in program planning and implementation through the establishment of a steering committee, 3) group and organizational goal-setting, and 4) environmental supports and prompts that publicized and facilitated physical activity. Group goal-setting was intended to promote social support, social networks, and competition, but these variables were not evaluated as mediators of the intervention.

We assessed participant perceptions of management support and employee involvement at three time points: baseline, mid-point of intervention, and at the end of the intervention period. Management support for employee physical activity was assessed using a five-item scale derived from the physical activity portion of Heart Check, a worksite health promotion assessment instrument [11]. This scale included items such as: "Management at my worksite directly supports my physical activity goals." Employee involvement was measured using a 4-item scale adapted from the high involvement work processes literature [22]. The scale was designed to capture the four components of PIRK framework of high involvement work processes: Power, Information, Rewards, and Knowledge [14], and feature items such as: "In general, employees at my worksite are actively involved in shaping practices, systems, or methods for enhancing greater physical activity and exercise while at work." Both measures used 5-point Likert-type scales ("strongly agree" to "strongly disagree") with a neutral midpoint. In the present sample, scores on each measure conformed to a single factor. Internal consistency (Cronbach α) was .92 to .94 for management support and .83 to .87 for employee involvement.

The LGM for management support provided acceptable fit to the data in the intervention and control groups. The fit of the LGM for employee involvement was good

Table 1. Means and standard deviations (SD) for perceived management support, employee involvement, and physical activity for control and treatment groups

	Measure		Time 1	Time 2	Time 3
Control	Perceived management support	Mean	3.16	3.13	3.05
		SD	0.93	0.92	0.96
	Employee involvement	Mean	2.74	2.92	2.94
		SD	0.78	1.08	0.99
	Physical activity (MET-minutes)	Mean	1552	1531	1848
		SD	1781	2002	2450
Treatment	Perceived management support	Mean	3.38	3.48	3.43
		SD	0.87	0.90	0.90
	Employee involvement	Mean	3.22	3.45	3.52
		SD	0.76	1.18	1.39
	Physical activity (MET-minutes)	Mean	1910	2562	2838
		SD	2294	2469	2811

in the intervention group but less acceptable in the control group. Groups did not differ on initial status (p > .05). There were linear increases in management support (p < .05) and employment involvement (p < .001) in the intervention group but a decrease in management support (p <.05) and no change in employment involvement in the control group. Results were not substantively different after adjustment for demographic variables.

In addition, management support and employee involvement were significantly correlated across all three time points (Time 1 r = .464, p < .001; Time 2 r = .526, p < .001; Time 3 r = .571, p < .001). Management support was significantly correlated with physical activity at all time points (Time 1 r = .101, p = .003; Time 2 r = .114, p = .001; Time 3 r = .071, p = .05). Finally, employee involvement and physical activity were significantly correlated but only at Time 1 (r = .066, p = .05). Table 1 contains treatment and control group means for each measurement period. Physical activity was assessed using the International Physical Activity Questionnaire (IPAQ) [14].

3 Worksite Weight Management Trial

This quasi-experimental cohort study was conducted with employees at nine treatment sites (n = 8,013) and three control sites (N = 2,269) of a major chemical manufacturing company. Again, following a social-ecological paradigm, two levels of intervention were designed to improve environmental and organizational supports for healthy eating and physical activity. The first level (moderate intensity) included a set of evidence-based environmental interventions (e.g., healthy vending options) that should be relatively easy and inexpensive to implement in a wide variety of work settings. The second level (high intensity) added in several additional components designed to reflect a high degree of management support for and engagement with weight management activities (worksite goal setting, reporting to senior management, etc.). The intervention period for this study was two years. As part of the formative research for this project [23], we developed two measures designed to assess different aspects of the management support: the LBE and the EAT.

3.1 The Leading by Example Questionnaire (LBE)

We sought to develop a brief, self-report instrument that could be used in two ways. The first use was to provide an overall global assessment of management support for health promotion within a variety of different types of workplaces. As such, a single administration of the LBE could be used to diagnose specific areas in which the health promotion climate might support or hinder programmatic efforts. The second use envisioned for the instrument was to assess or monitor change over time through repeated administrations.

In searching for a starting point for instrument development, we found the "Leading by Example" (LBE) questionnaire, which was developed by the Partnership for Prevention [17]. The questionnaire had been used as a descriptive/educational tool as part of the Partnership's broader Leading by Example initiative. With permission from the Partnership, we adopted their tool as the foundation for the current instrument. The original LBE provided a core of seven items directly related to management support, commitment, and engagement. Additionally, new items were generated, critiqued, and revised by the research team through a series of team meetings and conference calls. The new items addressed topics such as health promotion goal setting and alignment, leadership training, communication, culture building, and financial and other supports for health promotion. All items, both old and new, were edited for use with employees of all educational levels. These items were measured using a five-point Likert scale, with a neutral midpoint ("strongly agree" to "strongly disagree").

The adapted questionnaire was pilot tested using a small sample of employees at one of the control sites participating in the larger intervention study. Then, as part of formative research activities for the larger intervention study, the draft LBE was administered to groups of employees at the other 11 sites participating in the study. Reliability and validity were assessed using a combination of exploratory and confirmatory factor analyses. This sequence of procedures produced a 13-item scale consisting of four subscales: business alignment with health promotion objectives (e.g., "Our site health promotion programs are aligned with our business goals"), awareness of the economics of health and productivity (e.g., "Employees at all levels are educated about the true cost of health care and its effects on business success"), worksite support for health promotion (e.g., "This site offers incentives for employees to stay healthy, reduce their high risk behaviors, and/or practice a healthy life style"), and leadership support for health promotion (e.g., "The organization provides our site leadership training on the importance of employee health"). A more detailed explanation of the psychometric procedures used to develop this measure can be found in Della et al. [7].

LBE data were collected at four time points (baseline, intervention year one, intervention year two, and post-intervention) and biometric and other outcomes were

Table 2. Means and standard deviations (SD) for LBE factor scores for control and intervention groups at baseline (B), intervention year one (I – Yr 1), intervention year two (I – Yr 2), and post-intervention (PI)

	Measure		B	I – Yr 1	I – Yr 2	PI
Control	Business alignment	Mean	3.41	3.08	3.49	3.36
	with health objectives	SD	0.78	0.75	0.85	0.75
	Awareness of the	Mean	3.08	2.97	3.15	3.02
	economics of health	SD	0.66	0.82	0.95	0.90
	Worksite support for	Mean	3.32	3.23	3.62	3.65
	health promotion	SD	0.61	0.72	0.87	0.70
	Leadership support for	Mean	3.15	3.27	3.37	3.46
	health promotion	SD	0.53	0.74	0.83	0.91
Intervention	Business alignment	Mean	3.10	3.60	3.58	3.48
	with health objectives	SD	0.84	0.70	0.74	0.73
	Awareness of the	Mean	2.65	3.34	3.26	3.3
	economics of health	SD	0.73	0.84	0.78	0.8
	Worksite support for	Mean	2.99	3.44	3.53	3.52
	health promotion	SD	0.72	0.70	0.64	0.7
	Leadership support for	Mean	3.26	3.73	3.54	3.59
	health promotion	SD	0.72	0.68	0.72	0.69

collected at three time points (baseline, mid-intervention, and post-intervention). The LBE factor-scores (see Table 2) reflected changes over time across intervention levels, particularly for the business alignment with health objectives factor (p = .010), awareness of health economics of health and productivity factor (p = .060), and worksite support for health promotion factor (p = .085). Changes in LBE factor scores were also related to the primary study outcome of weight loss, with a 6.4% increase in the prevalence of employees who lost or maintained their weight per point increase in the total LBE score (p = .060)

3.2 The Environmental Assessment Tool (EAT)

This measure is essentially an audit tool that can be used to assess workplace supports for healthy eating, weight management, and physical activity. The EAT was developed in three stages: contextual analysis and literature review, prototype development, and pilot testing [6]. The contextual analysis involved working cooperatively with corporate staff to become familiar with the specific work and operational environments and the broader site and location characteristics of the facilities participating in the project. The EAT integrated the physical characteristics of the worksite, features of the information environment, and characteristics of the immediate neighborhood around the workplace from the previously developed CHEW (Checklist of Health Promotion Environments at Worksites) instrument [16], as well as characteristics of employer and administrative support from the Heart Check instrument [11]. Questions for the EAT were developed around these concepts as they applied specifically to environmental physical activity and obesity management interventions. These questions addressed the job factors, physical and social-organizational work environment, and socio-cultural and economic/legal environment variables found in DeJoy and Southern's [4] social-ecological model for workplace environmental interventions.

The final EAT prototype consisted of two sections, one completed by site staff and the other by independent observers who toured the site and recorded their observations. The portion to be completed by site staff consisted of questions that could best be answered by those closely affiliated with the site, and included such topics as work rules and requirements, current health promotion programs and services, and formal policies that support or facilitate healthy eating and/or physical activity participation. The EAT instrument has three subscales, pertaining to 1) Physical Activity, 2) Nutrition and Weight Management, and 3) Organizational Characteristics and Support.

A 100-point scoring system was developed to permit quantitative comparisons of environmental supports across control and treatment sites and to monitor changes over time. A weighting exercise was performed to assess the relative importance of each component in terms of supporting nutrition and weight management and physical activity in the workplace context.

As with the LBE, EAT data were collected at four time points (baseline, intervention year one, intervention year two, and post-intervention). The EAT sub-scores (see Table 3) reflected the environmental changes implemented as part of the intervention. Intervention sites demonstrated significantly greater changes in EAT scores, from baseline to intervention year two, compared to control sites for the nutrition and weight management (β = 8.28, p = .012) and organizational support (β = 6.59, p = .010) scales as well as the total EAT score (β = 16.10, p = .002). Changes in the total EAT scores were also related to the primary study outcome of weight loss, with a 0.4% increase in the prevalence of employees who lost weight per point increase in the total EAT score (p = .013). Changes in the EAT organizational support, physical activity, and nutrition and weight management scales demonstrated similar trends. Table 3 shows EAT sub-scores for each of the four measurement periods for the three treatment groups.

Table 3. Means for EAT sub-scales for control, moderate and intense treatment groups at baseline (B), intervention year one (I − Yr 1), intervention year two (I − Yr 2), and post-intervention (PI)

	Measure	B	I − Yr 1	I − Yr 2	PI
Control	Access to physical activity (32 possible points)	12.0	13.3	10.4	10.0
	Nutrition and weight management (32 possible points)	2.5	3.6	2.8	2.7
	Organizational characteristics and support (36 possible points)	21.0	15.0	17.0	14.0
Treatment	Access to physical activity (32 possible points)	9.3	10.4	11.4	12.4
	Nutrition and weight management (32 possible points)	8.7	15.9	14.5	18.9
	Organizational characteristics and support (36 possible points)	18.6	18.7	21.2	18.9

4 Discussion

At a very fundamental level, no worksite health promotion programming occurs without at least some basic level of support from management. After all, management sets the policies, determines goals and priorities, and allocates budget and other resources. The findings summarized in this paper suggest that the level of management support for health promotion can be assessed and tracked across time using both perceptual and observational measures. Brief questionnaires such as the LBE can be used to assess employee or stakeholder perceptions of management support. The factor or subscale scores from the LBE can be used to provide basic diagnostic information concerning the organization's strengths and weaknesses. Observational tools such as the EAT can be used to gauge the degree to which management support translates into work environments that support and reinforce positive health behaviors. Both types of measures can serve as process evaluation measures of implementation fidelity or as checks on the effectiveness of manipulations and, therefore, can be used to determine whether intended changes related to management support have actually occurred.

The longitudinal results from the two intervention studies suggest that interventions designed to reflect increased management support result in changes in employee perceptions of support, as well as actual changes in work and organizational environments consistent with management support. These results also provide someinitial evidence that increased levels of management support can contribute to producing beneficial changes in health-related behaviors and outcomes. These results, however, are preliminary and more in depth and sophisticated analyses are clearly needed.

As argued at the beginning of this paper, management support for health promotion is a reflection of organizational climate. In the organizational behavior and management literatures, positive effects associated with increased management support have often been ascribed to a recalibration of the exchange relationship or the psychological contract, which exists between employers and employees [19, 21]. In simple terms, if your employer does more for you or otherwise demonstrates that you are valued by the organization, you are likely to reciprocate by expending more effort to help the organization reach its goals. This additional effort may extend beyond mere job performance and include other extra-role or citizenship behaviors. Citizenship behavior is not always completely altruistic, in that, some employees may see such behavior as a good way to increase their visibility within the organization or to impress their bosses with their initiative and team spirit [13]. Employee participation in health promotion programming itself fits the definition of organizational citizenship behavior. It is seldom a job requirement to participate in a worksite health promotion program. It follows, then, that demonstrations of management support may be quite important in boosting employee acceptance and participation in these programs.

Employers have a variety of motives for offering health promotion programs to their employees, including cost containment, productivity enhancement, absenteeism reduction, and improved recruitment and retention. Offering a health promotion program to employees is, by itself, a reflection of some level of management support for the health and well-being of the workforce. But how well this message is conveyed depends on the extent to which the message is consistent with other messages in the organization. A health promotion program is basically a human resource management (HRM) strategy and part of the organization's overall HRM system. Broad-based employee acceptance of health promotion efforts will likely depend on the extent to which the health promotion initiative is perceived as being congruent with other components of the overall HRM system. Employees will perceive enhanced management support for health promotion and respond appropriately only if this message is consistent with other messages and sources of evidence at their disposal [21,2]. In creating an organizational climate that values good health practices, there must be consistency in messages and the various HRM programs and practices should complement each other and make logical sense to employees. Too often, the health promotion message within organizations is fragmented, indistinct, and largely inconsistent with other apparent priorities. A strong climate for health promotion will exist when there is a high level of agreement among employees that health promotion is important and supported by the organization.

Acknowledgments

Preparation of this paper was supported in part by grants from the Centers for Disease Control and the National Institutes of Health.

References

1. Barrett, L., Plotnikoff, R.C., Raine, K., Anderson, D.: Development of measures of organizational leadership for health promotion. Health Edu. and Behav. 32, 195–207 (2005)
2. Bowen, D.E., Ostroff, C.: Understanding HRM- firm performance linkages: The role of the "strength" of the HRM system. Acad. Manage. Rev. 29, 203–221 (2004)
3. Craig, C.L., Marshall, A.L., Sjöström, M., Bauman, A.E., Booth, M.L., Ainsworth, B.E., Pratt, M., Ekelund, U., Yngve, A., Sallis, J.F., Oja, P., the IPAQ Consensus Group and the IPAQ Reliability and Validity Study Group: International Physical Activity Questionnaire (IPAQ): 12-country reliability and validity. Med. Sci. Sport Exer. 35, 1381–1395 (2003)
4. DeJoy, D.M., Southern, D.J.: An integrative perspective on worksite health promotion. J. Occup. Med. 35, 1221–1230 (1993)
5. DeJoy, D.M., Wilson, M.G.: Organizational health promotion: Broadening the horizon of workplace health promotion. Am. J. Health Promot. 17, 337–341 (2003)
6. DeJoy, D.M., Wilson, M.G., Goetzel, R.Z., Ozminkowski, R.J., Wang, S., Baker, K.M., Bowen, H.M., Tully, K.J.: Development of the environmental assessment tool (EAT) to measure organizational physical and social support for worksite obesity prevention programs. J. Occup. Environ. Med. 50, 126–137 (2008)
7. Della, L.J., DeJoy, D.M., Goetzel, R.Z., Ozminkowski, R.J., Wilson, M.: Assessing management support for worksite health promotion: Psychometric analysis of the Leading by Example instrument. Am. J. Health Promot. 22, 359–367 (2008)
8. Dishman, R.K., DeJoy, D.M., Wilson, M.G., Vandenberg, R.J.: Move to improve: A randomized trial to increase physical activity. Am. J. Prev. Med. 36, 133–141 (2009)
9. Flin, R., Mearns, K., O'Connor, P., Bryden, R.: Measuring safety climate: Identifying the common features. Safety Sci. 34, 177–192 (2000)
10. Goetzel, R.Z., Schechter, D., Ozminkowski, R.J., Marmet, P.F., Tabrizi, M.J., Roemer, E.C.: Promising practices in employer health and productivity management efforts: Findings from a benchmarking study. J. Occup. Environ. Med. 49, 111–130 (2007)
11. Golaszewski, T., Fisher, B.: Heart Check: The development and evolution of an organizational assessment of support for employee heart health. Am. J. Health Promot. 17, 132–153 (2002)
12. Guldenmund, F.W.: The nature of safety culture: A review of theory and research. Safety Sci. 34, 215–257 (2000)
13. Kidder, D.L., Parks, J.M.: The good soldier: Who is s(he)? J. Organ. Behav. 22, 939–959 (2001)
14. Lawler III, E.E.: The ultimate advantage: Creating the high-involvement organization. Jossey-Bass, San Francisco (1992)
15. Neal, A., Griffin, M.A.: Safety climate and safety at work. In: Barling, J., Frone, M.R. (eds.) The psychology of workplace safety, pp. 15–34. American Psychological Association, Washington (2004)
16. Oldenburg, B., Sallis, J., Harris, D., Owen, N.: Checklist of health promotion environments at worksites (CHEW): Development and measurement characteristics. Am. J. Health Promot. 16, 288–299 (2002)
17. Partnership for Prevention.: Leading by example: Improving the bottom line through a high performance, less costly workforce. Author. Washington, DC (2004)
18. Reichers, A.E., Schneider, B.: Climate and culture: an evolution of constructs. In: Schneider, B. (ed.) Organizational climate and culture, pp. 5–39. Jossey-Bass, San Francisco (1990)

19. Rhoades, L., Eisenberger, R.: Perceived organizational support: A review of the literature. J. Appl. Psychol. 87, 698–714 (2002)
20. Ribisl, K.M., Reischl, T.M.: Measuring the climate for health in organizations: Development of the worksite health climate scales. J. Occup. Med. 35, 812–824 (1993)
21. Roussseau, D.M.: Psychological contracts in organizations: Understanding written and unwritten agreements. Sage Publications, Thousand Oaks (1995)
22. Vandenberg, R.J., Richardson, H.A., Eastman, L.J.: The impact of high involvement work processes on organizational effectiveness. Group Organ. Manage. 24, 300–339 (1999)
23. Wilson, M.G., Goetzel, R.Z., Ozminkowski, R.J., DeJoy, D.M., Della, L., Chung Roemer, E., Schneider, J.H., Tully, K.J., White, J.M., Baase, C.M.: Using formative research to develop environmental and ecological interventions to address overweight and obesity. Obesity 15(suppl.), 37–47 (2007)

Usage of Office Chair Adjustments and Controls by Workers Having Shared and Owned Work Spaces

Liesbeth Groenesteijn[1,2], Merle Blok[1], Margriet Formanoy[1],
Elsbeth de Korte[1], and Peter Vink[1,2]

[1] TNO Work and Employment, Polarisavenue 151,
2130 AS Hoofddorp, The Netherlands
[2] Delft University of Technology,
Industrial Design Engineering, The Netherlands
liesbeth.groenesteijn@tno.nl

Abstract. In this study two seats were used by workers having shared and workers having owned work spaces. 51 subjects (22 female, 29 male) participated in a six week experiment in a naturalistic setting. The chairs were different with respect to adjustability options, design of controls and external design. Most of the subjects adjusted the office chairs the first time for seat height, arm rest height and back rest inclination. Adjustment times of seat height and armrest height were shorter for chair A. Back rest pressure adjustment takes much time and it is difficult to adjust this without instruction. The workers having shared desks adjust their chair more often and are faster in the adjustment of the backrest pressure compared with workers with an owned work space. The quality of adjustments of seat height, arm rest and back rest pressure was improved by an instruction for 32% of the subjects.

Keywords: office chair, shared workspace, chair controls, adjustment time.

1 Introduction

Of all EU work, 47% is white collar work, which is predominantly done in offices and this percentage is still growing [9]. The consequence of a growing service sector is that more people use office chairs. Of course it is of importance that this population can work productive, comfortable and without complaints. A couple of studies has shown that a good adjustable chair in combination with an ergonomic training increases the productivity and reduces musculoskeletal complaints [6], [9]. On the other hand a Dutch-Spanish study showed that the number of persons adjusting their chair is very low. 30-60% of the working population never adjusts their chair [12]. The 30% was in the Spanish group where seats were less complex to adjust. So, a possible explanation for not adjusting could be the complexity of the control system. The question is "what is a good adjustable chair"? A good design of the controls is important, but what is a good design? When the controls are in a logical intuitive position and the adjustment time are low usability increases, but is that enough? [7]. From the functionality perspective it is important to take the work task into account as different work tasks cause different body dynamics [2], [3], [4], [6], [11], and therefore different tasks might need

B.-T. Karsh (Ed.): Ergonomics and Health Aspects, HCII 2009, LNCS 5624, pp. 23–28, 2009.
© Springer-Verlag Berlin Heidelberg 2009

different chair adjustability options. In this context a study showed that different chair preferences were found in relation to different function types [8].

In this study the user type in terms of work tasks and mobility in combination with the fit with particular adjustment properties was carried out. As there is a number of organizations that move from conventional offices with owned work spaces to more open and transparent offices with shared workplaces [10] the differences between workers using one workstation and users that do not have a fixed work station is becoming of importance. Therefore, in this study these two groups (a group having owned work spaces and a group having shared work spaces) are taken into the study population. The effects of chair characteristics and user type on number of adjustments made, adjustment times and adjustment quality are presented in this paper.

2   Methods

The study was carried out in a real office environment of an international consultancy company for Information Technology. Out of the 60 subjects that start the experiment, 51 subjects (22 female, 29 male) participated the whole 6 weeks during experiment. The mean ages were 42.5 years (SD 10.9 years). One group of 17 subjects had an owned work space and one group of 34 subjects used shared work spaces. Sometimes this is called hotelling. The "owned work space users" had mainly administrative functions and secretary work. About one third of their function consisted of call centre work. The "shared work space users" had mainly consultancy functions. Initially the user type groups were more equal in number, but nine flexible work stations users could not complete the experiment. Due to the consultancy work they were no longer at work in their own office environment.

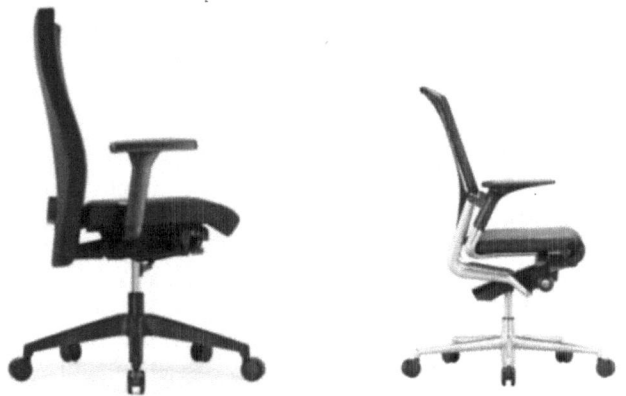

Fig. 1. The experimental chairs A (left) and B (right)

The two types of office chairs, chair A and B, of this study differed with respect to adjustability options, design of controls and external design (see fig. 1). The original chairs normally meet the European standard, but for this experiment chair A was supplied with fewer options (see table two for adjustability options). So, chair A was seen as the easy adjustable chair and chair B as the more complex adjustable chair. None of the subjects was familiar with the chairs before the experiment. They were used to an office chair meeting the Dutch and European standards. The subjects used each chair for three weeks in a systematically varied order (30 subjects started with chair A and 30 subjects with chair B).

Initial chair adjustments by the subjects were observed. After two weeks of getting used to the chair the subjects were one by one invited to a separate meeting room with their 'own' test chair.

The following measurements were performed:

1. To define user adjustments; seat height, seat depth (chair B only), arm rest height, space between arm rest (chair A only), backrest angle, backrest height (chair A only), use of the dynamic mode and back rest pressure.
2. Time to adjust seat height, arm rest height, seat depth and back rest pressure by use of a stopwatch. From a default chair setting (lowest position armrest, seat, backrest, maximum upright and fixed back rest, minimum seat depth and lowest back rest pressure) the subject adjusted the chair in a fixed order to his/her personal location and each subject was encouraged to get comfortable in the chair. This was repeated two times.
3. Chair related body dimensions; lower leg length, upper leg length and height between posterior seat surface and elbow bone (table 1).
4. Quality of the adjustments before and after instructions. This is a combination of chair adjustment and chair related body dimensions.
5. A questionnaire to define user characteristics,   work task characteristics, user-friendliness of the chair in terms of adjustability, functionality, task suitability, work related musculoskeletal disorders and comfort

Table 1. Chair related body dimensions of the subjects in centimeters

	Lower leg length	Upper leg length	Seat surface-elbow height
Mean	47.6	48.2	20.7
Std. Deviation	2.7	3.5	2.5
Minimum	43.0	42.0	16.0
Maximum	55.0	57.0	27.0

At the end of the third week the adjustments the users made were measured again to define whether and how the chair was adjusted in the last week. Then the second chair was presented to the subject and the protocol was repeated.

3 Results

Chair Adjustments Made

No significant differences between chairs are found from the questionnaire in how often the subjects do adjustments their chair. The majority (62%) only adjusted the chair when they received the chair at the start of the three weeks. 16% adjusted it more than once a week. Weekly adjustments were made by 11% of the subjects. Table 2 shows which parts of the chair were adjusted when the subjects received the chair. There are no significant differences between the comparable chair parts of chair A and B in the observed (and questioned) adjustment numbers. Seat height and armrest height are most often adjusted followed by back rest inclination. Space between armrests and the dynamic mode are the least adjusted chair options.

Table 2. Adjustment of the chair element when subjects received the chair (% yes)

	Seat height	Seat depth	Armrest height	Inter armrest space	Dyna -mic mode	Back rest pressure	Back rest inclina- tion	Lumb ar support
Chair A	95%	-	83%	10%	15%	18%	70%	-
Chair B	92%	31%	90%	-	21%	33%	42%	28%

Adjustment Times

The first time the adjustment time was shorter for chair A compared with chair B concerning armrest height adjustment and seat height adjustment. The second time only the arm rest height adjustment time was significantly shorter. The first time adjustments were significantly faster than the second time with exception of the armrest of chair B. The back rest pressure (used in dynamic mode) was very difficult to adjust. In the first attempt 62% of the subjects were not able to find or adjust de backrest pressure of chair A in a proper way. For chair B 36% of the subjects didn't do it in a proper way.

User type

Chair use of the experimental chairs for one work station users is 85% of the total work time and 65% for the flexible work stations users. Flexible workspace users adjusted their chair significantly more often (weekly - more than once a week) than the one station workers (when receiving chair – weekly). Chair height was adjusted by significantly more (96%) of one work station users compared to flexible workspace users (87%). Significantly less one work station users workers (8%) changed the chair into dynamic mode compared to flexible workspace workers (39%).

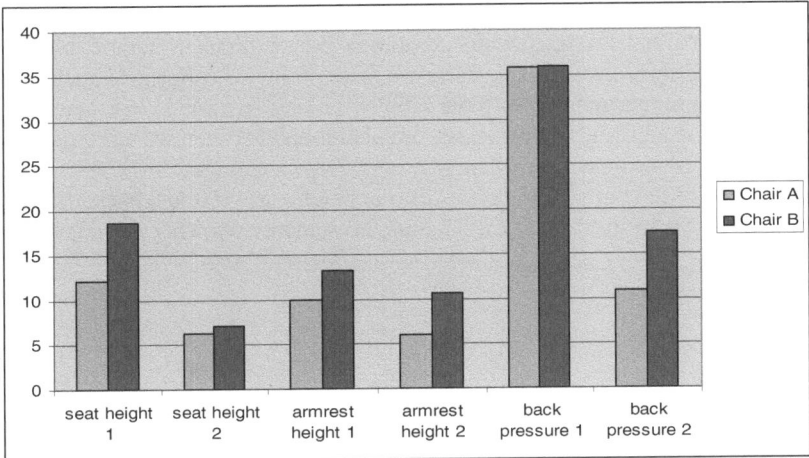

Fig. 2. Average adjustment times (sec) for chair A an B in the first (1) and second time (2) measurements

The work tasks of "one work station users" consist significantly more of reading and writing, calling, archiving and filing than the "flexible workspace users". The two user types perform the same level of intensive computer work 4-8 hours a day.

Flexible workspace workers value operation of the backrest height control and space between armrest controls lower (on average a little worse) than fixed workers (a little good). Flexible workspace users faster adjusted the backrest pressure of chair A the second time. Lower leg length of flexible workspace users was significantly longer (average 0.49 m) compared fixed (average 0.47 m).

Instruction
After an instruction the average seat height is significantly lower than before for both chairs. 32% of the subjects made after instruction a substantial change in seat height of at least 2 cm in comparison to their initial adjusted seat height. The variation range in comparison to their lower leg length is -3 < 0 > 3 to lower leg length. 43% made a substantial change in armrest height after instruction of at least 2 cm in comparison to their initial adjustment. The range is -2 < 0 > 2 cm in relation to seat surface – elbow height. The backrest pressure felt for 79% of the subjects comfortable after instruction. For 19% there was no comfortable feeling achieved after instruction.

4 Conclusions

Most office chair elements were only adjusted once during use. When subjects do adjust the chair mostly the seat height, arm rest height and back rest inclination is adapted. Space between arm rests and the dynamic mode are the least used chair adjustment options.

Adjustment times of seat height and armrest height were shorter for the simple chair (chair A). There was no relationship with the number of adjustments, showing that adjustment time was not the most crucial factor. Back rest pressure adaptation takes much time and for many subjects it was very difficult to adjust this without instruction. The shared work space users are faster in the adjustment of backrest pressure the second time compared with the subjects having an owned work space.

Differences in adjustment frequencies are also found between worker types. Shared workspace workers adjust more often.

The quality of the initial adjustments of seat height, arm rest and back rest pressure was improved by an instruction for 32% of the subjects, showing the importance of instructions.

References

1. Amick, B.C., Robertson, M.M., Derango, K., Bazzani, L., Moore, A., Rooney, T., Harrist, R.: Effect of office ergonomics intervention on reducing musculoskeletal symptoms. Spine 28(24), 2706–2711 (2002)
2. Adams, M., Dolan, P., Marx, C., Hutton, W.: An electronic inclinometer technique for measuring lumbar curvature. Clinical Biomechanics 1, 130–134 (1986)
3. Babski-Reeves, K., Stanfield, J., Hughes, L.: Assessment of video display workstation set up on risk factors associated with the development of low back and neck discomfort. International Journal of Industrial Ergonomics 35, 593–604 (2005)
4. Commissaris, D.C.A.M., Reijneveld, K.: Posture and movements during seated office work; results of a field study. In: Veiersted, B., Fostervold, K.I., Gould, K.S. (eds.) Proceedings of the 37th Annual Conference of the Nordic Ergonomics Society. Ergonomics as a Tool in Future Development and Value Creation. NES and NEF, Oslo, Norway, October 10–12, 2005, pp. 58–61 (2005)
5. Derango, K., Amick, B., Robertson, M., Palacios, N., Allie, P., Rooney, T., Bazzani, L.: The productivity consequences of office ergonomics training and an ergonomically designed chair. In: Luczak, H., Cakir, A.E., Cakir, G. (eds.) WWDU 2002 - World Wide Work. Proc. 6th Int. Scientific Conf. on Work with Display Units, ERGONOMIC Institut fur Arbeits- und Sozialforschung, Forschungsgesellschaft mbH, Berlin, pp. 368–370 (2002)
6. Ellegast, R., Hamburger, R., Keller, K., Krause, F., Groenesteijn, L., Vink, P., Berger, H.: Effects of Using Dynamic Office Chairs on Posture and EMG in Standardized Office Tasks, pp. 34–42. Springer, Berlin (2007)
7. Groenesteijn, L., Vink, P., Looze, M., de Krause, F.: Effects of differences in office chair controls, seat and backrest angle design in relation to tasks. Applied Ergonomics 40, 362–370 (2009)
8. Legg, S.J., Mackie, H.W., Milicich, W.: Evaluation of a prototype multi-posture office chair. Ergonomics 45(2), 153–163 (2002)
9. Parent -Thirion, A., Fernández, M.E., Hurley, J., Vermeylen, G.: Fourth European Working Conditions Survey. In: Dublin: European Foundation for the Improvement of Living and Working Conditions (2007)
10. Van der Voordt, D.J.M., Van Meel, J.: Psychologische aspecten van kantoorinnovatie (Psycho-logical aspects of office innovation). Delft/Amsterdam: BMVB & ABN AMRO (2002)
11. Van Dieën, J.H., De Looze, M.P., Hermans, V.: Effects of dynamic office chairs on trunk kinematics, trunk extensor EMG and spinal shrinkage. Ergonomics 44(7), 739–750 (2001)
12. Vink, P., Porcar-Seder, R., Page de Poso, A., Krause, F.: Office chairs are often not adjusted by end-users. In: Proceedings of the Human Factors and Ergonomics Society (HFES) 51st Annual Meeting, Baltimore, October 1-5 (2007) (CD-ROM)

Health Promoting Leadership: The Mediating Role of an Organizational Health Culture

Jochen Gurt and Gabriele Elke

Ruhr-University at Bochum, Universitätsstraße 150, 44780 Bochum, Germany
Tel.: +49-234-32-24608 {Jochen Gurt}
jg@auo.psy.rub.de

Abstract. Drawing from the findings within the safety literature, the present study identifies the effects of leadership on an organizational health culture and strain. The importance of leadership for the development of a corporate health culture is demonstrated as well as the positive effect of health culture on employee strain level. Empirical data from a longitudinal study in the German tax administration is presented. Leadership has a positive impact on the development of a corporate health culture, which in turn reduces employees' strain level. Discussion addresses the similarities of health and safety leadership regarding effects and mediating processes.

1 Introduction: From Health and Safety Management to Worksite Health Promotion

Health and safety in organizations have often been treated as a single subject in the literature [28]. In Germany the classical domain, which dealt with employee health, has been that of occupational health and safety management. Primary focus of this approach was to protect workers and employees health from dangers and hazards originating from work or the working environment (e.g. accidents, contamination). A lot of research concerning health and safety management was carried out in production sites, power plants and military settings, where technical and organizational configurations served as barriers for the protection of employee health. A second approach to employee health is worksite health promotion [10]. Studies here take place more often in office-settings. They build on the findings of health and safety management, but shifted the focus to employee health: Along with the World Health Organization (WHO) health is understood as "a state of complete physical, mental and social well-being" [25], health promotion as a "process of enabling people to increase control over, and to improve their health" [25]. Worksite health promotion, particularly coping with stress therefore rests on a Job Demands-Resources Model JDR, [4], which draws from the salutogenetic approach of Antonovsky [1]. At the core of this model is the idea that employee health (and strain) is affected by two factors: First, job demands originating from the task, the workplace, the organization or the physical surroundings, which can induce strains and may have a negative effect on health and well-being. Second, job

B.-T. Karsh (Ed.): Ergonomics and Health Aspects, HCII 2009, LNCS 5624, pp. 29–38, 2009.

resources (physical, social, psychological and organizational job characteristics), which have a buffering effect within this process by reducing job demands and strains as well as stimulating personal growth and development. Resources are categorized into internal (personal) and external. Personal resources are personality characteristics or qualifications like coping strategies, attribution styles or skills. External resources refer to the organizational and off-the-job settings and include amongst others factors of workplace design and work organization, work autonomy, social support from friends, family, but also colleagues and supervisors. Following an organizational management approach, top-management commitment and leadership (supervisor) support are seen as key resources for successful worksite health promotion [29]. Leadership qualities have shown to be an important explanatory psychosocial factor with regard to sick leave, employee health and well-being [8]. In addition to their direct influence on employee health, leaders are also seen as promoters of a supportive organizational climate and culture. Support of this view comes from findings within the safety promotion domain [31], [33]. Safety climate/ culture are seen as important outcomes of all health and safety initiatives [7]. However, empirical studies identifying leadership behaviors and culture together influencing health related variables within worksite health promotion are rare. The present study tries to empirically support the claim of the prominent role of leadership and organizational health culture within clerical work. Data is presented from a longitudinal study in the German tax administration.

2 The Role of Leadership and Organizational Culture in Safety and Health Management

The impact of leaders on safe and healthy behavior of employees is twofold: First, management and leaders (to some extent) shape organizational processes and management sub-systems (e.g. human resource management). Through these systems they exert control over a variety of health-related physical and psycho-sociological characteristics of work and the working environment e.g., the individual workload and amount of responsibilities, technical equipment, but also the organization of work like working hours or breaks [6]. As shown, within the JDR model these factors impose demands upon the employee, which in turn could lead to strains [4]. Numerous studies underscore this relationship (e.g. review by Sonnentag & Frese, [19]). It could also be demonstrated that leadership has an impact on the design of these work characteristics, and acts as a buffering resource for health relevant outcomes [16], [26]. In these studies work characteristics can also be regarded as mediators through which leadership behaviors affect employee outcomes. For example the study by Wilson et al. [26] linked organizational attributes (e.g. policies and practices to facilitate employees' abilities to balance work and non-work issues) to climate (which included involvement with supervisor) and job design, which comprised workload, work scheduling, and physical work conditions.

Second, leaders also influence safety behavior and health of employees through day-to-day direct and personal interaction and communication. Two distinct ways of influence can be identified:

1. The direct approach to immediate modification of behavior functions via behavior control through training, personnel appraisal and reward systems. Behavior control has its origins in the operant perspective of role behavior and the connected ABC framework (i.e. antecedents-behavior-consequences; Stajkovic & Luthans,[21]. Mainly two kinds of antecedents were used - goal setting and training - and three kinds of consequences, namely feedback, incentives, and social recognition. Antecedents have mostly been used in combination with positive consequences of some kind [9]. Modification of safety behavior by the ABC-framework received impressive empirical support in particular on individual and group level [7], [22].
2. The second (indirect) influence of leadership interaction on health and safety behavior is through mediating variables. Strong evidence comes here from safety literature for the important role of safety climate and culture as important mediating variables [12]. Drawing from social cognitive learning theory, employee behavior is (among other factors) a function of perceived behavior of their environment. Leaders serve as role-models. Norms and values develop from this learning process, which may serve as leadership substitutes to guide employee behavior. While also operant and transactional leadership behaviors are expected to have a beneficial effect on safety culture [7], ethical and transformational leadership seem to contribute even more to a supportive safety culture. These leadership styles rest on value-based behavior, charisma and authenticity of the leader. Various studies confirm their direct positive impact on organizational safety culture/ climate and safety [3], [14], [32].

However, reverse effects or additional mediators between leadership and safety like safety consciousness, safety communication, safety programs and initiatives as well as safety commitment have been examined. Other studies show even moderating effects of safety climate, safety priority or transformational leadership. In sum, the studies draw attention to the fact that leadership is a crucial variable to improve workplace safety. Safety climate is the most important mediator, but the mechanisms behind the effects are highly complex and yet not fully understood.

Concerning health promotion, the direct leader employee interaction is also seen to be crucial for the success of organizational health promotion programs [29]. So far, only a few studies within the health promotion literature have addressed this issue. One study on a health promotion program on tobacco and alcohol use in the armed forces reported that successful implementation and retention of this program was largely dependent on leadership engagement for the program [27]. Another indication comes from a Swedish study at municipally human service organizations [8]. The impact of workplace health promotion initiatives was dependent on various leadership behaviors, such as participation, the attitude towards the cause of sick leave as well as respect, trust and open discussion. This finding also underpins the importance of a participative approach, which is seen as an important prerequisite for successful health [19], [28]. Westermayer and Stein [24] identified reliability and trust as the core factors of leadership influencing stress level and absenteeism. Transformational and ethical leadership, which rest on value-based behavior, charisma and authenticity, have proven to have a direct positive impact on the perception of work characteristics and employee well-being (e.g. Nielsen et al.[16] Arnold et al., [2]) and are negatively related to stress symptoms and burnout (e.g. Hetland, Sandal, & Johnsen, [13]; Sosik & Godshalk,[20]). In some studies also reciprocal effects were found, indicating that well-being of employees at the first time of measurement had an effect on leadership behavior measured at the second point of time. This indicates that employee well-being (and probably behavior) also impacts leader behavior [16],[23].

Summarizing the findings, culture is seen as a prominent mediator in both health and safety leadership in order to increase safety performance and health. Within health promotion, engagement of the leader for health promotion seems to be of relevance for the success of health initiatives. While in the safety literature especially the studies of Zimolong and Elke [29] and Zohar and colleagues (e.g. Zohar & Tenne-Gazit, [32]) addressed the issue of the importance of safety climate as a mediating variable, there are only few studies identifying leadership behaviors and culture together influencing health related variables. Longitudinal studies separating concurrent and long-term effects are also rare (Nielsen et al., [16]). Based on the empirical findings in the safety literature, this analysis aims to identify the impact of leadership on strain in a longitudinal design, including corporate health (OH) culture as a mediating organizational resource.

3   Method

3.1   Design and Participants

The sample consisted of 265 employees in four local tax offices in the German tax administration in North Rhine-Westfalia. Tax office size ranged from 188-293 employees. The 265 respondents represented 31.4% of all 982 employees in the four locations. Survey questionnaires were administered online during a two-week period with a six-month interval between the two sampling points. Questionnaire responses were completely anonymous, and participation was encouraged via emails but voluntary. Frequency of participation at t_1 was 487 and 350 at t_2. Participation rates in the tax offices ranged from 51.3% to 65.2%, at t_1 from 36.5% to 53% at t_2. Individuals were tracked by an individual code. In the analysis only data from employees were included, who responded at both sampling points, which led to the reduced sample size for the analysis of 265 employees. Socio-demographic data showed that 4.9% were younger than 30, 68.8% between 30 and 50 years, and 28.3% older than 50 years. About 72.1% of participants were female and 57.4% employed full-time. These figures mirror the actual distribution of the socio-demographic profile in the four tax offices.

3.2   Instruments and Measures

Study participants were provided an inventory comprising different questionnaires. Strain captured the level of irritation of the individual employee. It was measured using three items ($\alpha = .71/.76$) from the irritation scale by Mohr et al. [15]. A sample item reads "I have problems to relax, even in my leisure time".

Healthy leadership behavior and cultural scales are drawn from a short version of the Organizational Health and Safety (OHS) questionnaire (FAGS, [11] in press). The Organizational Health (OH) questionnaire follows the Job Demands–Resources Model (JDR) and addresses three different areas: Demands, individual resources of the employee, external resources provided by the organization, including leadership performance and assessment of OH culture.

OH culture refers to the degree to which "health" is already integrated in the organizational norms and values. It was measured with two items (α = .64/.66), such as "Health initiatives in my organization are either insufficient or inadequate" (reverse coded).

Leadership behavior is measured in terms of general healthy leadership behaviors (HLB) and the engagement in health promotion of the leader (EHP). While HLB captures routine behaviors that have shown to have beneficial effects on employee health and well-being, such as setting objectives, giving feedback and recognition, employee participation and information (8 items, α = .87/.88, sample item: "My achievements are recognized by my supervisor"), EHP specifically captures the degree of engagement of the leader regarding health promotion (7 items, α = .91/.92, sample item „My supervisor asks me to contribute my experiences to the implementation of the health project"). These scales are not regarded as leadership styles or types, but rather as an index for a set of leadership behaviors that have been identified to be related to health outcomes in the past. Exploratory factor analysis yielded the two main factors HLB and EHB, extracting 64% of the variance. Confirmatory factor analysis revealed a deeper second-order factor structure with the two factors each having two sub-factors: relationship and performance orientation, χ^2 (101, N=265) =333.5; GFI = .92; CFI= .94; RMSEA= .069. All factor loading were psychological substantial (>.30) except for one item, which was dropped from the scale. For the further analysis we used the second-order factors without taking into account the particular sub-orientation.

Employees were asked to state their degree of agreement to various statements. Scales ranged from 1 to 5, 1 indicating "totally untrue" and 5 "exactly true".

3.3 Computational Methods

In order to test concurrent and time-lagged direct and mediated effects, structural equation modeling (SEM) with manifest variables was applied using AMOS 16. Three different models were tested. The first model (M1) assumed full-mediation of the effect of EHP and HLB on strain (irritation) through OH culture. Synchronous mediation effects at each point of time were included as well as time-lagged mediation effects, i.e. that EHP/ HLB at t_1 influenced OH culture at t_2. The second model (M2) assumed only partial-mediation and in addition to the mediated effects allowed for direct effects. The third model (M3) integrated the findings of Van Dierendonck et al. [23] and allowed for reciprocal effects of irritation at t_1 on leadership variables behavior at t_2.

4 Results

Table 1 shows the descriptive values and correlations among all study variables.

Table 1. Means, standard deviations, alphas, and correlations among study variables

Scale (# of items)	Means		SD		1	2	3	4
	t_1	t_2	t_1	t_2				
1 Healthy Leadership Behavior (HLB, 8)	3.14	3.15	(.81)	(.83)	**.87/.88**	.656**	.227**	-.137*
2 Engagement for Health Promotion (EHP, 7)	2.17	2.23	(.89)	(.94)	.630**	**.91/.92**	.310**	-0.041
3 OH Culture (2)	3.30	3.37	(1.00)	(.98)	.264**	.307**	**.66/.64**	-.215**
4 Strain/ Irritation (3)	2.77	2.65	(.88)	(.88)	-.194**	-0.065	-.171**	**.71/.76**

⁺Cronbach's Alphas are on the diagonal, correlations above represent t_2 data, below t_1 data;
*≤.05, **≤.01, ***≤.001

Table 2. Fit indices for longitudinal models testing for mediation

Models	χ^2	$\Delta \chi^2$ (df $_{\Delta, p}$)	NC (χ^2/df)	GFI	AGFI	CFI	RMSEA
M 1	13.819 (df=13; p=.387)		1.06	.987	.963	.999	.015
M 2	9.053 (df=8; p=.338)	4.76 (df $_\Delta$ = 5; n.s.)	1.13	.992	.962	.998	.022
M 3	6.274 (df=5; p=.280)	7.58 (df $_\Delta$=2; n.s.)	1.25	.994	.958	.999	.031

Means of all scales are rather stable over time, exhibiting only marginal changes. HLB means exceed at both times EHP. With means of 3.14 and 3.15 HLB lies slightly above the scale mean, while EHP lies clearly below (2.17/ 2.23). At both sampling points t_1 and t_2 correlations among the variables are as expected, indicating positive relationships between leadership and OH culture. Negative correlations are found for irritation and the remaining scales. The only correlation that neither became significant at t_1 nor t_2 is between EHP and irritation. Table 2 lists the fit indices for each model derived from the SEM. Although all models indicate satisfactory fit, M1 (as indicated by the RMSEA and standardized chi-square (NC)) best fits the empirical data indicating that the effects of leadership on irritation are fully mediated via OH culture. Models M2 and M3 do not help the model indicated by a non-significant change of Chi-Square ruling out reciprocal and direct effects. Coefficients of the added paths in M2 and M3 also fail to reach significance with the exception of HLB, which shows a significant direct relationship with irritation of -.11 (but only at t_1). Figure 1 shows the M1 model with standardized path coefficients (non-significant paths are indicated by dotted lines). Stability paths ($t_1 - t_2$) of the measures indicate that rank order of subjects in respect of the measures remains rather stable (coefficients between .61 and .74). The two leadership scales (HLB and EHP) correlate around .60, indicating that engagement for health promotion (EHP) often comes together with (routine) healthy leadership behavior (HLB).

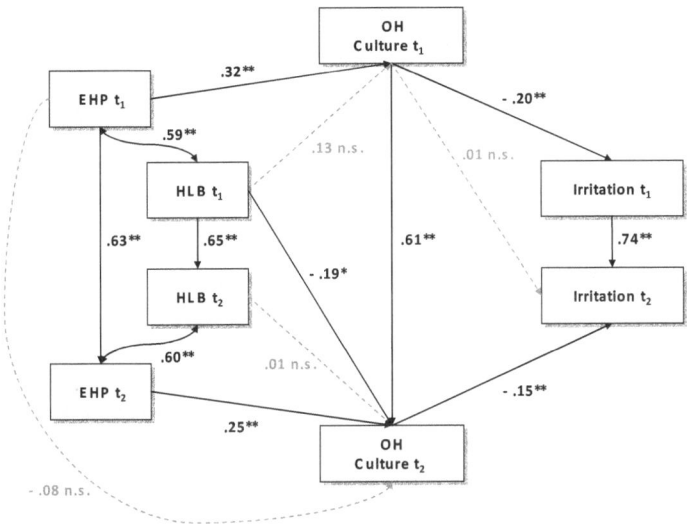

Fig. 1. Standardized maximum likelihood estimates for model M1

For the impact of OH culture on irritation we only find concurrent effects at t_1 and t_2, but no lagged effects from t_1 to t_2. EHP is a strong predictor of OH culture at both t_1 (.32) and t_2 (.25), while we do not find this effect for HLB concerning the routine leadership tasks. What we do find is a surprisingly negative time-lagged effect of -.19 from HLB at t_1 on OH culture at t_2.

5   Discussion

The aim of the study was to identify the role of leadership and OH culture with regard to their impact on employee strain level within the context of health promotion in a clerical setting.

Considerable previous research had supported the association between transformational leadership behavior and various measures of strain, health and well-being (e.g. Nielsen et al. [16]). This study has given special attention to the specific engagement of the leader in health promotion. The results indicate that indeed the special leader engagement has a beneficial effect on employee strain level via higher values of corporate health culture. Culture works as a mediator for the beneficial effects of leadership, backing the claims within health promotion of corporate health culture being a central success factor [29].

Routine leadership behaviors (HLB) do not contribute to an OH culture, which indicates that employees did not attribute "good" general leadership behavior with underlying organizational values concerning health. In order to contribute to the perception of a supportive OH culture the leader has to show his specific engagement for health promotion. Correlations indicate a significant negative relationship with strain (irritation), which is partly supported by the significant effect found in M2. This hints in the direction that such leadership behaviors (like giving feedback and setting objectives) should either have a direct influence on strain or be mediated by other variables, e.g. lower levels of role ambiguity [17].

Effects seem to be rather concurrent. Except for the contra-intuitive effect of HLB, no time-lagged effect of leadership behavior on OH culture is found, which makes it impossible to resolve the question of causality. In this study, it seems to be the actual behavior of the leader at one point of time, which influences perceptions of culture. Also it is the "current perception of health culture", which leads to lower values of strain. Perceptions of culture at t_1 are irrelevant for level of strain at t_2.

The results of this study mirror the findings in the domain of safety culture, where leadership is an important predictor of safety culture (e.g. Zohar & Tenne-Gazit, [32]). Irrespectively from the domain (health promotion or safety) leaders serve as role models and their engagement in the respective domain seems to contribute a great deal to the development of the respective culture.

One limitation of the study might be the short time-lag between the two measurements. In the six-month study interval, long-term effects are not really captured by the study. There might also be seasonal effects, as workload within the tax administration is known to be seasonal. This indicates a confounding variable, which was not integrated in the model. Due to the missing time-lagged effects, no inferences on causality between the constructs can be made; all relationships might be of a rather reciprocal nature. Leadership might also be influenced by OH culture. In addition to that, there is an unresolved debate (also in safety and health management science) if the culture or the climate of an organization can be inferred from psychometric measures like a questionnaires [12], [18]. Nevertheless, it is widely agreed that both constructs serve as core indicators for safety and health within an organization [7], [28].

Practical implications from this study are that first by developing a visible OH culture the strain impact on employees can be reduced. Second, in order to establish an OH culture, the support of leadership should be ensured as they have a strong influence on the creation and development of a corporate health culture. Supervisors act as role models and should be regarded as a cornerstone for success of organizational health promotion activities. Therefore organizational health promotion practitioners should ensure that leaders are willing to assume responsibility, have the necessary qualification and play an active part within the process. In this context it is not sufficient that leaders have the general qualification for "good" leadership behavior; they also need to be aware of their function as role models and have the adequate strategies to show their willingness to take over responsibility for their subordinates health and safety. Only then will they be able to create a beneficial climate or culture. Regarding this issue healthy leadership and safety leadership seem to rely on comparable mechanisms.

References

1. Antonovsky, A.: Unraveling the mystery of health. How people manage stress and stay well. Jossey-Bass, San Francisco (1987)
2. Arnold, K.A., Turner, N., Barling, J., Kelloway, E.K., McKee, M.C.: Transformational Leadership and Psychological Well-Being: The Mediating Role of Meaningful Work. Journal of Occupational Health Psychology 12(3), 193–203 (2007)
3. Barling, J., Hutchinson, I.: Commitment vs. controll-based safety practices, safety reputation, and perceived safety climate. Canadian Journal of Administrative Sciences 17, 76–84 (2000)
4. Bakker, A.B., Demerouti, E., Euwema, M.C.: Job Resources Buffer the Impact of Job Demands on Burnout. Journal of Occupational Health Psychology 10(2), 170–180 (2005)
5. Böhnisch, W.R., Krennmair, N., Stummer, H. (eds.): Gesundheitsorientierte Unternehmensführung. Eine Werteperspektive [Health-oriented Management. A value based perspective]. DUV, Wiesbaden (2006)
6. Cox, T., Leather, P., Cox, S.: Stress, health and organizations. Occupational Health Review, 13–18 (February/March 1990)
7. DeJoy, D.M.: Behavior change versus culture change: Divergent approaches to managing workplace safety. Safety Science 43, 105–129 (2005)
8. Dellve, L., Skagert, K., Vilhelmsson, R.: Leadership in workplace health promotion projects: 1- and 2-year effects on long-term work attendance. The European Journal of Public Health 17(5), 471–476 (2007)
9. Geller, E.S.: Actively caring for occupational safety: Extending the performance management paradigm. In: Johnson, C.M., Redmon, W.K., Mawhinney, T.C. (eds.) Handbook of organizational performance. Behavior analysis and mangement, pp. 303–326. Haworth, New York (2001)
10. Goetzel, R.Z., Ozminkowski, R.J.: The health and cost benefits of work site health-promotion programs. Annu. Rev. Public Health 29, 303–323 (2008)
11. Gurt, J., Uhle, T., Schwennen, C.: Fragebogen zum Arbeits- und Gesundheitsschutz - Betriebliche Gesundheitsförderung [Health and Safety Management Questionnaire – Organizational Health Promotion]. In: Sarges, W., Wottawa, H. (eds.) Handbuch wirtschaftlicher Testverfahren, Pabst, Lengerich (in press)
12. Guldenmund, F.W.: The nature of safety culture: A review of theory and research. Safety Science 34, 215–257 (2000)
13. Hetland, H., Sandal, G.M., Johnsen, T.B.: Burnout in the information technology sector: Does leadership matter? European Journal of Work and Organizational Psychology 16(1), 58–75 (2007)
14. Hofmann, D.A., Morgeson, F.P.: The role of leadership in safety. In: Barling, J., Frone, M.R. (eds.) The Psychology of Workplace Safety, pp. 159–180. American Psychological Assoc., Washington (2004)
15. Mohr, G., Müller, A., Rigotti, T., Aycan, Z., Tschan, F.: Concerning the Structural Equivalency of Nine Language Adaptations of the Irritation Scale. European Journal of Psychological Assessment 22(3), 198–206 (2006)
16. Nielsen, K., Randall, R., Yarker, J., Brenner, S.-O.: The effects of transformational leadership on followers' perceived work characteristics and psychological well-being: A longitudinal study. Work & Stress 22(1), 16–32 (2008)
17. O'Driscoll, M.P., Beehr, T.A.: Supervisor behaviors, role stressors and uncertainty as predictors of personal outcomes for subordinates. Journal of Organizational Behavior 15(2), 141–155 (1994)

18. Ribisl, K.M., Reischl, T.M.: Measuring the climate for health at organizations: Development of the worksite health climate scales. Journal of Occupational Medicine 35, 812–824 (1993)
19. Sonnentag, S., Frese, M.: Stress in organizations. In: Borman, W.C., Ilgen, D.R., Klimoski, R.J. (eds.) Handbook of Psychology, Industrial and Organizational Psychology, pp. 453–491. J. Wiley & Sons, Hoboken (2003)
20. Sosik, J.J., Godshalk, V.M.: Leadership styles, mentoring functions received, and job-related stress: A conceptual model and preliminary study. Journal of Organizational Behavior 21, 365–390 (2000)
21. Stajkovic, A.D., Luthans, F.: Behavioral management and task performance in organizations: Conceptual background, meta-analysis, and test of alternative models. Personnel Psychology 56, 155–194 (2003)
22. Tuncel, S., Lotlikar, H., Salem, S., Daraiseh, N.: Effectiveness of behaviour based safety interventions to reduce accidents and injuries in workplaces: critical appraisal and meta-analysis. Theroretical Issues in Ergonomics Science 7(3), 191–209 (2006)
23. Van Dierendonk, D., Haynes, C., Borril, C., Stride, C.: Leadership behavior and subordinate well-being. Journal of Occupational Health Psychology 9, 165–175 (2004)
24. Westermayer, G., Stein, B.: Produktivitätsfaktor Betriebliche Gesundheit [Productivity factor: Organizational Health], Göttingen, Hogrefe (2006)
25. WHO, http://www.who.int/about/definition/en/print.html, http://www.who.int/about/definition/en/print.html
26. Wilson, M.G., DeJoy, D.M., Vandenberg, R.J., Richardson, H.A., McGrath, A.L.: Work characteristics and employee health and well-being: Test of a model of healthy work organization. Journal of Occupational an Organizational Psychology 77, 565–588 (2004)
27. Whiteman, J.A., Snyder, D.A., Ragland, J.J.: The Value of Leadership in Implementing and Maintaining a Successful Health Promotion Program in the Naval Surface Force, U.S. Pacific Fleet. American Journal of Health Promotion 15(6), 437–440 (2001)
28. Zimolong, B., Elke, G.: Occupational Health and Safety Management. In: Salvendy, G. (ed.) Handbook of Human Factors and Ergonomics, pp. 673–707. Wiley, New York (2006)
29. Zimolong, B., Elke, G.: Die erfolgreichen Strategien und Praktiken der Unternehmen [The successful strategies and practices of enterprises]. In: Zimolong, B. (ed.) Management des Arbeits- und Gesundheitsschutzes - Die erfolgreichen Strategien der Unternehmen, pp. 235–268. Gabler, Wiesbaden (2001)
30. Zohar, D.: The influence of leadership and climate on occupational health and safety. In: Hofmann, D.A., Tetrick, L.E. (eds.) Health and safety in organizations: A multi-level perspective, pp. 201–230. Jossey-Bass, San Francisco (2003)
31. Zohar, D.: The effects of leadership dimensions, safety climate, and assigned priorities on minor injuries in work groups. Journal of Organizational Behavior 23, 75–92 (2002)
32. Zohar, D., Tenne-Gazit, O.: Transformational Leadership and Group Interaction as Climate Antecedents: A Social Network Analysis. Journal of Applied Psychology 93(4), 744–757 (2008)
33. Zohar, D., Luria, G.: The use of supervisory practices as leverage to improve safety behavior: A cross-level intervention model. Journal of Safety Research 34, 567–577 (2003)

Increasing Information Worker Productivity through Information Work Infrastructure

Udo-Ernst Haner, Jörg Kelter, Wilhelm Bauer, and Stefan Rief

[1] Fraunhofer Institute for Industrial Engineering (IAO),
Nobelstr. 12, 70569 Stuttgart, Germany
{udo-ernst.haner,joerg.kelter,wilhelm.bauer,
stefan.rief}@iao.fraunhofer.de

Abstract. Deploying high-quality information work infrastructure leads to higher productivity levels of information workers, findings from empirical research show. Different types of information workers use different sets of technologies and devices. Knowledge workers with a high degree of autonomy depend on mobile and flexible work infrastructure. The OFFICE21® Information Worker's Workplace supports productive information work.

Keywords: information work, knowledge work, productivity, workplace, work infrastructure, technology profile, information and communication technology.

1 Introduction

The number of people working in offices keeps growing. For example, estimates say that some 45% of the working population in Germany work in office type environments where they process information, generate knowledge, or develop innovative products and creative solutions. Yet, it is not fully understood how to measure and increase the productivity of this increasingly valuable personnel. One lever for increasing productivity is to invest and provide better tools and work infrastructure including information and communication technology (ICT).

Investments in information technology lead to significant changes in the competitive environment and can increase the productivity of organizations. McAfee and Brynjolfsson [1] argue that not only the deployment of enterprise information technology (e.g. ERP and CRM systems, Web 2.0 applications etc.) leads to higher levels of productivity but also the usage of these technologies in particular for propagating business processes and innovations within an organization generates competitive difference. According to Vluggen and Bollen, IT investments have become a new competitive necessity [2] that organizations should embrace rather than simply accept.

To increase productivity on the individual level an active adoption and an appropriate integration of new equipment and applications is necessary. As Davenport [3] pointed out "companies load up knowledge workers with desktop and laptop computers, personal digital assistants, cell phones, wireless communicators, e-mail, voice mail, and instant messaging – then leave them to their own device." As a consequence companies should actively seek productivity increases through information

B.-T. Karsh (Ed.): Ergonomics and Health Aspects, HCII 2009, LNCS 5624, pp. 39–48, 2009.
© Springer-Verlag Berlin Heidelberg 2009

work systems by providing infrastructure that is appropriate for the type of information work to be performed.

As part of the project OFFICE21® at the Fraunhofer IAO in Stuttgart, Germany, the authors have conducted a series of studies – some conceptual [4], some empirical [5], [6] and [7] – in order to investigate information work and supportive infrastructures. Some results of this work are presented here.

2 Information Workers and Their Technology Profiles

To be precise about the terminology and the subject under investigation a characterization of information work profiles will be presented first. Subsequently, differences in the technological equipment as supportive infrastructure in form of selected technology profiles will be presented. The chapter closes with an assessment of the quality of the information and communication technology in use.

The findings presented here originate from an empirical study by Spath et al. [6]. It is based on the ongoing online-survey "Information Worker Check". The answers of 1020 German speaking respondents from January until December 2008 were considered and evaluated. The respondents were to 68.5% male and 31.5% female. The age of the respondents was well spread (age up to 29 years 12%, age 30-39 31%, age 40-49 37%, age 50 and older 20%). 22% of the respondents were in upper or middle management, 24% in lower management and 54% had no leadership position.

2.1 Knowledge Workers Are Information Workers – An Empirical Typology

Not all information work is knowledge work; however knowledge work is to a significant share information work. While seeking, handling, and acting upon information are general activities of both information and knowledge work, the distinctive characteristics of knowledge work are complexity with respect to the tasks, autonomy of the knowledge workers with respect to the work process they are engaged in, and newness with respect to the work results.

Focusing on these three constructs and accordingly formulated questionnaire items information workers have been surveyed for to learn about their characteristics, needs and current support through work infrastructure. The full sample of 1020 respondents displayed the following characteristics with respect to the indices computed based on the questionnaire items related to the three constructs: newness (average $\mu=4.87$, standard deviation $\sigma=1.14$, number of data sets considered with respect to this variable n=975), complexity ($\mu=5.48$, $\sigma=1.04$, n=979), and autonomy ($\mu=4.77$; $\sigma=1.31$, n=805) each based on a 7-level Likert-scale. All questions related to a construct had to be answered by a respondent for his data to be considered in computing the results.

Through performing a cluster analysis four different types of knowledge workers were identified. As can be seen in Figure 1, a first cluster of respondents – hereafter called Type A – is characterized by comparatively low values with respect to all three indices computed (newness, complexity and autonomy). This profile is best described as "knowledge-based" work where experience and knowledge may be important however where only little own decision-making is needed, where newness

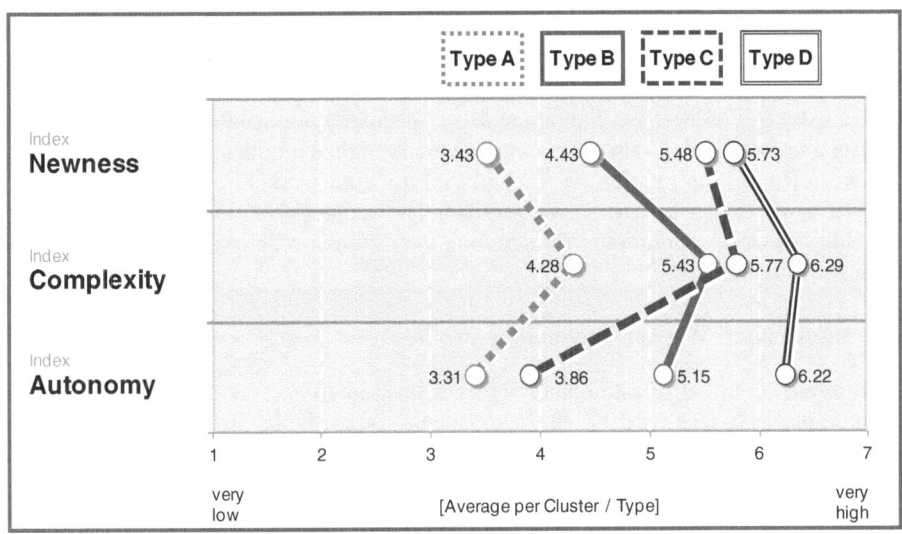

Fig. 1. Knowledge worker types and their profiles

is underrepresented with respect to the work results and where job complexity is below average. This profile relates to jobs with standardized processes and a significant share of routines (e.g. assistants).

The second cluster identified – Type B – represents respondents that perform knowledge work of average complexity and below average degree of newness with above average autonomy. This profile therefore stands for people performing "knowledge-intensive" work, i.e. tasks that require significant education and/or long-term experience in a particular field of work. This type B could for example be represented by a specialist in a particular occupation.

Type C – the third cluster identified – is characterized through high values with respect to the newness of the task and above average complexity but also through a below average autonomy. This profile also reflects "knowledge-intensive" work, however in contrast to Type B there is more newness with respect to the "what" and less autonomy with respect to the "when, where, and how" involved. Typical representatives of this cluster are for example engineers in development units who are bound to certain processes and laboratories.

The last cluster identified in this study – Type D – represents persons whose job profiles are to a very high degree characterized by newness and complexity of the tasks and who enjoy very high autonomy. The respondents in this cluster perform "knowledge" work in the narrowest sense possible. Their knowledge and experience needs constantly to be expanded, renewed, and revised in order find ever new solutions for the problems that arise. Representatives of this cluster are for example researchers but also consultants.

Returning to statement made earlier that not all information work is knowledge work however that knowledge work is to a significant share information work it becomes obvious that Type A and Type D are at different ends of the knowledge worker spectrum.

However, irrespective of their knowledge worker type all knowledge workers perform to a significant amount information work – with different purposes and different needs. It is this information work that can be supported directly by the work infrastructure, e.g. by ICT. Since this equipment serves primarily the handling and transmission of data and information rather than knowledge (which is a human trait) in the following we refer to "information work" and "information worker" as the encompassing terms for respective activities and persons. The typology introduced above will be sustained wherever appropriate for stressing the different requirements on information work infrastructures.

2.2 Information Worker Technology Profiles

A different group of questionnaire items addressed to the set of technologies and technological devices used by the respondents. In particular it has been of interest whether different types of information workers have access to different types of work infrastructure. At the same time potential differences in the daily use of the technologies and technological devices has been investigated.

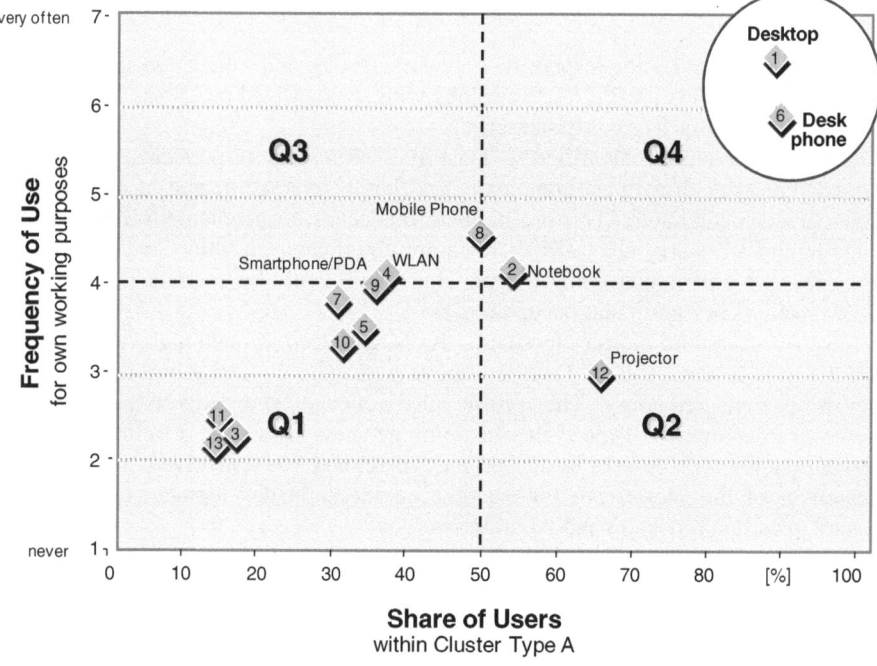

Fig. 2. Use of ICT available to information worker Type A

For this purpose typical technology profiles have been generated based on the data from the different clusters introduced above. These data sets have been evaluated with respect to the share of effective users of a particular technology or device and the frequency of its use. As a result portfolio have been generated, two of which will be presented here. The portfolio of Type A (Fig. 2) will be contrasted to the portfolio of Type D (Fig. 3).

Within the cluster of Type A 90% of all respondents have access to a desktop personal computer and a desk phone. These two ICT devices are also the most commonly used for own working purposes. In addition, about half of Type A respondents have a notebook, wireless network access, and a mobile phone available and in more frequent personal use. This set can be described as a "basic set" of ICT for performing information work. In contrast, within the cluster of Type D a quite extensive set of nine different technologies and devices is available and frequently used by the respondents. The core of this set consists of a notebook and a mobile phone, both available to about 95% of the respondents. It becomes obvious that the high autonomy of Type D knowledge workers implies the need for mobile devices and flexible technologies.

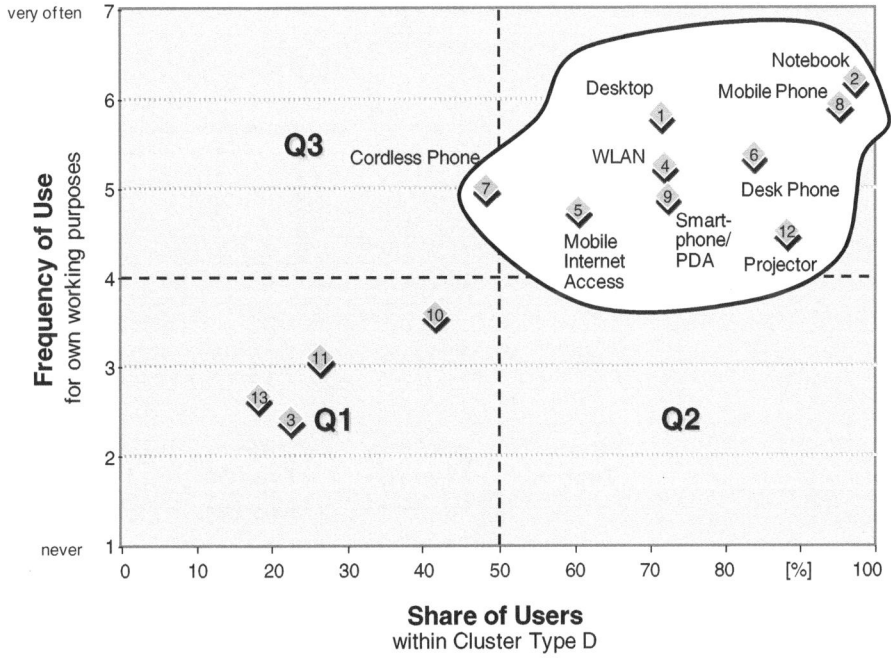

Fig. 3. Use of ICT available to information worker Type D

2.3 Quality of the ICT Set Available to Information Workers

For computing an index of ICT quality a set of questionnaire items has been evaluated that addressed different aspects of the technological work infrastructure. Particularly issues that are relevant to the general availability, functionality as well as the ease of use were investigated. Included were questions related to

- the accessibility of messages and documents irrespective of source and location;

- the reliability and stability of the ICT infrastructure;
- the availability of seamless solutions and general media consistency;
- the fulfillment of individual technological requirements;
- the general satisfaction level with the ICT equipment.

For the total sample the index of ICT quality demonstrates significant room for improvement (average μ=4.84, standard deviation σ=0.99). Highest scores were achieved with respect to the reliability and stability of the ICT infrastructure. On the low side, missing seamlessness and a rather low availability of the technological work infrastructure were the most important quality deficiencies.

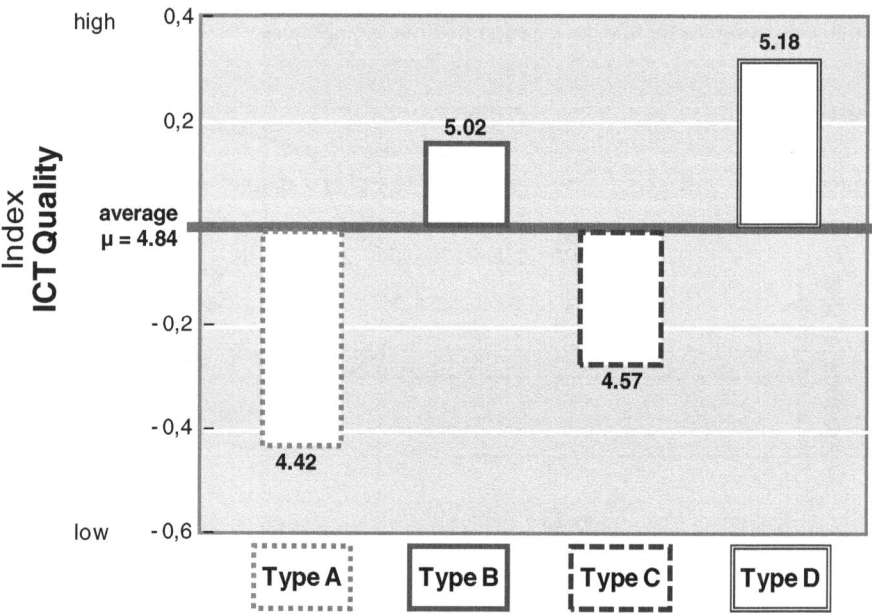

Fig. 4. ICT Quality Index for the different types of information workers

In a more detail analysis, the data shows a variation of the ICT quality index by the different clusters of respondents. While knowledge workers of Type A display the lowest quality of their technological work infrastructure, respondents of Type D have access to ICT of comparatively highest quality (Fig. 4).

3 OFFICE21® Information Worker's Workplace

As the results of the survey in the previous chapter show the higher the need for autonomy and consequentially for flexibility of the workforce, the more mobile and of higher quality the technological equipment becomes. In the same vein, the rollout of ever smaller and flexible devices in combination with increasing needs for communication and collaboration and supportive applications (e.g. e-mail push) changes the way people work and how organizations function. For example, why should some-body still go to the office, if the ICT set allows for location independent work? In spite of the availability of high-end video conferencing systems, e.g. telepresence solutions, the need for formal or informal face-to-face interaction with colleagues and collaborators will rather increase than decline due to the nature of concurrent work processes. Unfortunately, the technological solutions designed for mobility and flexi-bility, are not optimized for co-located collaboration.

For better supporting information workers in this respect a workplace has been conceptually designed and prototypically implemented within the OFFICE21® project at Fraunhofer IAO that addresses the needs of flexible knowledge workers when in the office. The so-called Information Worker's Workplace (IWWP) provides a better work infrastructure for individual work as well as for small team or project meetings.

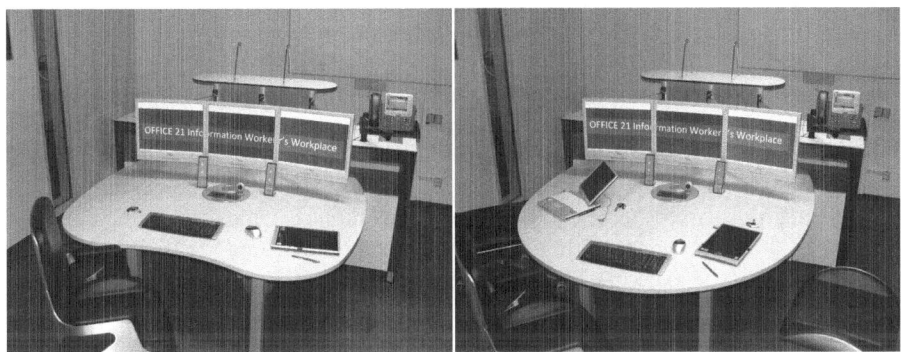

Fig. 5. a. /b. OFFICE21® Information Worker's Workplace – The original prototype [5]

As the pictures (Fig. 5) illustrate the most obvious characteristic of the IWWP is the triple-display setting. For individual work it provides a significantly enlarged desktop and for small meetings – whether co-located or distributed – it allows for parallel visualizations of different application windows. It is this simultaneous interaction with several applications (e.g. e-mail, browser, instant messaging, web conferencing, text document, presentation etc.) that to a large extent describes today's computer-based information work. Beyond that the IWWP supports an RFID-based login for personalization of the work environment – both physical (e.g. desk height or light brightness) and virtual (e.g. automated call-rerouting or personal settings of the pe-riphery devices). A special functionality of the IWWP is its physical adaptability (compare Fig. 5.a. and Fig. 5.b.) for supporting informal communication and sponta-neous interaction at the workplace. It abolishes the frequent search for a small meet-ing room or a projector by allowing connectivity for several persons at once.

4   Increasing Information Worker Productivity

Investing in better information work infrastructure – and particularly in ICT – is required to raise the productivity level of individuals and consecutively that of organizations. Several studies conducted at Fraunhofer IAO, e.g. [5], [6] and [7], prove a positive relationship between the quality of the personal technology set of information workers and their individual performance and productivity.

4.1 Multi-display-Settings Increase Productivity

To prove that the investment into higher quality work infrastructure like the IWWP presented in the previous chapter are worthwhile a laboratory experiment has been undertaken at Fraunhofer IAO [7]. The study is based on the results of 67 information workers. About two thirds of the participants were male and one third female. The average age of the sample was 32.5 years. Participants were required to extract information from different sources, think of the right solution and produce a textual result. Participants who used a three-display workplace completed this task faster, i.e. more efficient, and more accurately, i.e. more effective, than in a conventional one-display setting. This is particularly relevant for information workers who often need to process multi-source digital information, e.g. scientists, engineers or administrative staff. At first for all study participants an individual productivity benchmark was calculated based on the time required and the points achieved for correctly solved partial tasks. In a second step, the participants were divided into different groups: one group completed the next task continuing using a single-display-setting. One other group contrasted here was given a workplace with three interconnected displays of the same type to form one single desktop – matching the IWWP setting.

The results of the experiment were in their clarity surprising. The group that continued using a single-display setting increased its productivity at this task on average by 1.9 percent. This outcome can be explained by the regular learning effect. The group using a triple-display setting was significantly more productive. On average the participants in this group raised their productivity level by 35.5 percent. These statistically highly significant results were achieved without any previous training or indications how to make best use of the triple-screen setting.

The users' reaction to the triple-screen setting was also very positive. In a post-test survey the participants reported on average considerably higher satisfaction levels with the increased display system in comparison to the single display users. A similar result has been produced by the Information Work Study by Spath et al. [6]: A statistically significant linear positive correlation between monitor size and user satisfaction has been identified.

4.2 Information Work Performance

For not mistaking the different measures and methodologies used in the different studies here the term performance is used to indicate that the measure "Information Work Performance" is like "ICT Quality" an index based on several questionnaire items [7]. It consists particularly of items referring to effectiveness (using the right means to achieve the goals set), efficiency (the effort made to achieve these goals), task-related communication (effort and intensity), collaboration quality and organisational process efficiency.

The computed full sample Information Work Performance Index ($\mu = 4.32$; $\sigma = 1.02$) shows that there is a lot of improvement potential. In addition, the data shows, that information workers rate their effectiveness with respect to right means and processes highest while they rate their efficiency with respect to time and effort to reach their goals lowest. Interestingly, also in this case, similar differences among the clusters of information workers become visible (Fig. 6). Again, information workers Type A scored lowest while those of Type D highest.

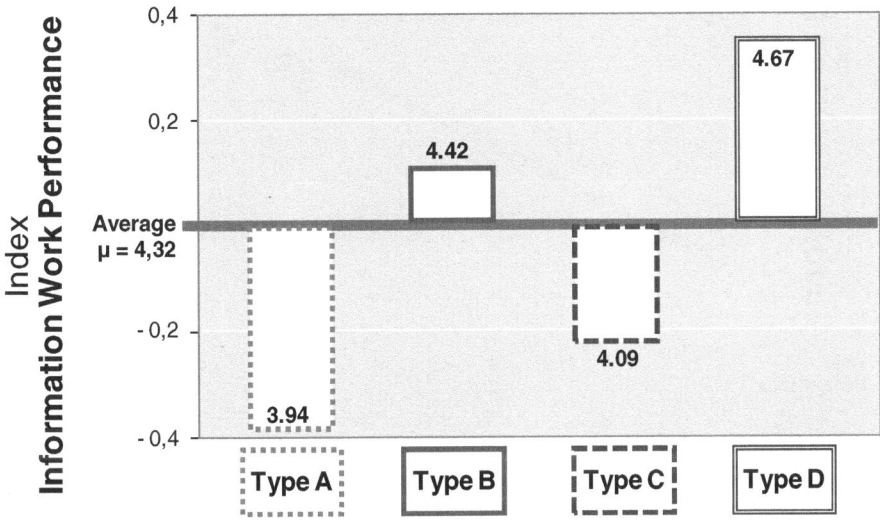

Fig. 6. Information Work Performance Index for the different types of information workers

5 Summary and Conclusion

The empirical findings presented here show that different types of knowledge and information work can be distinguished; that for different types of information work different sets of technologies and devices are in use; and that the ICT Quality and the Information Work Performance vary with the different types of information work. In addition, the OFFICE21® Information Worker's Workplace was presented. Based on a laboratory experiment it was proved, that productivity can be significantly increased by providing a multi-display setting similar to the IWWP.

In conclusion: Productivity of information workers is increased by providing supportive information work infrastructure. The statistically significant positive correlation between ICT Quality and Information Worker Performance (Figure 7) proves that one lever to higher productivity levels is information work infrastructure. Referring to Davenport's comment [3], deployment of appropriate and high-quality infrastructure for information workers is not a fad but a clear necessity.

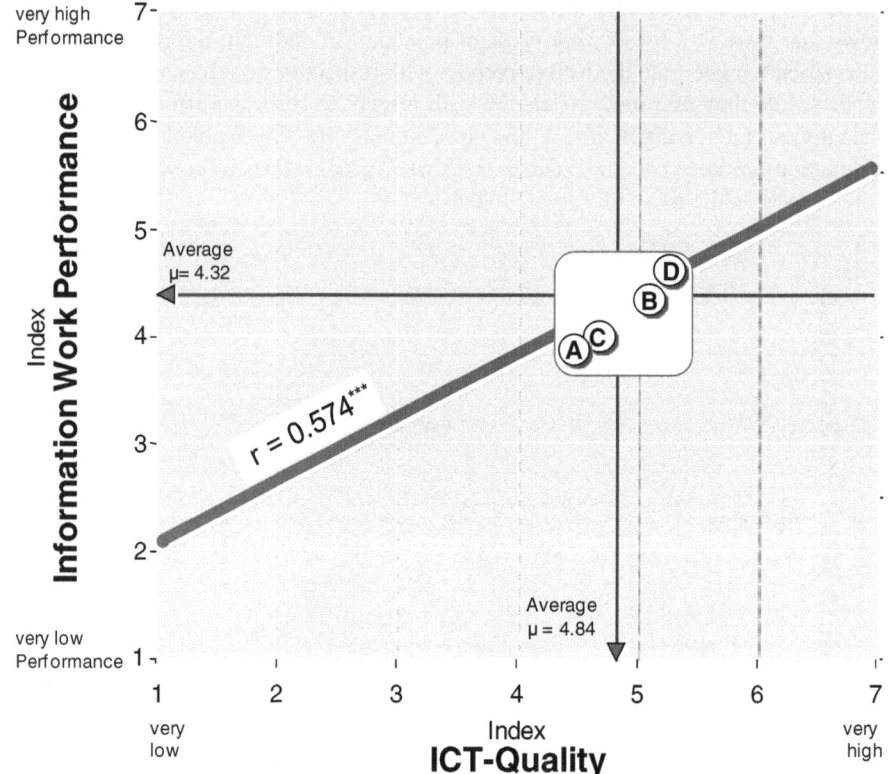

Fig. 7. ICT Quality correlates to Information Work Performance

References

1. McAfee, A., Brynjolfsson, E.: Investing in the IT That Makes a Competitive Difference, Harvard Business Review, 98–107 (July-August 2008)
2. Vluggen, M., Bollen, L.: A reply to [1]. Harvard Business Review, 110 (January 2009)
3. Davenport, T.H.: Let them all be power users. The HBR List: Breakthrough Ideas for 2005. Harvard Business Review, 41–42 (February 2005)
4. Kern, P., Bauer, W., Haner, U.-E.: Optimierte Infrastruktur für Wissensarbeit. Mensch und Büro 2, 36–37 (2007)
5. Greisle, A.: User-Study E-Work II – Information Worker Performance. Research Report. Fraunhofer IAO, Stuttgart (2006)
6. Spath, D., Kelter, J., Rief, S., Bauer, W., Haner, U.-E.: Information Work 2009. Fraunhofer IRB, Stuttgart (2009)
7. Haner, U.-E., Leuteritz, J.-P., Bauer, W., Hoffmann, S.: Knowledge Work Productivity and Multi-Monitor-Settings (in publication)

Merging Virtual and Real Worlds – Holistic Concepts for the Office of the Future

Hermann Hartenthaler

Deutsche Telekom Laboratories, Ernst-Reuter-Platz 7, 10587 Berlin, Germany
hermann.hartenthaler@telekom.de

Abstract. Information, communication, media, building and security technologies are growing together. The key to the integration of all infrastructure systems is the use of IP in all technical systems. The real and the virtual worlds are merging. This means that the real world around us and the world of IT systems are connected to one another. This paper shows how these concepts can be implemented in an innovative office infrastructure to increase the efficiency in the office.

Keywords: Virtual and Real World; All-IP; Office of the Future; Location-based Services; Building Automation.

1 Introduction

In future, office work will be much more flexible as teams distributed around the planet work together on projects. Knowledge workers will not just be productive in the office, but also when out and about and when at home. Working hours will be managed more flexibly, as what was previously a more rigid separation between professional and private life takes on new forms. Information has to be pervasively available (everywhere and at any time).

To provide better support for these new professional and private lifestyles, at Deutsche Telekom Laboratories a whole range of well-matched systems is being developed and tested to help knowledge workers. This work is based on earlier activities at other offices of Deutsche Telekom (see [1] and [2]).

Infrastructure components which have previously been inflexibly fixed in the real world are being virtualized and thus made accessible to optimization by IT systems. This can increase the efficiency of knowledge work while at the same time permitting more sustainable use to be made of the necessary resources. Intuitive usability is achieved by a consistently ergonomic user interface concept.

2 Holistic Concepts for the Office of the Future

The newly developed modules for the office of the future are based on a holistic approach. Information, communication, media, building and security technologies, which used to be separate, are growing together. This means that the organizational structures

B.-T. Karsh (Ed.): Ergonomics and Health Aspects, HCII 2009, LNCS 5624, pp. 49–55, 2009.

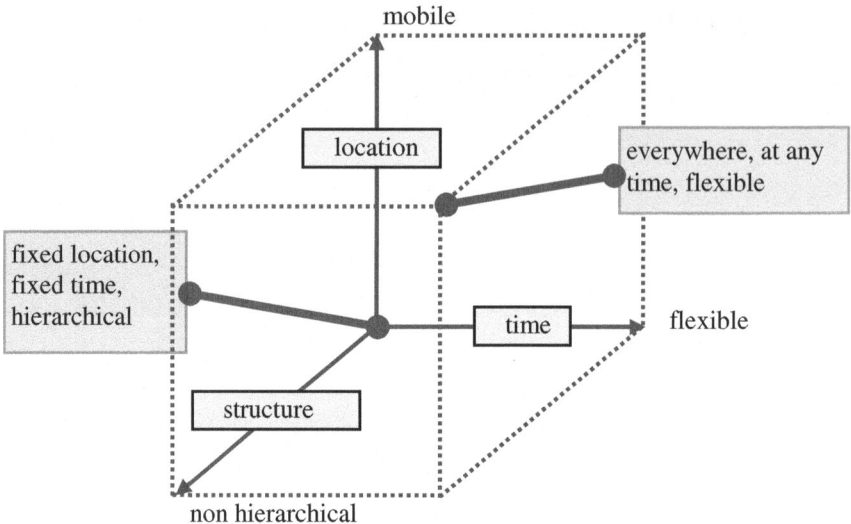

Fig. 1. Collaboration in three dimensions: mobile, flexible and non-hierarchical work environment

responsible for IT, for telecoms and for facility management can also be combined in future. The complete solution results in efficiency savings, despite the higher investment costs involved. This is because of the operational aspects, which can now be optimized as a whole, and because of the use of ideas such as desk sharing, which make best use of resources.

The key to the integration of all infrastructure systems is the use of IP in all technical systems. Not just the data network and the telephone system are based on this, both building services and media technology components also communicate via IP. This allows applications to be implemented which use several systems as well as permitting all infrastructure components to be managed and operated with unified processes.

The real and the virtual worlds are merging. This means that the real world around us and the world of IT systems are connected to one another so that procedures in the real world can be made more efficient by the use of processes supported by IT. To this end, more and more sensors, actuators and output devices will be installed in the office environment, such as interactive door-signs, RFID readers and intelligent, personalized building automation solutions.

Being able to locate people inside and outside of office buildings permits new, sophisticated functions. Several sensor systems are used to detect the last position of people: RFID cards are used to open doors, to book a workplace or to receive information at an information screen. Whenever a RFID card is used, the position of the user is determined. Whenever a phone is used, the system assumes that the user of the phone is at the known location of the phone. Additionally an experimental system component uses WLAN localization [6].

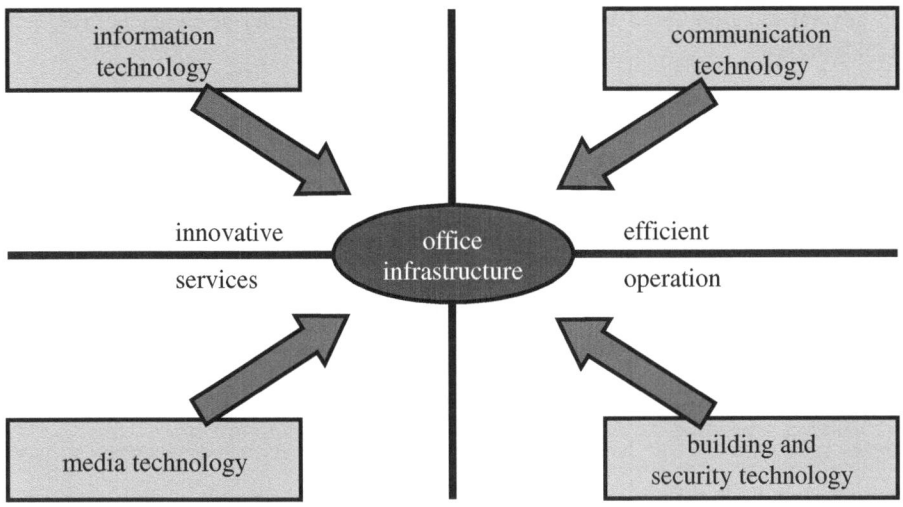

Fig. 2. Integrated services and an innovative office infrastructure for more efficient Information Workers

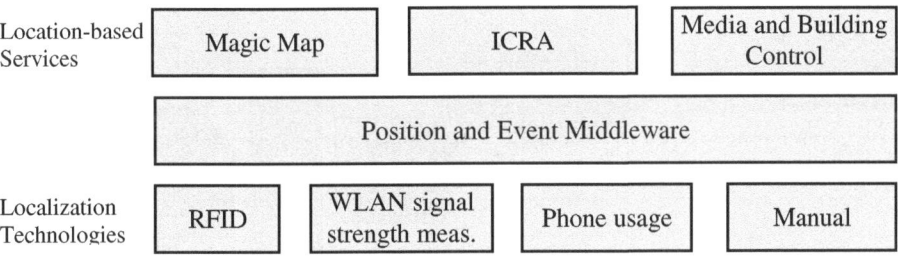

Fig. 3. Location-based services (LBS) are used to take advantage of location to automate services

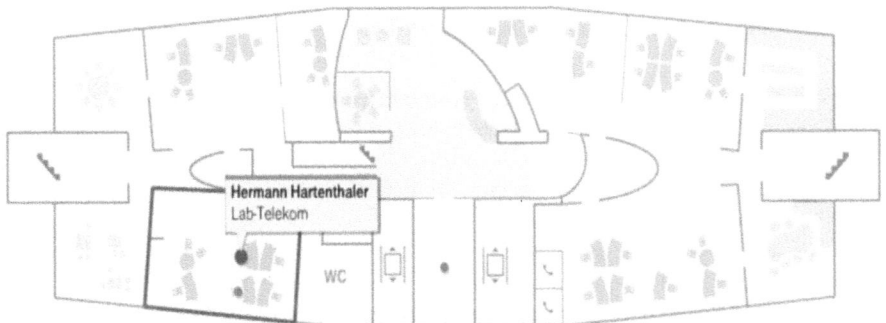

Fig. 4. The Magic Map shows the last monitored position of colleagues

Several location-based services were deployed and tested at Deutsche Telekom Laboratories:

- Magic Map – display the current location of colleagues
- ICRA – Intelligent Call Routing Agent to automatically redirect incoming calls
- Media & Light control – control features provided only where the user is currently located.

The geographic separation of company locations loses some of its drawbacks if all of the infrastructure services can be offered whatever your location is. Even home offices can become an integral part of the corporate infrastructure due to ubiquitous, high bandwidth connections to the Internet.

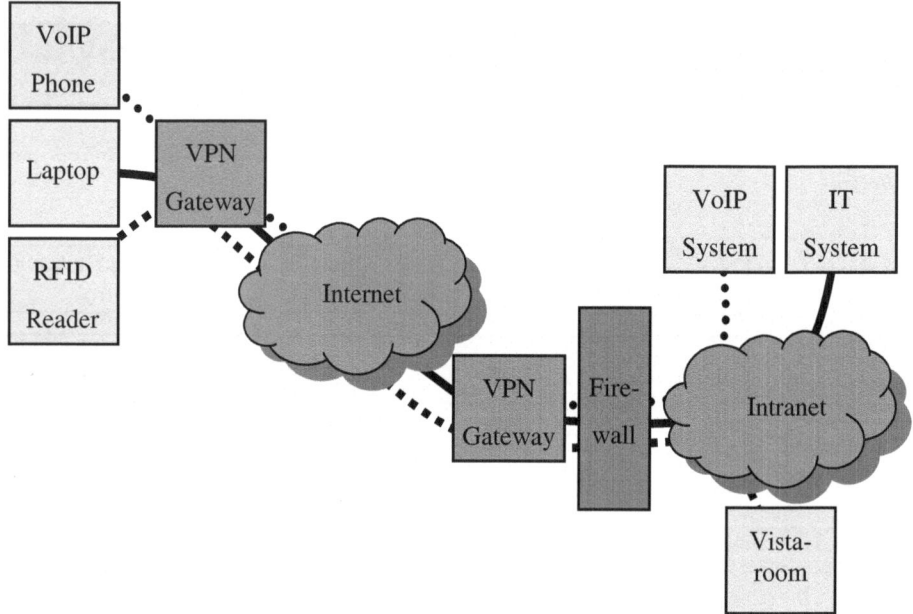

Fig. 5. Home offices can be connected to the intranet of the company

Mobile work in and out of the office is supported by WLAN and UMTS technologies. Even physically connected data networks can be flexibly used by dynamically assigned virtual networks. The use of virtual LANs (VLANs) means that current restrictions, when assigning IP networks with differing security guidelines to the computers concerned, can be loosened up.

The use of desk sharing is supported by a workplace booking system [7], where the workplace booked can be customized to your personal preferences via an RFID card. This is detected at the desk concerned and configures the IP phone for your personal phone number and programs the buttons with your settings, as well as activating your own scenario for the building services at the location. To make this work, the building automation system is integrated into the infrastructure management system via IP.

This means that the use of energy can be optimized as, in contrast to conventional building automation systems, the control system can take account of the planned use. Traditional administration of building automation services regards them as having a confined scope, operating in isolation or tightly coupled and providing only minimal support for an overall coordination and a holistic management approach. IP-based building automation components and services can be integrated more easily.

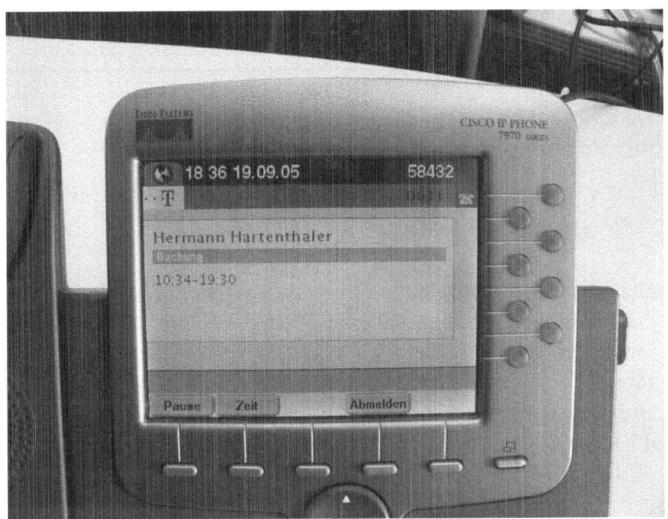

Fig. 6. Booking of workplaces and control of lights and blinds are possible using an IP-Phone or a browser application

The booking of items such as workplaces, rooms or even lockers for personal documents, always uses the same sequence of operations so that it is easy to get to know and then to use the system.

Paper mail is distributed via an electronic mailbox. If someone puts physical mail such as magazines or even contracts into a pigeon-hole for a user, they also activate a push-button, which triggers an email to the user saying "You have mail". Physical and electronic mail are thus linked together.

A video conference system at the workplace supports communication processes, which amongst other things is also compatible to UMTS picture phone applications. A video conference solution fixed to a particular room is also used, to protect the environment and to save travelling time and expenses. Here, a telepresence approach [8] is pursued, where all of the video conferencing rooms are identically equipped with very large HDTV monitors, creating the feeling for the participants in a meeting, that the physically separate rooms merge to a single, virtual conference room.

3 Increasing the Efficiency in the Office

When planning a meeting, the date is fixed, the room booked and the agenda is produced, all in virtual space (using Microsoft Sharepoint (MOSS) [9]). When the meeting

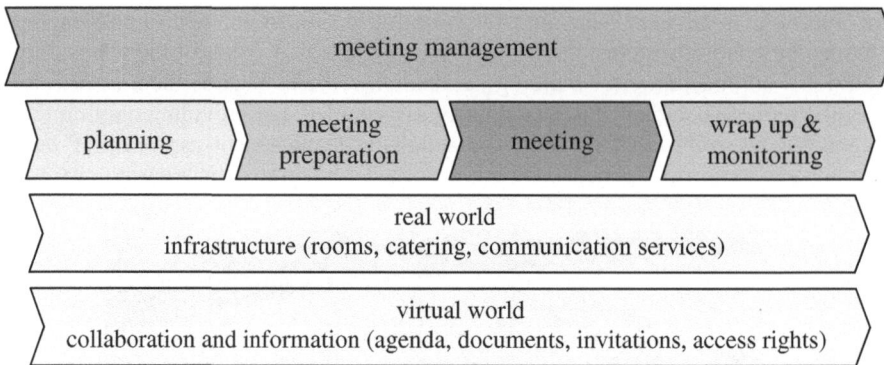

Fig. 7. Real and virtual world are interconnected in the process "Meeting Management" for more efficient meetings

starts, the interactive doorplate on the physical conference room will show the name of the meeting, the invited participants will have access to the room and the projector will show the agenda already.

In the conference rooms involved, interactive whiteboards are used on which presentations can be projected and on which special pens can be used to "write", and the writing then becomes a graphical object in the presentation. This makes the transition from "real" drawing on the board, to saving in a "virtual" document very easy.

4 Experience

The modules which have been implemented and integrated have now been used on a daily basis for three years in everyday work. About 160 employees are using 120 desk-sharing workplaces at two locations, one in Berlin, Germany, and another one in

Table 1. Advantages and Disadvantages of new office environment

Advantages	Disadvantages
Flexibility with the office organization allows dynamic change processes.	Excessive compaction of office space leads to strong work load.
Integration of all technical areas leads to more comfortable and efficient structures.	Higher complexity requires more broadly qualified infrastructure staff.
Open space office leads to more communication and fewer barriers.	Fewer walls mean more noise and more disturbances for employees.
Work at any time and everywhere by telepresence and flexible work models leads to increased efficiency.	Permanent accessibility and omission of unproductive working phases lead to higher load of the employees.
Knowledge management and central information systems lead to a better availability of information in the enterprise.	Inadmissible monitoring of the employees must be prevented.

Los Altos, California. Another 150 colleagues are using traditional workplaces at three other locations in Germany. The complete solution has led to very efficient use of office space and other resources; it has led to increased flexibility for the project teams and to a working atmosphere which is quite an inspiration.

References

1. Pfeifer, T., Micklei, A., Hartenthaler, H.: Internet-integrated Building Control: Leaving the Lab – Robust, Scalable and Secure. In: 26th IEEE Workshop on Local Computer Networks, LCN 2001, Tampa, Florida USA, November 14-16, pp. 306–315. IEEE Computer Society Press, Los Alamitos (2001)
2. Pfeifer, T., Hartenthaler, H.: Internet Embedded Control Networks – A Reality Check. In: Proc. of 6th World Multiconference on Systemics, Cybernetics and Informatics, SCI 2002, Orlando, Florida USA, July 14-18, 2002; International Institute of Informatics and Systemics (IIIS): Proc. SCI 2002/ISAS 2002, vol. XII (Industrial Systems and Engineering II) (2002) ISBN: 980-07-8150-1 (hardcopy), 980-07-8146-3 (CD)
3. Ray, S., Kwiat, K., Zhang, D.: Energy-efficient placement/activation algorithms for authorization servers in sensor network. In: Proceedings of Ninth International Symposium on Computers and Communications (ISCC 2004), June 28-July 1, vol. 1, pp. 312–317 (2004) ISBN: 0-7803-8623-X
4. Malatras, A., Asgari, A.H., Baugé, T., Irons, M.: A service-oriented architecture for building services integration. Journal of Facilities Management 6(2), 132–151 (2008)
5. Krishnamurthy, S., Anson, O., Sapir, L., Glezer, C., Rois, M., Shub, I., Schlöder, K.: Automation of Facility Management Processes Using Machine-to-Machine Technologies. In: Floerkemeier, C., Langheinrich, M., Fleisch, E., Mattern, F., Sarma, S.E. (eds.) IOT 2008. LNCS, vol. 4952, pp. 68–86. Springer, Heidelberg (2008)
6. Ekahau product RTLS, http://ekahau.com
7. Ivistar product Vistaroom, http://www.ivistar.de
8. Cisco product TelePresence, http://www.cisco.com
9. Microsoft product Sharepoint (MOSS), http://microsoft.com

The Relationship between Working Conditions and Musculoskeletal/Ergonomic Disorders in a Manufacturing Facility – A Longitudinal Research Study

Dennis R. Jones

Department of Technology
College of Engineering and Engineering Technology
Northern Illinois University
DeKalb, Illinois, USA
jones@ceet.niu.edu

Abstract. I have done research on the relationship between working conditions and musculoskeletal/ergonomic disorders in a manufacturing facility. I believe that the biomechanical and psychosocial aspects of work have a significant influence on the individual worker's health and well-being. The work organization at which I have evaluated the employee's health and well-being and collected a large amount of data; which I have analyzed; is at a large manufacturing facility. This research is based upon the Balance Theory Model of Smith & Carayon-Sainfort [2], [3]. This model specifies that the working conditions and other factors outside of work can create a stress on the individual. That stress can have physiological and psychological consequences. If the stress exceeds the individual's capacity, the stress can produce a negative effect on the individual which could result in a strain. This is a bad fit between the individual resources and the work demands. If the stressful exposure continues for a prolonged time period, then this can result in serious musculoskeletal disorders.

Keywords: Human Factors, Ergonomics, Musculoskeletal Disorders, Psychosocial, Balance Theory Model, Applied Field Research, Manufacturing, Assembly, Production Processes.

1 Introduction

The Balance Theory Model is a system view concept for the various elements of a work system, it shows the stress that working conditions can exert on the individual. In the model the elements interact to determine the way in which work is done. At the center of this model is the individual with their physical characteristics, perceptions, personality and behavior. The task, technology, organization, and environment affect the content of the job and the physical demands the job makes on the individual.

2 The Research Purpose

The overall purpose of this research study was to identify the stressful working conditions and control them. Therefore the purpose of an intervention is to control

B.-T. Karsh (Ed.): Ergonomics and Health Aspects, HCII 2009, LNCS 5624, pp. 56–60, 2009.

musculoskeletal disorders, to reduce the stress load, and to eliminate strain. There are a variety of things that can be done in the workplace for eliminating or reducing the occurrence of occupational musculoskeletal disorders. These include engineering redesign, change in work method, administrative control, worker training, exercise, work hardening, and management to reduce exposures.

3 The Research

This research was performed by using a multiple paged questionnaire survey to evaluate three different assembly methods at a large manufacturing facility. Data was collected several times over a period of time; therefore a longitudinal research study design was conducted. These three different assembly methods were exhibited and displayed by these three distinct individual assembly lines. One of these assembly lines consisted of the employee subjects of interest (i.e. the study group). The other two assembly lines served as the control groups for the study group.

The overall aim of this research is to improve the long term health and well being of workers in a manufacturing facility. The overall purpose of this research is to identify the stressful working conditions and control them. Therefore the purpose of an intervention is to control musculoskeletal disorders, in order to reduce the stress load and to eliminate strain.

4 Research Contributions

One of the contributions of this research is to determine the relationship between working conditions and musculoskeletal / ergonomic disorders in a manufacturing facility. Generally the literature on this topic tends to be more heavily concentrated on the office worker, or service provider type of worker. Therefore the area of workers in a manufacturing facility needs further investigation. Generally, the combination of biomechanical and psychosocial working conditions on musculoskeletal pain / discomfort also needs further investigation.

A second contribution is to improve the research techniques and methodology which has been utilized in some previous scientific studies which attempted to control musculoskeletal disorders. Specifically the scientific evidence on interventions to control musculoskeletal disorders has some shortcomings. The lack of sound research methods and the lack of sound research designs are significant shortcomings in some of the existing literature. This position is supported by the National Academy of Sciences paper of Smith, Karsh & Moro [4]. Their paper investigated and reviewed the research on interventions to control musculoskeletal disorders.

A third contribution is that the results of this research study can assist engineers in designing the jobs of workers in a manufacturing facility. The incorporation of both biomechanical and psychosocial aspects on worker job design should reduce the worker's musculoskeletal / ergonomic disorders, and therefore improve the long term health and well being of workers in a manufacturing facility.

5 Literature Review – Summary

In summary, the National Research Council [1] concluded that there is theoretical evidence and some empirical evidence that links psychosocial factors and musculoskeletal discomfort. Stress appears to be a mediating variable that contributes to the development of musculoskeletal disorders. There also exists some theoretical evidence and some empirical evidence that links biomechanical factors and musculoskeletal discomfort.

In conclusion, more research studies need to be done in order to provide an answer to the existence of the link between biomechanical factors and psychosocial factors, and musculoskeletal disorders. Substantial research literature needs to be developed before a definitive answer could be given; yet the link seems very plausible.

6 The Study Design

The study was performed by using a multiple paged questionnaire to survey the three different assembly methods at the manufacturing assembly facility. Data was collected several times over a period of time; therefore a longitudinal study was conducted. These three different assembly methods were exhibited and displayed by three distinct individual manufacturing assembly lines. One of these manufacturing assembly lines consisted of the employee subjects of interest (i.e., the study group) which was called the study group. The other two assembly lines served as the control groups for the study group; these two areas were called the control group 1 and the control group 2.

7 The Data Collection

Data was collected from the three manufacturing assembly line area employee groups by utilizing a multiple page questionnaire survey. The multiple page questionnaire surveys were designed in order to obtain the information of desired pertaining to the research questions asked. The multiple page questionnaire surveys were given to both the study group and the control groups.

The multiple page questionnaire survey which was given to the study group and control groups was organized as follows:

1. Job Information (8 questions),
2. Characteristics of Work Environment (41 questions),
3. Quality of work Life (5 questions),
4. Health Information (23 questions),
5. Ergonomics and Physical Environment (28 questions),
6. Performance (11 questions),
7. Demographics (3 questions),
8. Implementation (3-5 questions) – this section was only given to the study group.

8   The Multivariate Analysis of Variance

I concluded from the results from the multivariate analysis of variance (MANOVA) that musculoskeletal discomfort is primarily influenced by psychosocial factors (such as anxiety, and uncertainty), and physical demands. As when psychosocial factors (such as anxiety, and uncertainty), and physical demands increased; musculoskeletal discomfort also increased. It could be implied that musculoskeletal discomfort and psychosocial factors (such as anxiety, and uncertainty), and physical demands are linearly related.

Therefore, when the physical demands are increased, the stress on the individual is increased, and the ergonomic musculoskeletal discomfort is also increased.

Also, when the anxiety and uncertainty are increased, the stress on the individual is increased, and the psychosocial factor discomfort (i.e., negative psychosocial factors) is also increased.

So, an increase in physical demands, results in increased ergonomic musculoskeletal discomfort. And, an increase in anxiety and uncertainty, also results in increased negative psychosocial factors.

9   The Discussion

The control groups appear to be stable over time in terms of musculoskeletal discomfort, neck/shoulder/back discomfort, hand/arm discomfort, and leg discomfort. The control group 2 consistently exhibits higher self reports of musculoskeletal discomfort, neck/shoulder/back discomfort, hand/arm discomfort, and leg discomfort than the control group 1, over the three rounds of data collection. This is to be expected since the human factors, ergonomics, and working conditions of the control group 2 is significantly worse than the control group 1.

The study group exhibited lower self reports of musculoskeletal discomfort, neck/shoulder/back discomfort, hand/arm discomfort, and leg discomfort than the control groups. This is to be expected since the human factors, ergonomics, and working conditions of the study group was significantly better than the control groups.

The control groups appear to be stable over time in terms of the physical aspects of work. The control group 2 consistently exhibits higher self reports of physical demands, repetitive motions, and loading on individual than the control group 1, over the three rounds of data collection. This is to be expected since the human factors, ergonomics, and working conditions on the control group 2 is significantly worse than the control group 1.

The study group exhibited lower self reports of physical demands, and repetitive motions than the control groups. This is to be expected since the human factors, ergonomics, and working conditions of the study group was significantly better than the control groups.

The control groups appear to be stable over time in some of the psychosocial aspects of work. The control group 2 exhibited lower self reports of task control, job control, resource control, and decision control than the control group 1, over the three rounds of data collection. This is to be expected since the human factors, ergonomics, and working conditions of the control group 2 is significantly worse than the control group 1.

The study group appears to be stable over time in some of the psychosocial aspects of work. The study group exhibited greater self reports of task control, job control, resource control, and decision control than the control groups. This is to be expected since the human factors, ergonomics, working conditions, and employee empowerment of the study group was significantly better than the control groups.

10 Conclusion

In summary, there is theoretical evidence and some empirical evidence that links psychosocial factors and musculoskeletal discomfort. Stress appears to be a mediating variable that contributes to the development of musculoskeletal disorders.

There also exists some theoretical evidence and some empirical evidence that links biomechanical factors and musculoskeletal discomfort.

In conclusion, more research studies need to be done in order to provide an answer to the existence of the link between biomechanical factors and psychosocial factors, and musculoskeletal disorders. Substantial research literature needs to be developed before a definitive answer can be given; yet the link seems very plausible.

References

1. National Research Council: Work-Related Musculoskeletal Disorders: Report, Workshop Summary, and Workshop Paper. Steering Committee for the Workshop on Work-Related Musculoskeletal Injuries: The Research Base. National Academy Press, Washington (1999)
2. Smith, M.J., Carayon, P.: New technology, automation, and work organization: stress problems and improved technology implementation strategies. The International Journal of Human Factors in Manufacturing 5, 99–116 (1995)
3. Smith, M.J., Carayon-Sainfort, P.: A balance theory of job design for stress reduction. International Journal of Industrial Ergonomics 4, 67–79 (1989)
4. Smith, M.J., Karsh, B., Moro, F.B.P.: A review of research on interventions to control musculoskeletal disorders. In: Work-Related Musculoskeletal Disorders: Report, Workshop Summary, and Workshop Papers, National Research Council, National Academy of Sciences, pp. 200–229. National Academy Press, Washington (1999)

Measuring Support for Health in Offshore Environments

Kathryn Mearns and Tom Reader

School of Psychology, University of Aberdeen, Aberdeen AB24 2UB, Scotland, UK
k.mearns@abdn.ac.uk

Abstract. Health and safety are often discussed in the same breath but the relationships between them are not clearly articulated. The current study was conducted in the UK offshore oil and gas industry – a physically and mentally
challenging work environment - where the well-being of personnel is important
for their performance. This paper will describe the development of scales for
measuring support for health offshore and report the results obtained from a
sample of 703 workers from 18 installations regarding the relationship between
perceived support for health and health and organizational outcome measures.

Keywords: Support for health, organizational commitment, organizational citizenship behaviour, health activities.

1 Introduction

The offshore environment is a 'rough, tough world' [3] where the fitness and well-
being of offshore workers can be a major factor in their survival. This applies both in
emergency situations and in the routine of living and working in this remote and in-
hospitable environment. Offshore workers are exposed to confined work and living
conditions, noise and other physical environment stressors (including a range of hazards) and dull, monotonous work [17]. Furthermore they must get along with very
different types of people in this claustrophobic environment and therefore employers
have a 'duty of care' to ensure that their employees experience optimal physical and
mental health. All offshore employees are required to pass a mandatory medical examination and there is a raft of health and safety regulation in place to ensure workers
are protected from both occupational and major process hazards. In addition, many oil
and gas organizations provide health promotion and surveillance activities over and
above those mandated by legislation. These include health promotion and health education, e.g. stress management, healthy eating, as well as 'health therapies' e.g. massage and exercise classes. These 'discretionary' organizational health investment
activities may indicate organizational support for well-being leading to perceptions of
psychological contract fulfilment and associated attitudes and behaviours such as
organizational commitment and organizational citizenship [4], [6], Perceived Organizational Support – POS [7], [20] reflects employees' beliefs about an organization's
support, commitment and care towards them, whereas the 'psychological contract'
refers to employees' beliefs about the mutual obligations that exist between them and
the organization. Both constructs are perceptual in nature and therefore can be interpreted very differently by different employees in the organization – thus they are

B.-T. Karsh (Ed.): Ergonomics and Health Aspects, HCII 2009, LNCS 5624, pp. 61–69, 2009.

individual-level rather than group-level in nature. Employees who experience POS, show higher levels of organizational commitment and more active participation and increased performance in job activities assigned by the organization and those that go beyond their job description, known as organizational citizenship behaviors [19].

A question that has not been fully addressed in the literature is the extent to which an organization's care and concern for the health and well-being of its workforce actually leads to employee engagement in health activities, organizational commitment, OCBs and other behaviors that benefit the organization. According to Grawitch, Gottshalk & Munz (2006) job satisfaction has been the focus of much of the previous research on employee well-being and organizational improvements, although job satisfaction is related to organizational commitment [26] and organizational commitment has been associated with lower turnover and higher performance [14]. The reinforcing link between employee well-being and organizational improvements serves to strengthen the positive impact of supportive organizational practices.

2 Organizational Support for Health and Employee Commitment and Behavior

The current study explores the possibility that investment in employee health and well-being is indicative of an organization's care and commitment to its workforce. This will be particularly relevant in safety-critical industries such as offshore oil and gas, where the workforce have to perform at their optimum in order to maintain good safety performance. In this context, employees would have expectations of organizational support for health and fitness in order to reduce the risks of psycho-social stress and make the rigors of offshore life more tolerable. Earlier research has shown that offshore installations where worker health is a priority tend to have lower lost-time injury rates than installations where health is not a priority [16], and Mearns and hope [15] found that organizational investment in health results in positive employee attitudes and behaviors. Evidence was found for the proposition that organizational investment in employee health helps to foster perceptions of company commitment and build worker loyalty in areas such as safety. Respondents on installations that reported lower health management scores reported significantly poorer scores on unrelated measures of climate and commitment when compared to installations with high scores. Furthermore, greater investment in health-related activities was also found to result in fewer risk taking behaviors and greater commitment at the installation level. The findings indicated that organizational investment in workforce health may not only be limited to health related benefits, but may also be associated with broader organizational benefits in the form of greater workforce commitment and improved safety behavior. This finding will be expanded upon in current study. In particular, the current study investigates the hypothesis that support for health by the organization, supervisors and workmates impacts upon personal health activities, organizational commitment and organizational behavior.

3 Method

The 'Health at Work 2004' questionnaire contained an introductory text and several sections each identified by a title bar and an opening paragraph explaining how to complete that section. Respondents were requested to answer the questions as accurately as possible and to carefully consider their responses in relation to the installation they work on. Respondents were instructed to return completed questionnaires in the addressed envelopes supplied with the questionnaires and were assured of the confidentiality of their responses.

3.1 Section 1: General Information

Respondents were asked to indicate the name of the installation they were currently working on, whether they were employed by an operating or contracting company, whether they were in a supervisory role, whether they were a member of the core crew and the number of years they had worked on the installation. Respondents were reassured that it would not be possible to identify anyone personally from the data they provided.

3.2 Section 2: Support for Health

Three scales were designed to measure support for health at the organizational, supervisor and workforce level. Respondents were required to indicate their agreement, on a 5-point Likert scale (1=Strongly Disagree / 5=Strongly Agree), with 19 statements, 5 referring to health support from the organization (in this case the organization operating the installation), 6 from supervisors and 8 from workmates. The organizational support for health scale was based on items developed by Basen-Engquist, Hudson, Tripp and Chamberlain [1] The supervisor items referred to the degree to which supervisors ensure that employee health is not endangered by work, that health rules are enforced, that health and safety issues can be discussed with supervisors and the sympathy afforded by supervisors for health problems. The workmates items referred to the support and encouragement that workmates would provide if respondents started dieting, exercising or stopped smoking, the degree to which workmates share health information and give help and support when asked. Items were taken from the scale developed by Ribisl & Reischl [21].

3.3 Section 3: Organizational Commitment

This section referred to the commitment that respondents felt with regard to the installation they worked on. Respondents were asked to indicate whether, on a 5-point Likert scale (1=Strongly Disagree / 5=Strongly Agree), they agreed with a range of statements describing feelings about working on the installation. In total 7 items describing feelings of organizational commitment were incorporated into section 10. Items referred to the sense of belonging respondents felt towards the installation, the contribution they make to the installation and the pride they feel working for the installation. The items were taken from a measure used by Coyle-Shapiro & Kessler [4].

3.4 Section 4: Health Activities

This section contained 7 statements indicating whether respondents could engage in various health and well-being activities on the installation. Examples included managing stress levels, participating in health promotion activities and relaxing when off shift. Respondents were asked to indicated their level of agreement with the statements on a 5-point Likert scale ranging from 1=Strongly Disagree to 5=Strongly Agree).

3.5 Section 5: Organizational Citizenship Behaviour

This section contained 9 statements concerning organizational citizenship behaviours which respondents had to evaluate on a 5-point Likert scale (1=Not at all / 5=To a great extent). These behaviors included making suggestions to improve and revise work procedures, taking action to improve the organization and the installation, informing management about unproductive or unsafe practices and speaking up about work issues or rules that do not contribute to the achievement of the installation goals. The items for this scale were taken from Coyle-Shapiro & Kessler [5] and Tsui et al.[25].

4 Results

4.1 Sample Characteristics

The 18 installations surveyed were representative of those operating on the UK Continental Shelf and included fixed production platforms, drilling rigs, well-service vessels and floating production storage and offloading vessels (FPSOs). A total of 703 useable questionnaires were received (overall response rate 35%, range 22% to 94%). The majority of respondents (84%) were core crew and 40% indicated that they were employed directly by an operating company, with 60% working for contractor or subcontractor companies.

The greatest proportion of respondents (37%) were aged 41–50 years; 26% were more than 51 years of age; 27% were aged between 31 and 40 years and 10% were aged 20–30 years indicating an ageing profile of the workforce. The main occupations included maintenance (23%); administration/ management (15%); production (13%), construction (11%) and catering (10%). Overall, 19% of respondents had worked on their installation for less than a year while 45% indicated they had worked on their installation between 1 and 5 years. 22% had spent 6–10 years on their installation while 14% had been on their installation for more than 10 years.

Table 1. Descriptives and Correlations between measures

	Mean	OHS	SHS	WHS	OrgCom	HealthAct	OCB
OHS	3.35	**.80**	.51	.40	.39	.48	.17
SHS	3.74		**.91**	.41	.18	.47	.20
WHS	3.52			**.87**	.19	.35	.19
OrgCom	3.06				**.93**	.25	.02
HealthAct	3.38					**.83**	.13
OCB	3.64						**.89**

OHS=Organizational health support, SHS=Supervisor health support, WHS=Workmate health support, OrgComm=Organizational Commitment, OCB=Organizational Citizenship Behaviour

Table 2. Regression analysis for organizational commitment, health activities and organizational citizenship

Outcome	Predictors	Beta	R	F
	Final model		.384	12.68***
Organizational Commitment	Installation	.003		
	Employed by	-.007		
	Supervisor	.022		
	Core Crew	.078		
	Years worked	.048		
	OHS	.395***		
	SHS	-.070		
	WHS	.029		
	Final model		.559	33.24***
Health Activities	Installation	.073*		
	Employed by	.144***		
	Supervisor	.049		
	Core Crew	-.043		
	Years worked	-.024		
	OHS	.290***		
	SHS	.247***		
	WHS	.130***		
	Final model		.438	17.36***
Organizational citizenship	Installation	.092**		
	Employed by	-.072		
	Supervisor	-.256***		
	Core Crew	-.151***		
	Years worked	-.009		
	OHS	.040		
	SHS	.119**		
	WHS	.128***		

*p<.05, **p<.01, ***p<.001

Overall, only 6% of respondents had been involved in an accident on that installation in the past year, indicating high levels of safety performance. The demographic data indicated that the survey sample was representative of the offshore workforce regarding their age, experience and type of job. Data was inputted and analysed using SPSS v. 12.

4.2 Relationships between Variables

Table 1 shows the relationship between the variables investigated in the study. All correlation coefficients are significant at the 0.01 level except the Organizational Commitment and OCB relationship, which is not significant. As can be seen from the table most of the correlation coefficients are small to medium in size. Scale reliabilities (Cronbach's Alpha) are shown on the diagonal. Mean values show that most respondents were giving neutral or slightly positive responses to the scale items.

Three regression equations were run investigating the effect of the three health support measures on the dependent measures of organizational commitment, health activities and organizational citizenship. Demographic variables were also entered into the equations as a control measure.

For Organizational Commitment only Organizational Support for Health was a significant predictor explaining 13.6% variance ($F_{(9,668)}=12.68$, $p<.001$; $t=9.11$). None of the demographic variables exerted an effect.

For health activities, all three health support measures plus installation and employee status were significant predictors explaining 30.3% of the variance ($F_{(9,667)}=33.24$, $p<.001$); $t(OHS)=7.45$; $t(SHS)=6.40$; $t(WHS)=3.58$; $t(Installation)=2.23$; t(employee status)$=3.93$). Obviously the capacity to engage in health activities will be affected on what facilities the installation can or does provide, hence this effect would be anticipated. Furthermore, operator personnel (who are direct employees of the organization) engaged in more health activities than contractors.

For OCB, Supervisor health support ($t=2.85$) and Workmate health support ($t=3.24$) were significant predictors as were Installation ($t=2.56$), supervisor status ($t=7.19$) and being a member of the core crew ($t=3.80$), ($F_{(9,667)}=17.36$, $p<.001$). These variables explained 18.1% of the variance.

5   Discussion

The results indicate that different types of health support exert differential effects on the outcome measures of interest in this study. Health support was chosen as the independent variable of interest since it is believed to reflect levels of care and concern for employees' well-being, particularly in the offshore environment where well-being can have important implications for organizational outcomes, such as safety. Higher levels of organizational health support predicted greater organizational commitment but supervisor and workmate support for health showed no significant effect. For engagement in health activities it would appear that support at all organizational levels is important and explains a reasonably high amount of variance in the outcome measure, thus higher levels of perceived support lead to higher levels of health engagement. Being a member of the operator staff also leads to higher levels of engagement. Finally, for organizational citizenship behaviors, organizational health support does not seem to play an important role but support from supervisors and workmates exerts a small but significant effect. Finally supervisory status and being member of the core crew also have significant effects with both groups being more likely to engage in this type of behavior.

The relationship between organizational support and organizational commitment is well-established in the literature [10] and is believed to be based on Social Exchange Theory [2] and norm of reciprocity [13]. The current study provides further support for this relationship and extends the POS work by focusing more specifically on POS for health and therefore practices that are implemented to encourage employee well-being. Whitener [27] found that high commitment human resource practices strengthened employees' trust and commitment to the organization when they perceived the organization to support them. Supervisor and workmate support for health probably did not show an effect because in both the commitment and support scales the 'organization' was the object of evaluation (in this case the organization referred to the installation the individual was working on). Eisenberger et al. [9] found that supervisors, depending on the degree with which they are identified with the organization, contribute to overall perceptions of operator support. Therefore supervisor support for the health and well being of employees may be perceived by the workforce as an indication of the organization's concern for the welfare of its employees.

Support from the organization, supervisors and workmates seemed to be necessary for employees to participate in activities designed to enhance their health and well-being. Sloan & Gruman [24] identified perceptions of control over work, supervisor support and work time flexibility to take part in healthy activities as dimensions of organizational climate that predicted employee participation in worksite health promotion programs. Ribisl and Reischl [21] identified 'a climate for health' subsumed under general organizational climate, which was strongly associated with exercise behaviors, smoking behaviors, nutrition, job stress and job satisfaction. Pender [18] suggests developing a 'health strengthening environment' which directly promotes and facilitates healthy behavioral norms. These results and the results of the current study seem to suggest that positive health norms are required at all levels of the organization in order to facilitate health behaviors. Even if the organization provides support for health, supervisors and workmates will have to be willing to accommodate the time and effort that their colleagues require in order to engage in these behaviors and group norms will be important for maintaining the activities.

Finally, the relationship between support for health and OCBs was mainly 'predicted' by demographic variables. Thus supervisors, core crew and operator employees were more likely to engage in these types of behavior. This makes sense as all these groups would be more motivated to engage in activities that led to the success of their workplace due to vested interests and their own job or career prospects with the organization. Supervisor support for health and workmate support for health also exerted a small significant effect but Organizational Support for Health did not. This relationship was hypothesized to exist due to care and concern for employees as demonstrated through health support would create a climate where support and assistance is provided for the organization, again reflecting the process of reciprocal exchange. Also, somewhat surprisingly there was no significant relationship between Organizational Commitment and OCB as anticipated (non-significant correlation). It would appear that a climate of care and concern for health and well-being is not necessarily responsible for motivating offshore workers to engage in OCBs and that demographic variables such as being a supervisor and being a member of the core crew on the installation exert more effect.

In general, the results of this study are supported by other evidence in the literature. For example, Shannon, Mayr & Haines [22] found that practices that reflected a 'genuine concern of management about their workforce' rather than 'tinkering' with policies and procedures tended to be more effective. Likewise, Mearns, Whitaker and Flin [16] found that installations with good health management practices had lower rates of lost-time injuries than installations with fewer health management practices. A further study by Mearns & Hope [15] found that greater investment in health-related activities resulted in fewer risk taking behaviors and greater commitment at the installation level. Discretionary activities related to health promotion and education at the workplace would seem to fit with a climate of care and concern, where the workforce feel obliged to reciprocate the altruistic actions espoused and enacted by their managers, in line with Social Exchange Theory [2] and the psychological contract [4]. Finally, the data appears to support Grawitch et al.'s [12] PATH model (Practices for the Achievement of Total Health), which proposes that healthy workplace practices such as work-life balance, employee growth and development, health and safety, recognition, and employee involvement has both direct and indirect links to positive employee and organizational performance, e.g. turnover, absenteeism, accidents/injuries. In conclusion, the evidence suggests that investing in workforce wellness and well-being delivers tangible benefits for both individual employees and the organization in general. However, there are limitations to drawing conclusions from this type of cross-sectional questionnaire design and future research should focus on examining the impact of a health promoting workplace on a range of outcome measures using quasi-experimental designs and incorporating control groups.

References

1. Basen-Engquist, K., Hudmon, K.S., Tripp, M., Chamberlain, R.: Worksite health and safety climate: Scale development and effects of a health promotion intervention. Preventive Medicine 27(1), 111–119 (1998)
2. Blau, P.: Exchange and Power in Social Life. Wiley, New York (1964)
3. Cox, R., Norman, J.: Some special problems. In: Raf, C. (ed.) Offshore Medicine: Medical Care of Employees in the Offshore Oil Industry. Springer, London (1987)
4. Coyle-Shapiro, J.: A psychological contract perspective on organizational citizenship behavior. Journal of Organizational Behaviour 23, 927–946 (2002)
5. Coyle-Shapiro, J., Kessler, I.: Consequences of the Psychological Contract for the Employment Relationship: A Large Scale Survey. Journal of Management Studies 37(7), 903–930 (2000)
6. Coyle-Shapiro, J., Conway, N.: Exchange relationships: examining psychological contracts and perceived organizational support. Journal of Applied Psychology 90, 774–781 (2005)
7. Eisenberger, R., Huntington, R., Hutchison, S., Sowa, D.: Perceived organizational support. Journal of Applied Psychology 71, 500–507 (1986)
8. Eisenberger, R., Fasolo, P., Davis-LaMastro, V.: Perceived organizational support and employee diligence, commitment, and innovation. Journal of Applied Psychology 75, 51–59 (1990)
9. Eisenberger, R., Stinglhamber, F., Vandenberghe, C., Sucharski, I.L., Rhoades, L.: Perceived supervisor support: contributions to perceived organizational support and employee retention. Journal of Applied Psychology 87, 565–573 (2002)

10. Fuller, J.B., Barnett, T., Hester, K., Relyea, C.: A Social Identity perspective on the relationship between perceived organizational support and organizational commitment. The Journal of Social Psychology 143(6), 789–791 (2003)

11. Geller, E., Roberts, S., Gilmore, M.: Predicting propensity to actively care for occupational safety. Journal of Safety Research 27, 1–8 (1996)

12. Grawitch, M.J., Gottschalk, M., Munz, D.C.: The path to a healthy workplace: A critical review linking healthy workplace practices, employee well-being, and organizational improvements. Consulting Psychology Journal: Practice and Research 58(3), 129–147 (2006)

13. Gouldner, A.W.: The norm of reciprocity. American Sociological Review 25, 165–167 (1960)

14. Mathieu, J., Zajac, D.: A review and meta-analysis of the antecedents, correlates, and consequences of organisational commitment. Psychological Bulletin 108, 171–194 (1990)

15. Mearns, K., Hope, L.: Health and well-being in the offshore environment: The management of personal health. Research Report 305. HSE Books, Norwich (2005)

16. Mearns, K., Whitaker, S.M., Flin, R.: Safety climate, safety management practice and safety performance in offshore environments. Safety Science 41, 641–680 (2003)

17. Parkes, K.: Human factors, shift work and alertness in the offshore oil industry. In: Part 1 A Survey of Onshore and Offshore Control-room Operators and Part 2 Alertness, Sleep and Cognitive Performance, HMSO, London (1993)

18. Pender, N.: Health promotion in the workplace: Suggested directions for research. American Journal of Health Promotion 3(3), 38–43 (1989)

19. Podsakoff, P.M., MacKenzie, S., Painea, J., Bachracha, J.: Organizational citizenship behaviors: a critical review of the theoretical and empirical literature and suggestions for future research. Journal of Management 26, 513–563 (2000)

20. Rhoades, L., Eisenberger, R.: Perceived organizational support: a review of the literature. Journal of Applied Psychology 87, 698–714 (2002)

21. Ribisl, K.M., Reischl, T.M.: Measuring the climate for Health at Organizations – development of the worksite health climate scales. Journal of Occupational and Environmental Medicine 35(8), 812–824 (1993)

22. Shannon, H., Mayr, J., Haines, T.: Overview of the relationship between organizational and workplace factors and injury rates. Safety Science 26, 201–217 (1997)

23. Simard, M., Marchand, A.: A multilevel analysis of organisational factors related to the taking of safety initiatives by work groups. Safety Science 21, 113–129 (1995)

24. Sloan, R., Gruman, J.: Participation in workplace health promotion programs: The contribution of health and organizational factors. Health Education Quarterly 15, 269–288 (1988)

25. Tsui, A.S., Pearce, J.L., Porter, L.W., Tripoli, A.M.: Alternative approaches to the employee organization relationship: does investment in employees pay off? Academy of Management Journal 40, 1089–1121 (1997)

26. Vandenburg, R.J., Lance, C.E.: Examining the Causal Order of Job Satisfaction and Organizational Commitment. Journal of Management 18(1), 153–167 (1992)

27. Whitener, E.M.: Do "high commitment" human resource practices affect employee commitment? A cross-level analysis using hierarchical linear modelling. Journal of Management 27, 515–535 (2001)

Understanding Patient User Experience in Obstetric Work Systems

Enid N.H. Montague

Industrial and Systems Engineering Department
University of Wisconsin-Madison3270 Mechanical Engineering
1513 University Avenue Madison, WI 53706
emontague@wisc.edu

Abstract. Patient user experiences with medical technology may be important predictors of patient ratings of satisfaction with health care systems and of acceptance of technologies used in their care. The purpose of this study was to understand how patients experience medical technology during medical events as passive users. 25 women were interviewed after the birth of their child about the technologies that were used to provide them care. Interviews were transcribed verbatim and reduced to codes in the qualitative data analysis tradition. Results show that patients have user experiences with technologies as passive users.

Keywords: Patients, Technology, User Experience, Health Care.

1 Introduction

Human computer interaction theorists have begun to explore new definitions of user experience that include concepts such as trust, engagement, fun and fidelity [1, 2]. This study used qualitative research methods to develop a typology of obstetric patients' user experiences with medical technology and proposes a socio-technical systems framework for measuring and understanding patients' total user experience with medical technology. We examined patients' user experiences with medical technologies during the birth of their child using open-ended interviews with 25 mothers after they had given birth. The decision to explore patients' experiences with the technologies used in their care, was based on our hypothesis that patients have experiences with technologies and the technologies affect patients' experiences, even when patients are not active users of the technologies, in the same sense that their care providers might be.

1.1 Definitions of User Experience

There are three major perspectives of user experience; 1) user experience as human needs beyond usability; 2) user experience includes emotional and affective aspects of human interactions; and 3) user experience is the deconstruction of what it means to have an experience [3]. This study examined the user experiences of patients in an obstetric work system to build upon theoretical perspectives of user experience that

B.-T. Karsh (Ed.): Ergonomics and Health Aspects, HCII 2009, LNCS 5624, pp. 70–77, 2009.

move user experience with technology beyond usability [3]. We were interested in how patients developed and expressed user experiences with technologies they might not use. We also wanted to understand the emotional aspect of user experience in health care, emphasizing how aspects of interactions with technologies and systems might lead to positive or negative user experiences. Lastly, we wanted to define user experience in the context of humans as both patients in a health care environment and as passive users of a technology.

1.2 User Experience Beyond Usability

Researchers have argued for the importance of including non-task related user needs in the design of products and systems, but gaps continue to exist in our collective understanding of the antecedents, factors and outcomes of emotional usability [3]. Researchers have explored constructs such as trust [4-6], fun [7-12] and happiness [13, 14] in relation to the creation of user experiences and perceptions of usability [15-17]. In health care work systems, trust and privacy are important for patients' interactions with technologies [18, 19]. We hypothesized that patients would expect their interactions with the technology and system to reflect their emotional experiences of happiness and excitement, which might affect their overall user experience.

1.3 Emotional User Experience

User experience research and health care research have recently adopted an emphasis on creating positive user experiences. In 2003 the Department of Health (DHS) found patient emotional experience to be an important predictor of overall patient satisfaction [20]. To work towards improved patient experiences the DHS issued a 'Patient Experience Statement' which summarizes how patients would like to experience the National Health System emphasizing emotional expectations rather than physical expectations [20]. Emotional experience is also important in user experience research; a major theme in this scholarship is understanding the relationship between design and emotional usability [15, 21-25]; specifically understanding how emotions lead to positive user experiences and how positive user experiences lead to emotions [3, 26, 27]. In this study we were concerned with the relationship between patients' user experiences with technologies and their resultant emotions; specifically how different aspects of the technology lead to different emotions.

1.4 Deconstructing User Experience

Users bring an array of individual characteristics such as emotions, values, experiences, and mental models for interpreting sounds, sight, and touch; each of these characteristics effects new and current experiences [28]. To design a user experience the designer must understand the user holistically, which is particularly important when designing technologies for a health care experience. The experience of being a patient is one of inherent vulnerability and consternation; which may be created at the moment of the medical event or over time as one prepares for the event with smaller medical events. An experience contains countless discrete experiences that are associated with various environments, individuals and objects [29]. The experience of having a baby is made of many small experiences such as the physical experience of being pregnant, having an ultrasound, visiting a hospital, interacting with a doctor and attending a childbirth class. A woman may have many key stakeholders in her experience, such as her friends and family who have had babies before her, her doctor, and her partner. The context of her interactions with her health care providers has the potential to create a type of experience for her; a warm homely doctors office creates a different experience from a sterile, clinic office. In this study we wanted to deconstruct the experiences patients were having with the technologies used in their care to understand how patients might fit in to the sociotechnical system as users.

2   Methods

2.1   Participants

Twenty-five new mothers represented the patient group. All mothers had given birth in a hospital and were between the ages of 19 and 35. Seventeen participants self identified as White or Caucasian, one participant identified as Asian and one as Hispanic, five participants identified as Black or African American. The total number of children a participant had ranged from one to four, 12 mothers had one child, nine had two children, four had three children and two had four children.

2.2   Procedure and Analysis

Qualitative research methods are effective at revealing meanings people assign to their experiences [30]. To explore patients' experiences with the technology they were interviewed about the kinds of technologies that were used in their childbirth experience, what they noticed about the technology and how the technology made them feel. Interviews were transcribed verbatim and data were analyzed using grounded theory methods, processes, actions and interactions involving many individuals were studied [31]. To clarify participants' understandings of their experiences with medical technology the methods used in this study involved: 1. Developing codes, categories and themes inductively rather than imposing predetermined classifications on the data [32]. 2. Generating working hypotheses or assertions [33] from the data. 3. Analyzing narratives of participants' experiences with medical technology [30].

3   Results

3.1   Technology Used

Patients reported the technologies that were used during the births of their children. These technologies were coded individually and then grouped into singular codes to describe technologies that were essentially the same. For example codes such as scalp electrode, vaginal fetal monitor, and internal fetal monitor were all coded as internal fetal monitor. These codes were then organized into larger categories. Larger categories labeled; low technologies, monitoring technologies and birth assistive technologies, were created to capture the purposes of the various technologies.

Low technologies were described as the sole technologies used in natural birth experiences; examples included adjustable beds and clamps. Monitoring technologies were divided into two categories, those that monitor the mother and those that monitor the baby. Maternal monitoring technologies included maternal heart monitor, blood pressure machines and contraction monitors, while fetal monitoring technologies included heart rate monitors and ultrasounds. Birth assistive technologies were those technologies that were used when natural birth did not occur and interventions were needed. These technologies ranged in invasiveness from forceps, vacuums, epidurals, induction, and c-sections. Three patients reported not remembering or knowing what was used.

3.2 See, Hear or Feel

Participants' responses to what they noticed about the technology were divided into what they could see, hear and feel. Thirty-three codes were derived from sight, 14 codes were derived from feelings and 13 codes from hearing. Example codes for seeing included being able to see the monitor, seeing alarms, seeing pulse rate, seeing graphical readouts, and seeing contraction graphs on the monitor. The group feeling, contained codes such as feeling the internal fetal monitor, feeling the monitor during contraction, feeling the oxygen mask, feeling straps of the monitor around the stomach area, feeling blood pressure cuffs, and feeling medications through veins. Hearing included codes such as hearing heart beats, hearing unidentified beeps, hearing unidentified noises, hearing the baby's heart beat, and monitor print outs.

Table 1. Code Families of Technology Attributes Associated with Positive and Negative Feelings

Positive feelings	Negative feelings
Technology was comforting	Immobility
Perceiving heart beat is comforting	Belt as the source of negativity
Having the technology equaled overall good feelings	More pain than necessary
Knowing when and how long contractions would be	Frustrated about IV
Monitors helped outsiders (partners and nurses)	Unreliability
Seeing and monitoring ones own blood pressure.	Machines were distracting
Keeping an eye on babies heart beat	Equipment didn't feel natural
Knowing more	Contraction monitor is unnecessary
Knowing that the mom and baby were being monitored	Depending on others
Knowing that the baby is ok	Dislike of blood pressure cuff
	Feeling like you're in a hospital
	Doctors pushing more medical Interventions

3.3 Positive and Negative Experiences

After open coding, patients' experiences with the technologies were categorized into ten positive experiences and twelve negative experiences (see Table 1). Positive feelings were characterized as feelings that were welcome and comforting. These feelings were the result of what the patient noticed from the technology and how it helped them feel positive about the technology and the process. Negative feelings were characterized by expressions of negativity towards the technology and the feelings that resulted from the feedback from the technology.

4 Discussion

The results show that patients have user experiences with technologies that are used in their care and translate the feedback they receive into positive and negative feelings. Positive feelings were the result of what the patient noticed from the technology and how it made them feel comforted or positive. Subcategories of positive experiences included:

1. Generally feeling that technology was comforting because it gave them more information about what was happening to them and their baby. Erin expressed positive feelings when she said, "It made me feel I guess more comfortable and relaxed knowing that you know my baby's heart rate was being monitored and they knew what was going on as far as my contractions when they developed and… it was more comfortable."
2. Hearing the simulated heartbeat from the fetal heart monitor gave mothers comforting feelings. Hearing the heart beat, gave them a sense of reassurance that the baby was healthy and that they were more connected to their baby.
3. Having the technology equaled overall good feelings for some mothers. The presence of the technology made them feel that they were receiving first class care and that the system would be prepared if anything were to go wrong.
4. Knowing when and how long contractions. Mothers described knowing about the contractions as a positive experience for themselves and for the information it provided to their partners and care providers. Knowing when they would have contractions helped them prepare for them and it also helped their partners empathize when they could see the intensity of contractions on the monitors.

Kelly expressed positive feelings about the technology when she said "I'd say it was comforting, to be able to hear that the babies were doing fine, and you know, to be able to know when you were having a contraction too, and how much longer you were going to have to endure it. So I would definitely say it was comforting."

Negative feelings were characterized by expressions of negativity towards the technology and the feelings that resulted from the feedback from the technology. These negative feelings were:

1. Immobility was described as a source of negatively; the presence of the technology changed participants' experiences as patients. With the fetal heart rate monitor, patients were not able to move freely without regard to how the movement would affect the monitors functioning. Nicole expressed negative feelings about immobility

and depending on others when she said "I didn't like having to wear the monitors. I mean they put them around and she... kind of... you're kind of on a leash, so if you are trying to turn around to get comfortable, you can't. You have to ask the nurse, to like, make sure everything is still hooked up when you go to turn on your side and stuff like that. And that was kind of a pain."

2. Participants described frustration about having to use intervention that they perceived to be unnecessary. These interventions included intravenous therapy, automated blood pressure cuffs, and points where doctors suggested they interventions that had not planned for such as induction and epidurals.

3. Unreliability was a salient theme in negative experiences as indicated by the number codes between and within interviews. Participants expressed negative feelings when they could not depend on the technology to accurately reflect the health and well being of their baby. Jennifer discussed how unreliability contributed to a negative experience when she said:

"It's a little nerve wracking when they are like okay you know uh you know we are suppose[d] to be able to monitor the baby's heart rate and we can't find it. Even the attitude of the nurses in the room, they were agitated when they couldn't find the heart rate so you know and then, you know, you hear the beeeeeep, the loud beeps of straight lines and things like that. So it is, you know, you know, having had a more consistent experience with my son, you know, having all that going on and having the nurses attitude be a little more agitated with the process you know it kind of it kind of sends you into a "okay what's going on? Why isn't this working? Is something wrong with the baby?" So it was a little, a little nerve wracking not knowing, you know, not knowing why alarms were going off or not knowing why their machines weren't working for me."

4. A final major theme in negative experiences included participants' feelings that the technology was unnatural in their experience. The unwanted presence of technology was expressed by codes that described the presence of the machines and their outputs as distracting, the technology as unnatural and feeling like they were "in a hospital" as an unwelcomed experience.

5 Conclusion

One of our objectives was to define user experience in the context of humans as both for patients in a health care environment. Our results provide evidence to support the notion that patients have experiences with technologies used in their care. We also hoped to understand the relationship between characteristics of the technologies and positive or negative user experiences. Emotional aspects of user experience were present in our findings in both positive and negative experiences. When technology worked well, it had the potential to create positive experiences and enhance the patients' connection with their babies. Examples of designs that enhanced the emotional experience were the audible simulated heartbeat; when patients could hear the heartbeat they felt reassured that their baby was ok. Negative experiences occurred when technology did not work well or when care providers could not get technologies to work properly. We hypothesized that patients would expect their interactions with the technology to reflect their expected emotional experiences. Patients identified mismatches between the experience the technology afforded them and their desired experience. These experiential mismatches were reflected in patients' desire not to feel like they were in a hospital or feeling the technology was an unnatural artifact in their experience. Patients also identified experiences where technologies met their expected needs, such as a need for more information or assurance that they were receiving high quality care.

Patients' experiences with technologies contributed to positive and negative experiences as individuals and the resultant co-experiences patients experienced with their birth partners and care providers [28]. Technologies that lead to positive experiences lead to positive co-experiences; seeing the contraction graph allowed partners and care providers to share patients experiences by showing them when contractions would occur, the intensity and how long they would last. Hearing the baby's heartbeat allowed both the patient and the birth partner to experience the baby. We found that patients' experiences were grounded in expectations and contexts such as feeling that the "technology gave more information" or "feeling the technology was unnatural."

This study was limited by its small sample size, study population. The qualitative methodology used, was not intended to build causal relationships but to generate hypotheses about patient user experiences. Future studies should explore patient user experiences in other health care contexts and the effects of patients' positive or negative user experiences on the health care work system. Understanding how to design technologies that create positive experiences for both patients and workers will lead to more effective health care systems.

Reference

1. Davis, M.: Theoretical foundations for experiential systems design. In: Proceedings of the 2003 ACM SIGMM workshop on Experiential telepresence. ACM Press, Berkeley (2003)
2. Blythe, M., Wright, P., McCarthy, J., Bertelsen, O.W.: Theory and method for experience centered design. In: CHI 2006 extended abstracts on Human factors in computing systems. ACM Press, Montreal (2006)
3. Hassenzahl, M., Tractinsky, N.: User experience—a research agenda. Behaviour & Information Technology 25, 91–97 (2006)
4. Cassell, J., Bickmore, T.: External manifestations of trustworthiness in the interface. Communications of the ACM 43, 50–57 (2000)
5. Corritore, C.L., Kracher, B., Wiedenbeck, S.: On-line trust: Concepts, evolving themes, a model. International Journal of Human-Computer Studies 58, 737–758 (2003)
6. Friedman, B., Kahn, P.H., Howe, D.C.: Trust online. Communications of the ACM 43 (2000)
7. Aboulafia, A., Bannon, L., Fernstrom, M.: Shifting Perspective from Effect to Affect: Some Framing Questions. In: Proceedings of The International Conference on Affective Human Factors Design, pp. 508–514 (2001)
8. Agarwal, R., Karahanna, E.: Time Flies When You're Having Fun: Cognitive Absorption and Beliefs About Information Technology Usage. MIS Quarterly 24, 665–694 (2000)
9. Bonner, J.V.H.: Envisioning Future Needs: From Pragmatics to Pleasure. In: Green, W.S., Jordan, P.W. (eds.) Pleasure with Products. Taylor & Francis, London (2002)
10. Carroll, J.M., Thomas, J.M.: Fun. Sigchi Bull. 19, 21–24 (1988)
11. Draper, S.W.: Analysing fun as a candidate software requirement. Personal Technology 3, 117–122 (1999)

12. Monk, A., Hassenzahl, M., Blythe, M., Reed, D.: Funology: Designing enjoyment. In: Conference on Human Factors and Computing Systems, CHI 2002, Minneapolis, Minnesota, USA (2002); Workshop description Funology: Designing enjoyment
13. Bruseberg, A., McDonagh-Philp, D.: New product development by eliciting user experience and aspirations. International Journal of Human-Computer Studies 55, 435–452 (2001)
14. Margolin, V.: Getting to know the user. Design Studies 18, 227–236 (1997)
15. Overbeeke, K., Djadjadiningrat, T., Hummels, C., Wensveen, S.: Beauty in Usability: Forget about Ease of Use? In: Green, W.S., Jordan, P.W. (eds.) Pleasure with Products, pp. 9–18. Taylor & Francis, London (2002)
16. Noyes, J., Littledale, R.: Beyond Usability, Computer Playfulness. In: Green, W.S., Jordan, P.W. (eds.) Pleasure with Products, pp. 49–59. Taylor & Francis, London (2002)
17. De Angeli, A., Lynch, P., Johnson, G.I.: Pleasure versus Efficiency in User Interfaces: Towards an Involvement Framework. In: Green, W.S., Jordan, P.W. (eds.) Pleasure with Products, pp. 97–111. Taylor & Francis, London (2002)
18. Dolan, G., Iredale, R., Williams, R., Ameen, J.: Consumer use of the internet for health information: a survey of primary care patients. International Journal of Consumer Studies 28, 147–153 (2004)
19. Ball, M.J., Lillis, J.: E-health: transforming the physician/patient relationship. International Journal of Medical Informatics 61, 1–10 (2001)
20. Opinion Leader Research for the Department of Health: Results from a programme of consultation to develop a patient experience statement High Holborn, London WC1V 7QG (2003)
21. Logan, R.J., Augaitis, S.: Design of Simplified Television Remote Controls. A Case for Behavioral and Emotional Usability (1994)
22. Bates, J.: The Role of Emotion in Believable Agents. Communications of ACM 37, 122–125 (1994)
23. Creusen, M., Snelders, D.: Product Appearance and Consumer Pleasure. In: Green, W.S., Jordan, P.W. (eds.) Pleasure with Products, pp. 69–75. Taylor & Francis, Abington (2002)
24. Jordan, P.W.: Designing Pleasurable Products. Taylor & Francis, London (2000)
25. Schenkman, B.N., Jönsson, F.U.: Aesthetics and preferences of web pages. Behaviour & Information Technology 19, 367–377 (2000)
26. Kim, J., Moon, J.Y.: Designing towards emotional usability in customer interfaces- trustworthiness of cyber-banking systems interfaces. Interacting with Computers 10, 1–29 (1998)
27. Desmet, P., Overbeeke, C., Tax, S.: Designing products with added emotional value: Development and application of an approach for research through design. The Design Journal 4, 32–47 (2001)
28. Forlizzi, J., Battarbee, K.: Understanding Experience in Interactive Systems. In: DIS 2004, Cambridge, Massachusetts, USA (2004)
29. Forlizzi, J., Ford, S.: The building blocks of experience: An early framework for interaction designers Systems 2000, New York, NY (2000)
30. Polkinghorne, D.: Two conflicting calls for methodological reform. The Counseling Psychologist 19, 103–114 (1991)
31. Creswell, J.W.: Qualitative inquiry and research design. SAGE, Thousand Oaks (2007)
32. Glaser, B.G., Strauss, A.L.: The discovery of grounded theory: Strategies for qualitative research. Aldine, Chicago (1967)
33. Erickson, F.: Qualitative methods in research on teaching, p. 147 (1985)

Unique Stressors of Cross-Cultural Collaboration through ICTs in Virtual Teams

Niina Nurmi

Stanford University
Center for Work, Technology & Organization (WTO)
210 Panama Street, Stanford, CA 94305-4101, U.S.A.
niinan@stanford.edu

Abstract. Geographically distributed virtual teams are increasingly prevalent in global organizations. Despite the growing attention to virtual teams, there is limited understanding of how cross-cultural collaboration and electronic dependence in communication affect virtual workers' psychological reactions and well-being. This qualitative multi-case study aims at understanding the different causes of stress in cross-cultural collaboration. An overarching analysis across seven case studies revealed that globally distributed team members experienced job stressors such as language challenges in English, or *lingua franca*, misunderstandings, and conflicts due to different mindsets, communication and behavior styles, and work-leisure orientations. Without adequate skills in *lingua franca*, or proper cultural and local awareness of distant team sites, coping was not successful, thereby stressors lead to distress.

Keywords: Virtual Teams, Cross-Cultural Collaboration, Stress, Coping.

1 Introduction

Within an increasingly global economy, more and more corporations engage multicultural, globally distributed, virtual teams. Such teams consist of individuals located in many different countries or geographical areas with a common goal, carrying out interdependent tasks, using mostly information and communication technologies (ICTs) for collaboration [3], [18]. This kind of global time-space compression of team functions facilitated by ICTs may result in collision of global, national and organizational attitudes. Cross-cultural virtual teams may face difficulties as they attempt to coordinate across distance, cultural differences and divergent mental models [22]. To facilitate collaboration across national and linguistic boundaries, global organizations are increasingly mandating that all employees use English as a common corporate language, a so-called *lingua franca*. Research suggests that such a language stipulation favors native English speakers and impacts negatively on collaboration in cross-cultural work teams [4]. For non-native English speakers, encountering the *lingua franca* may be anxiety-inducing [13], [15]. Prolonged communication-based anxiety, in turn, may lead to stress. According to a new common definition [8], stress is a state accompanied by physical, psychological or social complaints or dysfunctions, which

B.-T. Karsh (Ed.): Ergonomics and Health Aspects, HCII 2009, LNCS 5624, pp. 78–87, 2009.

results from individuals' feelings that their abilities are insufficient for the requirements and expectations placed upon them. This definition emphasizes the interaction between work stressors and a person's individual characteristics. Work stressors and stress in virtual work has rarely been studied [23]. Consequently, whether global virtual workers are a highly stressed group is not known. This study attempts to examine the characteristics and demands of cross-cultural collaboration through ICTs, and its contributions to stress, through an empirical investigation.

Lack of proximity, lack of face-to-face communication, ICT dependence, and cultural differences affect collaboration and communication in global virtual teams [5], [12]. Different sites of global organizations may appropriate the ICTs differently depending on their specific geographies, infrastructure, history, culture and languages. There might be different views of the relevance, applicability, and value of particular modes of working and use of ICTs which may produce conflicts in virtual teams, thereby leading to stress. Lean computer mediated communication (CMC) and language differences between the virtual team members can be an impediment for global collaboration. However, team members' diverse backgrounds and mindsets can lead to superior innovation performance, if the team invests in rich internal communication, e.g. defines goals well, develops work plans, prioritizes and coordinates work [1].

Despite the increasing attention to virtual teams, there is limited understanding of how cross-cultural collaboration through ICTs contributes to virtual team members' psychological reactions and well-being. Williams and O'Railey [24] argued that "diverse groups are more likely to be less integrated, have less communication, and have more conflict" (p.115). Scholars have consistently argued that conflicts are more extreme on geographically distributed as compared with collocated teams [1], [14]. In traditional, collocated organizations, interunit conflicts have been acknowledged to be a source of psychological stress for employees (e.g.[21]). However, there is a gap in research on stress and its antecedents in culturally diverse virtual teams, whose communication is mediated through ICTs. To fill this gap, I conducted an investigation designed to identify the job stressors of cross-cultural CMC that affect the well-being of virtual team members. Specifically, this research was guided by two key questions: (1) What are the job-stressors of cross-cultural collaboration through ICTs in virtual teams? and (2) How do employees cope with these job stressors to promote their well-being?

2 Methods

I applied qualitative, interpretive research methods [16] to study cross-cultural collaboration through ICTs in globally distributed teams. I used seven globally distributed teams for the comparative case design [7], [16]. Table 1 describes the seven distributed teams I studied. I applied respondent validation with the single case study results, enabling the informants to review the analysis before generalizing across cases [7], [16]. The focal teams employed people working and living in different geographical areas (North America, Europe and Asia), each with their own set of business conditions, cultural beliefs and history. The cases were selected from five globally distributed companies in the electronics and software industry. The teams called GlobEle, GlobTele and GlobTech were from the same electronics company, while the other teams were

Table 1. Stressors of cross-cultural collaboration through ICTs

Teams	Team member locations	Time difference between sites	Team size	Cultural backgrounds	Communication	FtF meetings
GlobEle Product development team Industry: Telecommunications	Dallas, Tx, USA Helsinki, Finland Tokyo, Japan	14 hours	29 persons 3 sub teams	American Chinese Finnish Japanese Iranian	e-mail video conference web conference teleconference telephone text messages	formal FtF every 6 months informal FtF every 6 months
GlobPro IT team Industry: Electronics	Tucson, Az, USA Boulder, Co, USA Boston, Ma, USA Vantaa, Finland	9 hours	19 persons 4 sub teams	American Finnish	e-mail telephone video conference discussion forum chat	formal FtF monthly informal F2F monthly on site
GlobSoft Customer Project Delivery team Industry: Software	Boston, Ma, USA Brussels, Belgium Stockholm, Sweden Helsinki, Finland	7 hours	36 persons	American Finnish Belgian Swedish	teleconference telephone e-mail document sharing system discussion forum text messages	formal FtF every 6 months informal FtF every 6 months
GlobTele Product development team Industry: Telecommunications	Boston, Ma, USA Helsinki, Finland	7 hours	4 persons	American Finnish Indian	e-mail telephone teleconference web conference	formal FtF every 6 months informal FtF every 6 months
GlobTech Product development team Industry: Telecommunications	Copenhagen, Denmark Helsinki, Finland Salo, Finland Tampere, Finland Tokyo, Japan	7 hours	7 persons	Danish Finnish Japanese	e-mail text messages telephone teleconference web conference	formal FtF every 6 months informal FtF every 6 months
GlobGate Global change project Industry: Electronics	Espoo, Finland Salo, Finland Pecs, Hungary Hong Kong, China Dongguang, China Tallin, Estonia	5 hours	12 persons	Finnish Hungarian Chinese Estonian	e-mail teleconference	formal FtF every 6 months informal FtF every 6 months
GlobOff Offering Team Industry: Software	Amsterdam, Netherlands Helsinki, Finland	1 hour	6 persons	Dutch Finnish	e-mail telephone teleconference	formal FtF every 6 months informal FtF every 6 months

selected from four different companies. All these companies' headquarters were located in Finland. In an effort to facilitate collaboration among co-workers across national and linguistic barriers, the focal organizations used English as their common language, *lingua franca.*

The team leaders and members (N = 65) were interviewed between March 2003 and July 2004 as part of a larger program of research on distributed and mobile teamwork. The interviews dealt with several aspects of virtual work, such as job demands and resources, cross-cultural collaboration, CMC, stress and well-being. 32 persons were interviewed in English and others in my native language, Finnish. Each semi-structured interview lasted 1-2 hours and was taped and fully transcribed, coded and analyzed qualitatively [7], [16] with a data analysis software. First, I broke down the data to extract key passages on expressions of felt stress or stress-related passages that could be identified as being of theoretical interest. Second, I continued the analysis by three linked subprocesses: data reduction (coding, teasing out themes), data display (making matrixes, lists) and drawing conclusions (noting regularities and patterns) [16]. In the data reduction phase, I coded the texts and extracted the passages related to stress and cross-cultural collaboration for further analysis. In the data display phase, I placed the coded passages in a matrix and monitored the internal cohesion of the codes. Thereafter, I recoded and analyzed the passages further to establish my results. In the next section, I present the results of an overarching analysis across all the seven case studies.

3 Findings

Language challenges, misunderstandings and conflicts caused stress to the studied team members who collaborated through ICTs. Table 2 shows the frequencies of the coded passages in my data expressing stress or stress-related negative emotions (such as overload, anxiety, nervousness, frustration) in cross-cultural collaboration. Cultural diversity affected the collaboration and communication in various ways in the focal teams. Some interviewees praised the diversity for arousing enriching viewpoints on design work. Still, most informants described cross-cultural collaboration as complicated and stressful due to language challenges and misunderstandings, which sometimes escalated to conflicts. Individuals felt stress when sufficient resources were not available for coping with these stressors.

Table 2. Stressors of cross-cultural collaboration through ICTs

Stressors of cross-cultural collaboration through ICTs	Frequences of the coded passages
Language challenges	89
Misunderstandings and conflicts due to:	
- different communication and behavior styles	89
- different mindsets	85
- different work-leisure orientations	28

3.1 Language Challenges

Language challenges in English, the *lingua franca,* was a major cause of stress in the studied cross-cultural teams. This language stipulation favored native English speakers. Less fluent English speakers felt inability and incompetence in expressing themselves and getting their point across in team communication. Some non-native English speakers reported that often they would rather withdraw from the conversation than continue fighting for their opinions. A Japanese interviewee described his coping mechanism: *"It's difficult if we have to discuss in English. [If we would have the] same problem but discuss in Japanese, I will try and get shared conclusion even if it takes time. If it's the same topic [and the] discussion [is held] in English, I will compromise a lot or just leave it to boss [and go] away."* Another Japanese interviewee was frustrated and anxious because he was unable to use his technical skills in cross-cultural team collaboration when English skills were required: *"I have these kinds of skills I need to accomplish my task. If it requires some English skills, I can't use my skills. The English reduces the opportunity to use my skills."* A couple of Chinese non-native English speakers, who worked for American managers, got nervous when they could not understand their manager's talk: *"My English is not good, if I did not get [my manager's] point I get nervous,"* one of them said.

Not only the non-native speakers became stressed but also the native English speakers found the language challenges and miscommunication stressful. The American manager of the Chinese team members mentioned above described his coping mechanism: *"Quite often you have to ask them to repeat what they said. I try to keep that to a minimum, because it can become insulting."* In some cases, written communication was used as a coping mechanism in bridging the language barriers between native and non-native English speakers. An American interviewee explained his communication strategy with non-native English speakers: *"Very often it is easier for me to communicate by writing to get a basic idea what we are talking about. Establish the thought and then ask specific questions and get answers. First we have to build a foundation for conversation in writing."*

However, some non-native English speakers experienced email as an especially stressful medium. E-mail communication in English was time-consuming and added to the sense of overload for a Japanese interviewee who was trying to cope with a busy work situation: *"Sometimes or always I've had difficulties in English. ... it is difficult to communicate ... if you send very long [e-mail message in] English, it takes time to read or go through."* In addition to e-mail, teleconferencing was also mentioned as a difficult communication medium for non-native English speakers because of the lack of body language. Even though e-mail was stressful for a Chinese interviewee, she still preferred written communication over talking in English: *"I [am] not good at English, so e-mail is pretty horrible. I can write English, but I'm not good at debate, talking. ... In case of teleconference we can not use body language. They don't wait for me to think in English. Q: Does that cause you stress? A: Yes."*

3.2 Misunderstandings and Conflicts

Different communication styles, mindsets and work-leisure orientations between the cross-cultural team members caused misunderstandings and sometimes conflicts in the studied teams. Interviewees described these misunderstandings and conflicts as stressful work events.

Different communication and behavior styles. Different communication and behavior styles, as well as language issues, created miscommunication in the studied teams when cross-cultural team members were not able to interpret each other correctly. An American leader described the collaboration as challenging and fragile as a house of cards: *"It takes weeks and months to set up the relationship and get it working well and one word can completely destroy it."* Another American interviewee related an example of destructive miscommunication between French and American collaborators: *"[After] four days of meetings and disclosures, a [native English-speaking] person wrote a summary of the meeting and a letter thanking [the French collaborators] for the meeting and so forth, and the last sentence was, 'Maria, we found this meeting to be invaluable.' And the whole thing collapsed, people were just furious that the perception was that they had come to the meeting and the whole thing was seen to be not valuable. In English invaluable means you can't do without it, it was very valuable. And in French, in means not, and it took weeks to undo and get that whole [collaboration] back on track again, so in language issues one word can completely destroy [everything]."*

ICT-mediated communicaton, in which non-verbal cues were minimized, caused the majority of miscommunication. Many interviewees said that e-mail messages were easily misunderstood and sometimes these misunderstandings escalated to conflicts in cross-cultural teams. An American interviewee warned: *"The written word can be very dangerous, when you're dealing at a personal level or interpersonal amongst the team. ... Especially if it's something that'll upset them, they'll read it again and again and every time they read it they will reinforce their own understanding which may be the incorrect understanding."* Another American interviewee reported that the most stressful problems in his teams occurred when e-mail messages were misinterpreted and taken personally: *"There are connotations in e-mail. The way things are written people may interpret them in incorrect manner. Especially going international, when there are different languages, different translations of words, and different meanings. On the sentence that I say in English to another person who is from America or an English speaking country, they would interpret it in one way whereas if you sent that same message to someone, say in Finland, and they read it, the context may mean something ELSE to them. And oftentimes, I think that's where we begin to have problems as a group, is when people begin to take messages personally or misinterpret them. That's when the biggest problems occur."*

In the studied teams, different cultures had different national traits, reactions and styles in communication. An American interviewee gave an example of stress exacerbating miscommunication between American and Finnish team members, who had different styles in reacting to stressful work situations: *"When [work] pressure gets extremely high, the American response will be an e-mail to Helsinki saying, [the] sky is falling, we have all these things to do, if all these things are not on the dock by next Thursday we all lose our jobs and millions of dollars and yada yada, whine whine whine... and then the Finnish response is, don't worry. And so the American gets that response and it's like, they don't understand, the world is falling and what do you mean, don't worry, of course I worry, like this.... so someone who has not been [in the Helsinki office] and not seen what that 'don't worry' really means will interpret that a little differently, and the Finnish response to that American [panicking] is stop whining and get some work done. It's the difference.* " Another American interviewee from Tucson described the aggressive "Bostonese" communication style, with which people from other cultures found hard to cope: *"Culturally people in Boston are hyper. They are intense. And they FIGHT to get to work, and they FIGHT to get to the grocery store. And they FIGHT to get to their club or their baseball game or their recreation, and then they go home and they start again the next day to FIGHT... So when they go to interact with people from a different culture they come off as being ignorant and boorish and too aggressive, and not considerate of others' needs... [the team member in Boston] just pissed everyone off by his attitude and actions. And he made it so that he was no longer welcome.* "

Many interviewees explained how Japanese and Chinese people became uncomfortable when communicating and negotiating with American and European colleagues, who expressed their ideas more aggressively than Asian people. Japanese interviewees emphasized how important it is in Japanese culture to consider other people's opinions and compromize. The direct western e-mail communication style was described to be offencive to Japanese: *"The style of e-mail is completely different [in Japan and Western countries]. It's difficult [for my Western colleagues] to see the situation of mine. Some [of their] e-mails look rude for Japanese.* "

Different mindsets. Different mindsets among people from different cultural backgrounds, i.e. different attitudes, ways of thinking and believing affected their responses to and interpretations of situations. An American interviewee said that conflicts occurred in cross-cultural collaboration if some people automatically assumed their way of thinking, or their way of doing things, was the only way or the "right" way and did not understand others' points of view: *"One side does not understand the scope or the gravity or the seriousness of the situation so [there is] a mismatch in perceptions of importance or significance, or one set of priorities does not align with another group's set of priorities. That's probably the single largest cause of some kind of dispute.* " A Dutch interviewee expressed his frustration against the Finnish mindset and considerate working style, and how he coped with it: *"Finnish people try to be very formal and structured. ... In practice, it leads to endless discussions and long delays in how things happen. If you want [to] really get things done, it's better to first do it and then ask permission, than first ask permission and then do it. I've worked for over two years [in this company] so I've kind of got used to this mentality and the fact that Finns are like this.* "

Different work and leisure orientations. Different work and leisure orientations between cross-cultural team members created misunderstandings and stressful surprises for those who were not culturally aware. Japanese people were described to be work-oriented and very flexible in their working time. They could be expected to work long hours, unlike Scandinavian people who were seen as more family-oriented, reinforcing their eight hour working schedule. A Japanese interviewee was frustrated about the different work orientations between Japanese and Finnish team members: *"When I need to do some work, I make sure that I finish the day's work before I go home... but Finnish people I think stop working when time hits 5pm or 6pm.* " He also told an example of a stressful event when he missed a major part of his human resources for a couple of months because he was not aware of Scandinavian holidays and could not prepare for the summer: *"I realized during the course of the project that people have differences in* *the weeks [of holiday] and they request the timing [for the vacation]. When the person is on a vacation, they actually do not work at all, so the project STOPS for that time. When there are many people consecutively taking vacation it could have been 2 or 3 months without any work done, which I wasn't expecting. Japanese companies' employees, we don't take this much vacation days."*

Major misunderstandings and conflicts were encouraged to be solved face-to-face in the studied teams. All companies invested in distributed team members' visits to the other team site. Exchange programs of two to three weeks were said to increase cultural understanding and decrease misunderstandings between the virtual team members: *"We solved [cultural issues] by exchanges, by group exchanges... it is actually through this exchange so that the person can begin to understand what each one of the priorities are. So that the misunderstanding[s] go away."* After a face-to-face encounter, virtual team members understood each other better in CMC, which made cross-cultural collaboration through ICTs less stressful.

4 Discussion

The potential of the virtual work environment to lead to adverse well-being and performance is high. As suggested by Armstrong and Cole [2] and Cramton [6], distributed teams often experience high levels of conflict; so did the cross-cultural virtual teams in this study. More importantly, I found that these conflicts, cross-cultural misunderstandings and language challenges in *lingua franca* contributed to virtual team member's stress in ICT-mediated collaboration if sufficient resources were not available for coping. I propose that the skills in *lingua franca*, and cultural and local awareness of distant sites help ensure that these potential sources of stress do not actually act as stressors for the virtual team members. It has been shown that particularly under high job demands, job resources may not only mitigate the negative impact of job demands on work engagement but more importantly even motivate and increase work engagement [9]. Therefore, it is also important to identify specific coping resources that may reduce job demands and stressors and support the work engagement of virtual workers. Earlier studies on competences in virtual teams suggests that these coping resources combine social and individual resources, such as goal and role clarity, common process compliance, commitment, intercultural sensitivity, language skills, mutual knowledge and understanding [17], [20].

Like any study, this has limitations. My data came from a relatively small number of individuals and teams. A larger sample drawing from more settings might reveal more job stressors and coping methods. Methodological triangulation, mixing quantitative and qualitative data, would have facilitated more comprehensive interpretations and strengthened the argumentation. Measuring the level of stress, job engagement, effectiveness and performance with survey methods might have complemented the qualitative analysis, maybe generated enriching viewpoints, and helped validate research results.

5 Conclusions

Despite these limitations, this study makes an important contribution to the literature on virtual teams suggesting that cross-cultural team members may experience stressors such as language challenges, misunderstandings and conflicts. Without adequate skills in *lingua franca*, or proper cultural and local awareness of distant sites, coping may be difficult, thereby causing distress. In the next phase of this research, I will measure these stress reactions directly and examine how they manifest themselves with respect to mental and physical disease. This is particularly important insofar as global expansion is making the management of cross-cultural employees in distant locations more critical than ever [19]. The present research provides a substantial base from which to launch such ambitious investigations. It also provides new viewpoints on management of global organizations, which should ensure that virtual workers are adequately prepared for the transition of the cross-cultural collaboration, ongoing monitoring of workers' perception of their health and well-being, and training of leaders to develop proper leadership and team practices that help in coping with the unique stressors of cross-cultural collaboration through ICTs in virtual teams.

References

1. Ancona, Caldwell: Bridging the boundary: external activity in performance in organizational teams. Administrative Science Quarterly 37, 634–665 (1992)
2. Armstrong, D.J., Cole, P.: Managing distances and differences in geographically distributed work groups. In: Hinds, P.J., Kiesler, S. (eds.) Distributed Work, pp. 167–190. MIT Press, Cambridge (2001)
3. Bell, B.S., Kozlowski, S.W.J.: A typology of virtual teams. Implications for effective leadership. Group and Organization Management 27(1), 14–49 (2002)
4. Beyene, T.: Fluency as stigma: implications of a language mandate in global work. Stanford University (2007)
5. Carcia, M.C., Canado, M.L.P.: Language and power: raising awareness of the role of language in multicultural teams. Language and intercultural communication 5(1), 86–104 (2005)
6. Cramton, C.D.: The mutual knowledge problem and its consequences for dispersed collaboration. Organization Science 12(3), 346–371 (2001)
7. Eisenhardt, K.M.: Building theories from case study research. Academy of Management Review 14(4), 532–550 (1989)
8. EUTC, UNICE, UEAPME, CEEP, Framework agreement on work-related stress (2004), http://ec.europa.eu/employment_social/news/2004/oct/stress_agreement_en.pdf
9. Hakanen, J.J., Bakker, A., Demerouti, E.: How Dentists Cope with Their Job Demands and stay Engaged: The Moderating Role of Job Resources. European Journal of Oral Sciences 113, 479–487 (2005)
10. Hakanen, J.J., Bakker, A., Schaufeli, W.: Burnout and engagement among teachers. Journal of School Psychology 43, 495–513 (2006)
11. Hinds, P.J., Bailey, D.E.: Out of sight, out of synch: Understanding conflict in distributed teams. Organization Science 14, 615–632 (2003)
12. Hinds, P., Kiesler, S.: Communication across Boundaries: Work, Structure and Use of Communication Technologies in a Large Organization. Organization Science 6(4), 373–393 (1995)
13. Knapp, K.: Approaching Lingua Franca communication. In: Knapp, K., Meierkord, C. (eds.) Lingua Franca Communication, Frankfurt Lang M.A, pp. 217–245 (2003)

14. Mannix, E.A., Griffith, T.L., Neale, M.A.: The phenomenology of conflict in virtual work teams. In: Hinds, P.J., Kiesler, S. (eds.) Distributed Work. MIT Press, Cambridge (2002)
15. Meierkord, D., Knapp, K.: Approaching Lingua Franca communication. In: Knapp, K., Meierkord, C. (eds.) Lingua Franca Communication, Frankfurt Lang M.A., pp. 2–28 (2003)
16. Miles, M.B., Huberman, A.M.: Qualitative data analysis: A sourcebook of new methods. Sage, Beverly Hills (1984)
17. Nurmi, N.: Coping Stress in Global and Finnish Virtual Teams. In: Proceedings of Global HRM Conference, Turku, Finland, August 27-29(2008)
18. Jarvenpaa, S.L., Leidner, D.E.: Communication and trust in global virtual teams. Organization Science 10, 791–815 (1999)
19. Kokko, N., Vartiainen, M., Hakonen, M.: Collective competencies in virtual organizations. In: Luczak, H., Zink, K.J. (eds.) Human factors in organizational design and management – VII. Re-designing work and macroergonomics – future perspectives and challenges, Proceedings of the Seventh International Symposium on Human Factors in Organizational Design and Management held in Aachen, Germany, October 2003, pp. 403–408 (2003)
20. Kokko, N., Vartiainen, M., Lönnblad, J.: Individual and Collective Competencies in Virtual Project Organizations. eJOV 8, 28–52 (2006)
21. Parasuraman, S., Alutto, J.A.: An Examination of the Organizational Antecedents of Sressors at Work. Academy of Management Journal 24(1), 48–67 (1981)
22. Powell, A., Piccoli, G., Ives, B.: Virtual teams: a review of current literature and directions for future research. The Data Base for Advances in Information Systems 35(1), 6–36 (2004)
23. Richter, P., Meyer, J., Sommer, F.: Well-being and stress in mobile and virtual work. In: Andriessen, J.H.E., Vartiainen, M. (eds.) Mobile virtual work. A new paradigm?, pp. 231–252. Springer, Heidelberg (2006)
24. Williams, K.Y., O'Reilly, C.A.I.: Demography and diversity in organizations: A review of 40 years of research. In: Staw, B.M., Cummings, L.L. (eds.) Research in Organizational Behavior, vol. 20, pp. 77–140. JAI Press, Greenwich (1998)

Examining the Effects of Workstation Design Satisfaction, Computer Usage, Supervisory and Co-worker Support on Perceived Physical Discomfort and Psychosocial Factors

Michelle Robertson[1], Emily Huang[1], and Nancy Larson[2]

[1] Liberty Mutual Research Institute for Safety, Hopkinton, MA
[2] 3M Corporation, Minnesota, MN

Abstract. This study examined the factors of computer use, job tasks, musculoskeletal and visual discomfort and organizational support to better understand the magnitude of their impact on the safety and health of computer work employees. A cross-sectional survey was administered to a large manufacturing company to investigate these relationships. Associations between these study variables were tested along with moderating effects framed within a conceptual model. Significant relationships were found between discomfort, computer use and psychosocial factors including supervisory relations moderating the relationships between workstation satisfaction and visual and musculoskeletal discomfort. This study provides guidance for developing recommendations in designing office ergonomic interventions with the goal of reducing musculoskeletal and visual discomforts while enhancing worker performance and their quality of worklife.

Keywords: Office ergonomics, computer workers, psychosocial factors, discomfort.

1 Introduction

The occurrence of Work-Related Musculoskeletal Disorders (WMSDs) and visual discomfort in computer workers continues to be of concern. Musculoskeletal disorders (WMSDs) in the US resulted in 375,540 occupational injury and illness cases involving days away from work (annual incidence rate 68.8 cases per 10,000 full time workers, accounted for 30% of total injury cases for 2005), and its prevalence is high among computer users (often 40 to 80%) [1-3]. Computer work is identified as a risk factor for WMSDs and visual discomfort in the working age population [4-6]. Upper extremity musculoskeletal symptoms among computer users are reported to be as high as 63% [4]. Critical computer and office work characteristics that have been found to be associated with WMSDs and visual discomfort are: workstation design, psychosocial factors, and daily hours working on a computer [7-10].

This study examines the relationships among the factors of satisfaction level regarding workstation design, computer use, relationships with co-workers and supervisors,

B.-T. Karsh (Ed.): Ergonomics and Health Aspects, HCII 2009, LNCS 5624, pp. 88–94, 2009.
© Springer-Verlag Berlin Heidelberg 2009

and various perceived musculoskeletal and visual discomfort levels (i.e., head, eye-strain, upper body, lower body and overall discomfort). Figure 1 presents the conceptual model for this study. These results would provide guidance in developing recommendations for designing office ergonomic interventions with the goal of reducing musculoskeletal and visual discomforts among intensive computer users as well as improving the overall safety of workers.

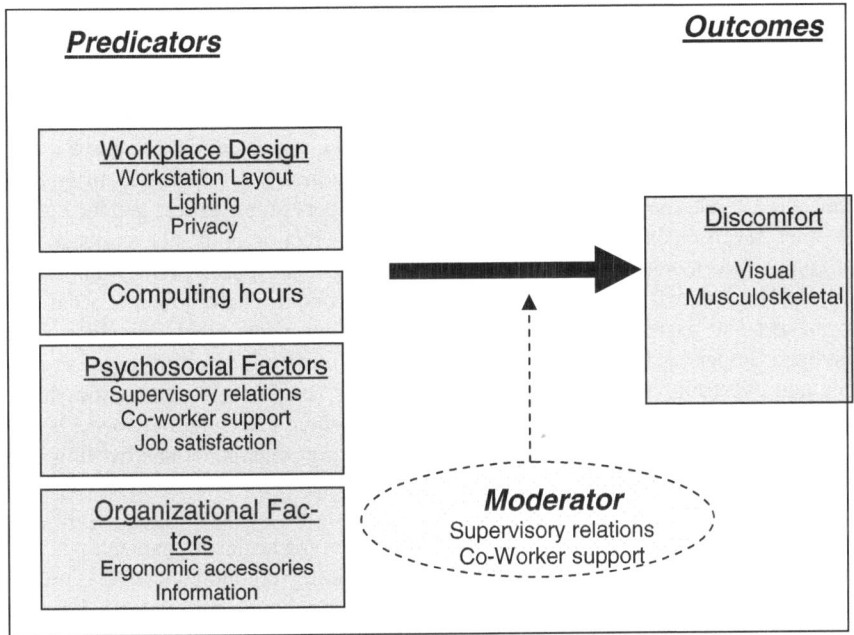

Fig. 1. Conceptual Model of the Study

2   Methods

2.1 Study Site

We conducted this study at a large U.S. manufacturing corporation whose offices consisted of multiple buildings, fairly similar in environmental design, workstation size, and workspace. There were differences, however, with regard to furniture and the computer tasks. The main computer tasks were word processing, data entry, and spreadsheet work. A few employees worked in design and used Computer Aided Design (CAD) computer equipment. The majority of workstations were not adjustable. There was a wide variety of chair styles and range of adjustability (a minimum of 3 adjustments). All employees had access to ergonomics information, accessory tools or, upon request, an individual ergonomics workstation evaluation.

2.2 Study Design

After approval by the Institutional Review Committee for Human Subjects, we administered a cross-sectional survey to a randomly selected sample of office computer users during work hours via Lotus Notes. An announcement about the study was made by the company's ergonomics manager. The survey was distributed to 20% of the company's population for a total distribution of 3,400 surveys.

2.3 Survey Design

The computer ergonomics survey was based on several previously validated computer ergonomics and discomfort questionnaires (11-12). The survey consisted of 52 items grouped in eight general categories. The first category consisted of demographic items: individual division, department, location, job categories (i.e., assistant, analyst, customer service, engineer, sales, staff, researcher, supervisor), tenure, gender and age. The other seven categories included self-reported perceptions of: (1) workstation design/layout (work surface area, surface height, storage space, privacy appearance, chair, lighting, glare); (2) organizational issues, (e.g., obtaining ergonomic accessories, information and assistance); (3) musculoskeletal discomfort (neck, shoulder, elbow, wrist/hand, upper back, low back, hip, knee, ankle/foot); (4) visual discomfort (headaches and eyestrain/vision); (5) psychosocial issues (co-worker support, job satisfaction, supervisory relations); (6) workload and computer use (hours at work, hours at home, time sitting); and (7) job tasks (mousing/keying, telephone, handwriting, meetings, office machine use, filing).

Respondents evaluated workstation design by rating satisfaction of eight workstation design features questions with 3-point Likert-type scales. Organizational issues were evaluated through questions on ease of obtaining ergonomics accessories, and accessible ergonomic information. Overall self-reported musculoskeletal discomfort experienced in the past three months was rated by responding to a Yes/No question. Additionally, musculoskeletal work-related discomfort was assessed for 9 different body parts and visual discomfort was assessed for 2 items (headache and eyestrain). Frequency and severity of symptoms during the preceding 3 months were evaluated using 5-point Likert-type scales. Productivity, as it relates to how often the discomfort interfered with the ability to perform the job, was rated with 5-point Likert-type scales for each of the 9 body parts and 2 visual items. Co-worker support was evaluated through five questions and was rated by a 3-Point Likert-type scale. Job satisfaction and supervisory support were evaluated through 2 questions and were rated by 3-point Likert-type scales.

Questions on workload, computer use and job tasks were rated by total computer use time, including computer work done both at work and at a home.

2.4 Data Analyses

Characteristics of the study population were summarized using relative frequency distributions and other descriptive statistics. Tests of bivariate associations were conducted to assess the relationships between the study variables. A series of multiple regressions were conducted to examine the effects of the predicators variables on the outcomes variables of visual and musculoskeletal discomfort as well as the moderating effects of supervisory relations and co-worker support. For the outcome variable of discomfort we created four composite scores of visual (1) and musculoskeletal discomfort (3) to be used in the testing of the model for overall visual and musculoskeletal discomfort.

3 Results

3.1 Participants

There was a response rate of 37%, where 1,259 surveys were completed. Of the survey respondents, 55% were male. There were nine job categories identified and the administration category represented the largest number of individuals (46%).

3.2 Musculoskeletal and Visual Discomfort

The survey findings revealed that for all job categories, the most frequent discomforts reported at least monthly were: eye strain (48%), neck pain (43%), headaches (45%), shoulder pain (40%), wrist pain (36%), and low back pain (35%).

Fifty seven percent of respondents reported experiencing discomfort while performing their job during the past three months, responding to a Yes/No question. Reporting discomfort over the past 3 months was positively correlated with more individual frequent reports of discomfort for all body parts: neck ($r = .34$), shoulder ($r = .33$), elbows ($r = .28$), wrists ($r = .38$), upper back ($r = .29$), lower back ($r = .27$), hip ($r = .16$), knee, ($r = .13$), and ankle ($r = .13$) as well as for headaches ($r = .23$) and eyestrain ($r = .27$) [all sig. at .01 level].

3.3 Computer Use and Musculoskeletal Discomfort

Seventy percent of the respondents reported spending four or more hours using the computer each day at work. Moreover, 35% of employees reported spending six or more hours using the computer each day at work. Participants in sales reported the highest percentage (67%) of overall musculoskeletal discomfort while performing their job, followed by analysts (64%), then assistants (58%).

Significant positive associations were found for all visual and body part discomfort frequency levels and the number of working computer hours. The correlation coefficients were: $r = .18$ (headache), $r = .23$ (eye strain), $r = .19$ (neck pain), $r = .18$ (shoulder pain), $r = .13$ (elbow pain), $r = .15$ (wrist pain), $r = .18$ (upper back pain), $r = .13$ (lower back pain), $r = .15$ (hip pain), $r = .15$ (knee pain), $r = .08$ (ankle pain) all significant at the .01 level.

3.4 Ergonomics Accessories and Musculoskeletal and Visual Discomfort

A significant negative correlation between obtaining ergonomic accessories and overall musculoskeletal discomfort ($r = -.18$, $p<.01$) was revealed. That is, the easier it was to obtain ergonomic accessories, the less frequently participants reported musculoskeletal discomfort over the three-month period. Further, significantly negative correlations were found between ease of obtaining ergonomic accessories and frequency of discomfort: headache (r = -.07), eye strain (r = -.10), neck pain (r = -.10), shoulder pain (r = .06), elbow pain, (r = -.08), wrists pain, (r = -.11), lower back pain, (r = -.10), knee pain (r = -.06), [all p's <.05]. Additionally, the finding that the more satisfied the respondent was with the workstation, the easier it was for them to obtain ergonomic accessories was positively significant (r = .27, p<.01).

A significant negative correlation was found between knowing how to request an ergonomic evaluation and less frequently reported musculoskeletal discomfort over the past 3 months (r = -.11, p <.01).

3.5 Work Environment Design

Only half the respondents reported making appropriate changes to their workstations or work habits to address their discomfort. Participants who did make changes to address their discomfort were associated with significantly less frequent discomfort over the prior 3 months (r = .21, p<.01).

3.6 Relationships among the Predicators and Outcomes

Predicators effects. The results from the multiple regressions showed that gender (being female), lower satisfaction level with the workstation design, higher number of hours of daily computer use, and poor relationships with co-workers and supervisors had significant effects on employees' various self-reported musculoskeletal and visual discomfort levels (all p's <.05).

Moderating effects. The psychosocial factor of supervisory relations partially moderated the relationships between satisfaction of workstation design and work environment lighting, as well as the number of hours of computer use on various musculoskeletal and visual discomfort levels (p <.05).

4 Conclusion

This study investigated the factors of computer use, musculoskeletal and visual discomfort and organizational support to more fully understand the impact of computer work on workers. Moreover, the moderating roles of supervisory support and co-worker support were examined. This study identified potential areas for designing office ergonomics interventions concerning workstation design, psychosocial issues, computer use, and organizational response.

Limitations of this study should be considered since these are baseline results representing a cross-sectional survey. Thus, temporal relationship between discomfort and the other study variables cannot be established. These study outcomes consisted of self-reported symptomatology which may not be a stable indicator of musculoskeletal disorder in the working population [6]. However, Hunting et al. [13] found that approximately one third of employees with complaints also had clinical findings associated with high muscle and tendon strain, suggesting that symptoms may be a sensitive indicator of musculoskeletal disorders.

Results of this study provide supporting and consistent evidence that musculoskeletal and visual discomforts of computer users are associated with a variety of physical, psychosocial and organizational factors such as working hours, job tasks, computer use, supervisory and co-worker support and ergonomics assistance [4-10]. These factors are to be considered as key indicators in designing and implementing corporate office ergonomics interventions [14-21] with the goal of reducing WMSDs and visual discomfort while enhancing worker performance and the safety of computer and office workers.

References

1. Katz, J.N., Amick, B.C., Carroll, B.B., Hollis, C., Fossel, A.H., Coley, C.M.: Prevalence of upper extremity musculoskeletal disorders in college students. Am. J. Med. 109(7), 586–588 (2000)
2. Schlossberg, E.B., Morrow, S., Llosa, A.E., Mamary, E., Dietrich, P., Rempel, D.M.: Upper extremity pain and computer use among engineering graduate students. Am. J. Ind. Med. 46(3), 297–303 (2004)
3. Zapata, A.L., Moraes, A.J., Leone, C., Doria-Filho, U., Silva, C.A.: Pain and musculoskeletal pain syndromes related to computer and video game use in adolescents. Eur. J. Pediatr. 165(6), 408–414 (1994)
4. Bernard, B., Sauter, S., Fine, L., Petersen, M., Hales, T.: Job task and psychosocial risk factors for work-related musculoskeletal disorders among newspaper employees. Scand. J. Work Environ. Health 20, 417–426 (1994)
5. Bergqvist, U., Wolgast, E., Nilsson, B., Voss, M.: Musculoskeletal disorders among visual display terminal workers: individual, ergonomic, and workorganizational factors. Ergonomics 38, 763–776 (1995)
6. Marcus, M., Gerr, F.: Upper extremity musculoskeletal symptoms among female office workers: associations with video display terminal use and occupational psychosocial stressors. Am. J. Ind. Med. 29, 161–170 (1997)
7. Hales, T.R., Sauter, S.L., Peterson, M.R., et al.: Musculoskeletal disorders among visual display terminal users in a telecommunications company. Ergonomics 37, 1603–1621 (1994)
8. Faucett, J., Rempel, D.: VDT-related musculoskeletal symptoms: interactions between work posture and psychosocial work factors. Am. J. Ind. Med. 26, 597–612 (1994)
9. Sauter, S.L., Schleifer, L.M., Knutson, S.: Work posture, workstation design, and musculoskeletal discomfort in a VDT data entry task. Hum. Factors 33, 151–167 (1991)
10. Demure, B., Luippold, R.S., Bigelow, C., Ali, D., Mundt, K., Liese, B.: Video display terminal workstation improvement program: I. Baseline associations between musculoskeletal discomfort and ergonomic features of workstations. J. Occup. Environ. Med. 42 (2000)
11. Caplan, R.D., Cobb, S., French, J.R., Harrison, R.V., Pinneau, S.R.: Job Demands and Worker Health, U.S. Government Printing, Washington, DC (1975)
12. Brill, M., Margulis, S., Konar, E.: Using Office Designs to Increase Productivity. Westinghouse Furniture Systems, New York (1984)
13. Bergqvist, U.O., Voss, M., Wibom, R.: A longitudinal study of VDT work and health. Int. J. Human-Computer Interaction 4, 197–219 (1992)
14. Hunting, W., Laubli, T., Grandjean, E.: Postural and visual loads at VDT workplaces. I. Constrained postures. Ergonomics 24, 917–931 (1981)
15. Knave, B.G., Wibom, R.I., Voss, M., Hedstrom, L.D., Bergqvist, U.O.: Work with video display terminals among office employees. I. Subjective symptoms and discomfort. Scand. J. Work Environ. Health 11, 457–466 (1998)

16. Daum, K.M., Clore, K.A., Simms, S.S., et al.: Productivity associated with visual staring among computer users. Optometry 75, 33–47 (2004)
17. Brisson, C., Montreuil, S., Punnett, L.: Effects of an ergonomic training program on workers with video display units. Scand. J. Work Environ. Health 25, 255–263 (1999)
18. Bayeh, A.D., Smith, M.J.: Effect of physical ergonomics on VDT workers' health: A longitudinal intervention field study in a service organization. International Journal of Human-Computer Interaction 11, 109–135 (1991)
19. Aaras, A., Horgen, G., Bjorset, H., et al.: Musculoskeletal, visual and psychosocial stress in VDU operators before and after multidisciplinary ergonomic interventions. Appl. Ergon. 29, 335–354 (1998)
20. Robertson, M.M., Huang, Y.H., Schliefier, L., O'Neill, M.: Applied Ergonomics. Flexible workspace design and ergonomics training: Impacts on the psychosocial work environment, musculoskeletal health, and work effectiveness among knowledge workers, Applied Ergonomics 39, 482–494 (2008)
21. Robertson, M.M., Amick, B., Bazzani, L., DeRango, K., Rooney, T., Harrist, R., Moore, A.: The effects of an office ergonomics training and chair intervention on worker knowledge, behavior and musculoskeletal risk. Applied Ergonomics, 124–135 (2009)
22. Henning, R.A., Jacques, P., Kissel, G.V., Sullivan, A.B., Alteras-Webb, S.M.: Frequent short rest breaks from computer work: effects on productivity and well-being at two field sites. Ergonomics 40, 78–91 (1997)

Defeating Back Pain at the Workplace: Results of the "Healthy Back" Program

Christian Schwennen and Bernhard Zimolong

Ruhr University Bochum, Department of Work- and Organizational Psychology
Universitaetsstr. 150, 44780 Bochum, Germany
christian.schwennen@rub.de

Abstract. A holistic occupational health management system was implemented at the German tax administration. It integrates a multi-component health program that focuses on back pain prevention. The present study reports results from the evaluation of the program. It consists of a health screening (N =1043) which measured 13 risk factors followed by tailored interventions. One half of the participants exhibit moderate to high risk for future back pain. Participation-rate of the program is 48.46%. Results reveal a significant increase in physical activity. Results of the pre-post-test evaluation show moderate changes in the psychological variables, except for a decrease in catastrophising. In addition, a substantial decrease in back pain frequency, -intensity and impairment through back pain could be observed. The results of the interventions are discussed with regard to participation issues of work site health programs.

Keywords: worksite health promotion program, multilevel program, back pain, health management.

1 Introduction

In Western countries musculoskeletal disorders are widespread and constitute a major problem that may affect a person's quality of life, including the ability to work, family life, and psychosocial well-being [20]. Musculoskeletal disorders are with 26.7% the number one cause of disability and sick-leave in Germany [31], causing Germany's health system at least 10-15 billion Euro each year on direct medical costs [10]. Due to the serve of musculoskeletal disorders, extensive research has focused on the aetiology, prevention and treatment of musculoskeletal disorders, expecially lower back disorders (LBDs). Winkel and Mathiassen [28] differentiated possible risk factors for LBDs into three groups: individual/socio-demographic, biomechanical and psychosocial. This distinction could be verified empirically (e.g. [7]). Based on these risk factors, researchers have conducted many interventions designed to reduce the prevalence and/or incidence in different occupational settings [21]. In recent years worksites have often been viewed as optimal settings for health promotion programs. Not only do worksites provide a good longitudinal access to a large number of employees, they also offer the possibility to conduct multi-component interventions, directed at individual, organizational, and environmental determinats of health. Tuncel et al. [23] categorized these

B.-T. Karsh (Ed.): Ergonomics and Health Aspects, HCII 2009, LNCS 5624, pp. 95–104, 2009.
© Springer-Verlag Berlin Heidelberg 2009

interventions into six main groups: (1) organizational environment changes, (2) job design, (3) job placement (worker selection), (4) education/training, (5) physical exercise, and (6) back supports.

Empirical data on the effectiveness of these interventions shows that many documented interventions to reduce occupational musculoskeletal disorders have been unsuccessful [26]. In spite of the reduction in occupational exposure level over time, musculoskeletal disorders still constitute a significant problem. Disorders may even occur frequently at workplaces offering ergonomic work station and tool design. One reason could be that interventions generally focus on a minor fraction of the problem, for instance concentrating on individual factors, or workstation and tool design, but neglect the basic assumption that LBDs are determined multi-causal.

1.1 Worksite Health Programs

Comprehensive and multi-component worksite health programs are able to face the multicausal causation of several disorders [16], [29]. Nine core elements of holistic health programs are described, repeatedly [9], [22], [30]: (1) decision about the strategy for health-promotion, (2) development of a healthy organizational culture, (3) implementation of health-screenings, (4) provision of a menu-approach, (5) recommendations for employees about health-promoting interventions and activities, (6) offer of personal counseling and follow-up support, (7) health-events to support activities, (8) networking with communal healthcare providers, and (9) evaluation and continuous improvement of the program.

The success of health programs depends on several program determinants and is to some extent program specific, but it is possible to specify super-ordinate factors that have of crucial influence on the success of occupational health programs [11], [18]. First, the topic „employee health" must be positioned in the organizational culture and the health program must be integrated in the human resource strategy of the organization, in order to be accepted as an obligatory norm [17]. The psychosocial work environment is of a significant relevance for the success of the program. Employees need to perceive that their senior management, supervisors, and co-workers have positive attitudes towards "health at the workplace" since these factors have been associated with improved employee health status [3]. Changes in the work environment could serve as an observable sign for importance of health issues in the organization.

Second, an anticipatory program planning is necessary to minimize organizational barriers and to maximize supporting organizational conditions. That needs a flexible design of the work processes in order to enable the employees to attend the program and to remain in it. As a basic principle it appears to be beneficial to include anticipated program participants as well as management at an early stage. An early strategy development is essential for a successful collaboration with the employees and an adequate supervision (intensity, length, frequency). The continuous contact to the employees, through for example regular monitoring of the follow-ups, individual counselling and support, are promising predictors for a successful program [8].

Third, it could be shown that programs have to be conducted with a run-time of a minimum of one year to decrease employees' health risks. Additional follow-ups and support offered after the end of the program showed positive effects, too. In general, for a program to be effective in reducing overall morbidity, it needs the sustained involvement of high risk employees. An individualized counselling concerning individual risks and risk behavior combined with risk specific intervention that focuses primarily on high risk employees offers the possibility of both clinical effectiveness and cost-effectiveness in a relatively short time period [6], [17].

Finally, comprehensive programs incorporating all activities, policies, and decisions related to the health of employees, their families, the communities in which they reside, and the company's customers are seen as beneficial for the participating and reaming in programs and for the behavioral change process. These strategies have proven to be effective if they are linked to the offering of a menu of interventions [8], [16], [29].

2   Initial Situation

Within the implementation of a holistic health management system (HMS) in a German tax administration[1] [4] the multi-component health program Healthy Back was realized, which focuses on back pain prevention. The aim of INOPE is the implementation of a holistic health management system in order to systematize, coordinate, evaluate and advance the occupational health promotion activities of the tax offices. Starting point of the one year Healthy Back program was the current health situation in the tax offices: Data of the yearly health survey showed that 40-50% of the employees suffer on back pain, several times a week to almost every day with an increasing trend over the years [19].

2.1   The Health Program "Healthy Back"

The Healthy Back program started with a kick-off event for all participating and non-participating tax offices in North Rhine-Westphalia. Subsequently, back health screenings (called "Back-Check") were conducted in all nine pilot tax offices. The Back-Check tested for 13 risks, e.g., previous back pain episodes, depression, pain handling, physical fitness, work satisfaction which are linked to back pain, empirically, were tested [14]. Participants were allocated to a low, medium, or high risk group for future back pain depending on the total score of the back check. They were offered a risk group specific intervention menu. Participants at low risk got a menu of preventive interventions to choose from (e.g. Nordic walking, relaxation, preventive back pain training, fitness, massage, promotion of mental health). Participants at medium and high risk were offered three additional behavioral change programs: "posture in motion", "back support for every day", or "e-back coach" [12]. The program *"back support for every day"* is a behavioral change program with the main training elements "information and knowledge", "self-management", and "trying and practicing". These elements all center on participants learning relaxation/recovering (simple exercise for every day: balance), getting instructions for activities (muscle formation), and learning coping strategies (coping with back pain, health behavior). The program *"posture in motion"* aims mainly on changes at the behavioral and physical level. Core elements are the

---

[1] INOPE (Health promotion and prevention through Integrated Network, Organizational, and Personnel development) is a project funded by BMBF (federal ministry of education and research. (www.inope.de)

development of movement-experiences and perception-abilities, recognition of habitual behavior, testing of alternative ways to act, improvement of physical performance, and integration of alternative ways to react with back pain in work and everyday-life. The *"e-back coach"* is a web-based self-management tool similar to classical behavioral trainings. It consists of knowledge transfer, behavior modification, workaday support, animation for activity and exercise. Figure 1 shows the three main intervention areas of the Healthy Back program.

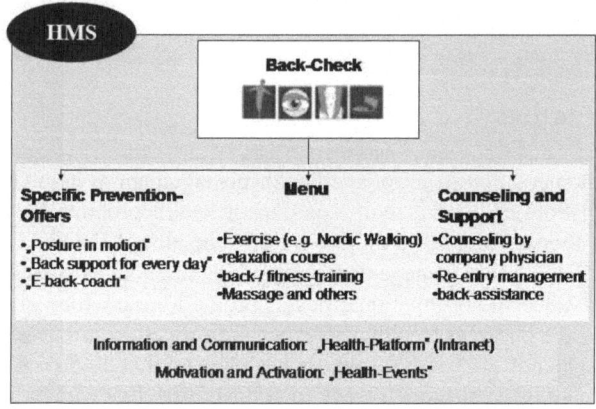

Fig. 1. Intervention areas of Health Back program

3   Evaluation of the "Healthy Back" Program

3.1   Objective of Evaluation

The objectives of the evaluation of the Healthy Back program was to examine the participation rate of the employees, and the outcomes on changes in health promoting activities, of psychological risks (vitality, well-being, catastrophizing, health perception, and health condition), and in back pain intensity, frequency und impairment. Furthermore, changes in sick leave caused by musculoskeletal disorders were calculated.

3.2   Method

A pre-post comparison was conducted. The measurement variables were arranged into 3 categories „physical activities, "well-being", and "back health".

Multivariate analysis of variance (MANOVA) with repeated measures were conducted in order to examine the longitudinal changes of the interval-scaled (psychological and back health) variables [2]. Ordinal-scaled variables (activities) were tested of changes over time with the Wilcoxon-Test.

3.3   Setting

The German fiscal authority provides 645 local tax offices in all federal states in Germany. North Rhine-Westphalia consists of 137 local tax offices with more than

30.000 employees. The Healthy Back program within the project INOPE took place in nine pilot local tax offices in North Rhine-Westphalia with 2.136 employees. Every tax office employs between 155 and 367 employees in 10-15 departments. The tasks of the tax offices are the administration of community-taxes (e.g., income- and wage income-tax) as well as state-taxes (e.g., property- and road tax), and federal taxes.

3.4 Participants

1039 employees (67.1% women, 32.9% men) of the 9 pilot tax offices volunteered to participate at the first time of measurement (s. figure 2).

These are 48.46% of the employees of the nine pilot tax offices. The age of the participants ranges from 19 to 65 years (M = 44.27 years, SD = 9.82). Participants were primarily high school (39.6%) and middle school (30.2%) alumni. The sample of the second point of measurement consisted of 406 employees, 70.2% women and 29.8% men between 19 and 62 years (M = 43.08, SD = 9.53). Concerning gender (χ^2 (1, 1039) = 1.70, p = .19) and educational degree (χ^2 (1, 1039) = 7.76, p = .35) the participants of both measurement times did not differ (s. table 1). However, concerning age they did: The participants of the post sample were younger (t (1037) = -3.12, p < .01).

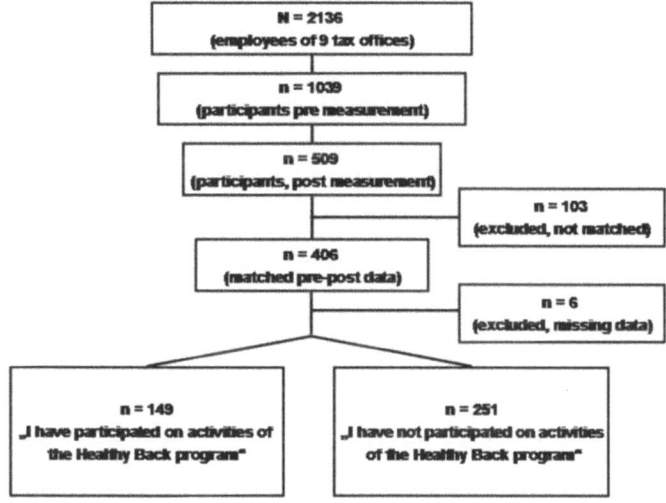

Fig. 2. Flowchart of clusters and participants through the surveys

3.5 Measures

In order to measure *participation rate in health-promoting activities* we used two items at point 2 that differentiated between tax office intern versus private activities (e.g. "In which health promoting activities did you participate?"). Response categories were: 1 = do not participate, 2 = participated already before implementation of HMS, 3 = participate since implementation of HMS, 4 = participate due to Healthy Back program. *Physical activity* was measured with one item „How often do you work

Table 1. Socio-demographic data of the participants of both investigations

Time of Measurement I	Time of Measurement II
1039 persons - *697 (67,1%) women* - *342 (32,9%) men*	406 persons - *285 (70.2%) women* - *121 (29.8%) men*
44.27 (SD = 9.82) years	43.08 (SD = 9.53) years
Level of education - *middle school 30.2%* - *high school, vocational deg. 20.7%* - *High school 39.6%*	Level of education - *middle school 32.4%* - *high school, vocational deg. 21.9%* - *High school 37.8%*

out?" (Lühmann, Müller, & Raspe, 2004). Response categories were: 1 = no physical activities, 2 = less than one hour per week, 3 = 1-2 hours a week, regularly, 4 = 2-4 hours a week, regularly, 5 = more than 4 hours a week, regularly.

Vitality was assessed with four items of a subscale of the SF 36 (e.g. „How often have you been full of energy during the last 4 weeks?"; [25], [1]. Response categories for these items were: 1 = never, 2 = rarely, 3 = sometime, 4 = frequently, 5 = mostly, 6 = always. Estimated Cronbach's alpha at time 1 was .85 and .88 at time 2, respectively. *Well-Being* was measured with five items of a SF 36 subscale. Estimated Cronbach's alpha at Time 1 was .84 and .87 at Time 2, respectively. *Health-Perception* was surveyed with a subscale of the SF 36, too. The scale comprises four items (e.g. „I seem to get ill more easily than others." Estimated Cronbach's alpha at time 1 was .59 and .57 at time 2, respectively. In order to assess *catastrophizing* we used a nine item subscale from the FSS (e.g. „When I suffer pain, I'm thinking that I cannot stand it any longer"; [5]. The 6-point scale was at its end verbally fixed (1 = almost never, 6 = almost always). The estimated Cronbach's alpha for this scale was .91 for time 1 and .93 for time 2. *General state of health* was measured by the item "How would you describe your health in general?" [14]. Response categories for all items were: 1 = bad, 2 = suboptimal, 3 = good, 4 = very well, 5 = excellent.

Back pain frequency, -intensity and impairment through back pain (BP) were measured with one item for each construct following von Korff, Ormel, Keefe, and Dworkin [24]. An example-item is: „How intense was your average BP in the last 4 weeks?" Response categories for these items were: 1 = never, 2 = every few month, 3 = every few weeks, 4 = every few days, 5 = almost daily (BP frequency), 1 = no pain, 2 = light pain, 3 = moderate pain, 4 = severe pain, 5 = very severe pain (BP intensity), 1 = no impairment, 2 = light impairment, 3 = moderate impairment, 4 = severe impairment, 5 = very severe impairment (impairment trough BP). *Sick leave* was measured with the single item "On how many days were you on sick leave due to back pain in the last 12 months?".

4   Results

50.74% of all employees attended the Back-Check. About one half of the participants were allocated into the medium or high risk group. They have an increased risk of suffering from back pain in the future (51.45%). This group were offered the risk-group-specific behavior programs. 125 (27.90%) employees of these target-groups participated on these trainings. Regarding the participation rate in health-promoting activities in the tax offices, 42% attended overall. 6% of the respondents had already been active before the implementation of the health management system. 18% have been active since the HMS was implemented, another 18% got active due to the Healthy Back program.

Concerning the physical activity, a significant increase in time spent for work out was found ($Z = -.14.85$, $p < .01$). The amount of time for regularly (2-4 hours a week and more than 4 hors a week) activities increased about 11%.

Comparing participants with non-participants (s. table 2), two MANOVAs show different trends in the two groups over 6 months period. Whereas non-participants did not change in catastrophising ($F (1, 250) = .45$, $p = .50$) and health perception ($F (1, 250) = .54$, $p = .46$), a significant decrease in vitality ($F (1, 250) = 26.64$, $p < .01$, $\eta^2 = .10$), well-being ($F (1, 250) = 11.13$, $p < .01$, $\eta^2 = .04$) and general state of health ($F (1, 250) = 8.27$, $p < .01$, $\eta^2 = .03$) was found. Participants of the interventions did not show these impairments. Vitality ($F (1, 148) = 3.57$, $p = .06$), well-being ($F (1, 148) = .98$, $p = .33$), health perception ($F (1, 148) = 1.17$, $p = .28$) and the general state of health ($F (1, 148) = 1.94$, $p = .17$) did not change over time. Moreover, a decrease in catastrophising was found ($F (1, 148) = 5.85$, $p < .01$, $\eta^2 = .04$).

Concerning the back health variables significant changes over time were found. Back pain frequency decreased, significantly (pre: $M = 3.19$, $SD = 1.19$; post: $M = 3.07$, $SD = 1.15$; $F (1, 1190) = 6.49$, $p < .05$, $\eta^2 = .003$) as well as back pain intensity (pre: $M = 2.37$, $SD = 1.03$; post: $M = 2.24$, $SD = .98$; $F (1, 964) = 6.15$, $p < .01$, $\eta^2 = .003$) and the impairment trough back pain (pre: $M = 2.13$, $SD = 1.07$; post: $M = 1.95$, $SD = .97$; $F (1, 964) = 11.34$, $p < .01$, $\eta^2 = .005$).

Furthermore, the decrease in back pain frequency led to an estimated reduction of sick days caused by musculoskeletal disorders about 540 days per year (12.32%).

Table 2. Pre-/post-treatment mean and within-group change on psychological variables

Variable (range)	participant (treatment, n = 149)			non - participant (control, n = 251)		
	Pre-treatment, mean (SD)	Post-treatment, mean (SD)	Change, mean	Pre-treatment, mean (SD)	Post-treatment, mean (SD)	Change, mean
vitality (1-6)	3.82 (.68)	3.72 (.91)	- .11	3.89 (.77)	3.66 (.90)	- .23
well-being (1-6)	4.41 (.84)	4.36 (.86)	- .05	4.54 (.71)	4.41 (.86)	- .13
catastrophizing (1-6)	.80 (.83)	.66 (.85)	- .14	.62 (.74)	.59 (.83)	- .03
health-perception (1-5)	3.64 (.76)	3.71 (.71)	+ .07	3.82 (.70)	3.79 (.78)	- .03
general state of health (1-5)	3.03 (.62)	2.97 (.71)	- .07	3.20 (.68)	3.08 (.78)	- .12

5 Discussion

The health program Healthy Back was developed, implemented and evaluated on the basis of the current health-situation in the financial administration. The results of the evaluation point to a positive development: Participation-rates are auspiciously high, compared to the reported rates of 20-30% of attained employees in worksite health-programs by Dishman et al. (1998). The physical activities of the employees increased within Healthy Back over time. Moderate changes in the psychological variables of well-being can be observed, especially in the variable "catastrophising", which is an important risk factor for future back pain, a decreasing trend over time can be stated. The success of the health-program is substantiated by an increase of back health and a decrease of absenteeism due to musculoskeletal problems.

Regarding the enduring effect, it has to be analysed if the structures and networks with local health providers that were established through the HMS can ensure the intended sustainable success of the health-program.

A general problem health programs have to face is the participation bias. The characteristics of program participants are generally different from non-participants. [15] stated that about 90% of program participants had self-reported low back diseases, whereas the information of this important predictor for future back pain is missing for non-participants in many studies which may lead in sum to a underestimation of the effect sizes [23]. Post-data of the present study support this suggestion. Participants of the initial health screening reported a lower general health status than non-participants (t (1049) = -2.68, p < .01). In addition, pre-data reveals that participants of the health program show a lower general health status, too (t (335) = 2.42, p < .05).

Notably, participants and non-participants did not differ in physical activities (Z = .66, p = .51) at the first time of measurement. This is a promising result because usually, preventive and exercise interventions and appeal only to healthy workers or those who have healthy habits [13]. This may be an effect of the HMS.

References

1. Bullinger, M., Kirchberger, I.: Der SF-36 Fragebogen zum Gesundheitszustand - Handbuch für die deutschsprachige Fragebogen-Version [The SF-36 health status inventory – handbook for the German version]. Hogrefe, Göttingen (1998)
2. Cohen, J., Cohen, P., West, S.G., Aiken, L.S.: Applied multiple regression /correlation analysis for the behavioral sciences, 3rd edn. Erlbaum, Mahwah (2003)
3. Della, L.J., DeJoy, D.M., Goetzel, R.Z., Ozminkowski, R.J., Wilson, M.G.: Assessing management support for worksite health promotion: Psychometric analysis for the leading by example (LBE) instrument. American Journal of Health Promotion 22, 359–367 (2008)
4. Elke, G., Zimolong, B., Schwennen, C., Gurt, J.: Betriebliche Kompetenz- und Ge¬sundheitsförderung durch integrierte Netzwerk-, Organisations- und Personalentwicklung – Forschungsprojekt INOPE [Occupational competence and health promotion through integrated network-, organisation- and personnel development – project INOPE]. In: Streich, D., Wahl, D. (eds.) Innovationsfähigkeit in einer modernen Arbeitswelt, pp. 101–108. Campus, Berlin (2007)
5. Flor, H., Turk, D.C.: Rheumatoid arthritis and back pain: Predicting pain and disability from cognitive variables. Journal of Behavioral Medicine 11, 251–265 (1988)
6. Goetzel, R.Z., Jacobson, B.H., Aldana, S.G., Vardell, K., Yee, L.: Health care costs of worksite health promotion participants and non-participants. Journal of Occupational and Environmental Medicine 40, 341–346 (1998)

7. Haldorsen, E.M., Indahl, A., Ursin, H.: Patients with low back pain not returning to work. A 12 month follow-up study. Spine 23, 1202–1208 (1998)
8. Heaney, C.A., Goetzel, R.Z.: A review of health-related outcomes of multi-component worksite health promotions programs. American Journal of Health Promotion 11, 290–308 (1997)
9. Heirich, M.A., Erfurt, J.C., Foote, A.: The core technology of work-site wellness. Journal of Occupational Medicine 34, 627–637 (1992)
10. Hildebrandt, J., Müller, G., Pfingsten, J. (eds.): Lendenwirbelsäule - Ursachen, Diagnostik und Therapie von Rückenschmerzen [Lumbar spine – causes, diagnostic, and therapy of back pain]. Elsevier, München (2005)
11. Kreis, J., Bödeker, W.: Gesundheitlicher und ökonomischer Nutzen betrieblicher Gesund-heitsförderung und Prävention: Zusammenstellung der wissenschaftlichen Evidenz [Health related and economic benefit of occupational health promotion: summary of scholarly evidence]. IGA-Report 3. BKK Bundesverband und HVBG (2003)
12. Lehnhoff, B.: Entwicklung, Umsetzung und Evaluation eines präventiven MSE-Verhaltensprogramms [Development, implementation, and evaluation of a preventive behavior program for musculoskeletal diseases]. In: Schwennen, C., Elke, G., Ludborzs, B., Nold, H., Rohn, S., Schreiber-Costa, S., Zimolong, B. (eds.) Psychologie der Arbeitssi-cherheit und Gesundheit. Perspektiven – Visionen, pp. 181–184. Asanger, Kröning (2008)
13. Lewis, R.J., Huebner, W.W., Yarborough, C.M.: Characteristics of participants and non-participants in worksite health promotion. American Journal of Health Promotion 11, 99–106 (1996)
14. Lühmann, D., Müller, V.E., Raspe, H.: Prävention von Rückenschmerzen [Prevention of back pain]. Unveröffentlichter Projektbericht (2004)
15. Mooney, V., Kron, M., Rummerfield, P., Holmes, B.: The effect of workplace based stren-ghthening on low back injury rates: a case study in the strip mining industry. Journal of Occupational Rehabilitation 5, 157–167 (1995)
16. Pelletier, K.R.: A review and analysis of the clinical- and cost-effectiveness studies of comprehensive health promotion and disease management programs at the worksite: update VI 2000-2004. Journal of Occupational and Environmental Medicine 47, 1051–1058 (2005)
17. Pelletier, K.R.: A review and analysis of the clinical- and cost-effectiveness studies of comprehensive health promotion and disease management programs at the worksite: 1998-2000 update. American Journal of Health Promotion 16, 107–116 (2001)
18. Richardson, K.M., Rothstein, H.R.: Effects of occupational stress management interven-tion programs: A meta-analysis. Journal of Occupational Health Psychology 13, 69–93 (2008)
19. Schwennen, C., Zimolong, B.: Evaluation of the "Healthy Back" program in a tax admini-stration. Paper presented at the 29th International Congress of Psychology, Berlin, Germany, July 20-25 (2008)
20. Sjöström, R., Alricsson, M., Asplund, R.: Back to work - evaluation of a multidisciplinary rehabilitation programme with emphasis on musculoskeletal disorders. A two-year follow-up. Disability and Rehabilitation 30, 649–655 (2008)
21. Smedley, J., Trevelyan, F., Inskip, H., Buckle, P., Cooper, C., Coggon, D.: Impact of ergo-nomic intervention on back pain among nurses. Scandinavian Journal of Work Environ-ment and Health 29, 117–123 (2003)
22. Tones, K., Green, G.: Health Promotion: Planning and Strategies. Sage, London (2004)

23. Tuncel, S., Iossifova, Y., Ravelo, E., Daraiseh, N., Salem, S.: Effectiveness of controlled workplace interventions in reducing lower back disorders. Theoretical Issues in Ergonomic Science 7, 211–225 (2006)

24. Von Korff, M., Ormel, J., Keefe, F.J., Dworkin, S.F.: Grading the severity of pain. Pain 50, 133–149 (1992)

25. Ware, J., Kosinski, M., Gandek, B., Aaronson, N., Apolone, G., Bech, P., Brazier, J., Bullinger, M., Kaasa, S., Leplège, A., Prieto, L., Sullivan, M.: The factor structure of the SF-36 Health Survey in 10 countries. Results from the IQOLA-Project. Journal of Clinical Epidemiology 51, 1159–1166 (1998)

26. Westgaard, R.H., Winkel, J.: Ergonomic intervention research for improved musculoskeletal health: A critical review. Intern. Journal of Industrial Ergonomics 20, 463–500 (1997)

27. Wilson, M.G., Holman, P.B., Hammock, A.: A comprehensive review of the effects of worksite health promotion on health-related outcomes. American Journal of Health Promotion 10, 429–435 (1996)

28. Winkel, J., Mathiassen, S.E.: Assessment of physical work load in epidemiologic studies: concepts, issues and operational considerations. Ergonomics 37, 979–988 (1994)

29. Wilson, M.G., Holman, P.B., Hammock, A.: A comprehensive review of the effects of worksite health promotion on health-related outcomes. American Journal of Health Promotion 10, 429–435 (1996)

30. Zimolong, B., Elke, G.: Occupational Health and Safety Management. In: Salvendy, G. (ed.) Handbook of Human Factors and Ergonomics, pp. 673–707. Wiley, New York (2006)

31. Zimolong, B., Elke, G., Bierhoff, H.-W.: Den Rücken stärken. Grundlagen und Programme der betrieblichen Gesundheitsförderung [Strengthening the back. Basics and programs of occupational health promotion]. Hogrefe, Göttingen (2008)

Using the 'Balance Model' for Occupational Safety and Health Promotion

Michael J. Smith and Pascale Carayon

Department of Industrial & Systems Engineering,
Center for Quality and Productivity Improvement
University of Wisconsin-Madison 1513 University Avenue, Madison, WI 53706 USA

Abstract. The 'balance model' of job design was introduced in 1989 [1] and expanded to the enterprise level later [2 - 7]. The main idea of this model is that various components of the workplace interact to increase and decrease workplace safety and health risk, and that careful 'balancing' of the components can produce reduced risk and improved employee safety and health. In this paper we discuss how the 'balance model' can be used to promote occupational safety and health.

Keywords: balance, design, hazard, health, risk, safety, system, wellness.

1 The Balance Model

Smith and Carayon [1-4], Smith, Karsh, Carayon and Conway [6], Carayon and Smith [5] and Carayon [7, 8] conceptualized the work system as comprised of five interacting components: employees, tasks, technology, work environment, and the organization (corporate processes). The proposition was that each of the components produced risks for employee safety and health; for example the work environment had hazards and the employees engaged in unsafe acts. These risks could be controlled by working with each component to make improvements. In addition there were safety and health risks that occurred because of the interactions among the various components; for example the organizational component's failure to notify employees about the risks of new materials, or the employees' failures to notify the organization about transient and temporary hazards. Smith, Carayon and Karsh [9], Smith, Karsh, Carayon and Conway [6] and Smith and Carayon [4] have discussed various hazards of each component of the work system and some hazards due the interactions among system components. In essence there is a need to be aware of and deal with the hazards that occur within a component and from the interactions among the components.

2 Organizational Considerations

Cohen [10], Smith, Cohen, Cohen and Cleveland [11], Cleveland, Cohen, Smith and Cohen [12] and Cohen and Cleveland [13] found that successful occupational safety program performance occurred in those companies that had a commitment to reducing

B.-T. Karsh (Ed.): Ergonomics and Health Aspects, HCII 2009, LNCS 5624, pp. 105–114, 2009.

workplace risks, good communication between the workforce and management, good human relations, structured activities for assessing and controlling hazards, and adequate resources for controlling hazards. The "safety culture" of the company has been identified as a critical element in the frequency rate for occupational injuries of a company [14, 15].

This illustrates the essential role that corporate commitment and involvement has in effective occupational safety and health programs. Conversely, without a strong corporate commitment and involvement it would be unlikely that a company would have a good safety record. Corporate (management) commitment and involvement is a foundation upon which effective occupational safety and health promotion is built.

The first element of a corporate commitment is a policy statement in support of occupational safety and health promotion that comes from the top of the company. This statement spells out the roles of each component of the company, the rewards and punishments for performance, and the resources available for achieving good occupational safety and health performance. It provides the "philosophy" of safety and health that promotes active participation by all employees from the top position to the shop floor employees and everyone between. Cleveland, Cohen, Smith and Cohen [12] found that the safest companies had greater participation by all employees and better human resource relations among managers, supervisors, shop floor employees and unions. Top management plays an important role in providing direction (vision) and resources for setting up the systems and processes related to safety and health promotion.

The importance of a strong culture with a corporate commitment to safety and health is in danger of reduced attention to safety and health when the economy becomes weak and a company's profits decline. Reduced attention to safety and health and cut backs in safety and health resources at such times undermine the corporate culture and are likely to increase the risk for greater hazards and subsequent injuries and illnesses among employees. A strong occupational safety and health corporate culture will reduce the likelihood that cut backs in occupational safety and health resources will occur.

Zimolong and Elke [16] concluded from a review of safety management research and theory that there are three consistent factors that emerge for ideal safety management considerations. These are (1) genuine and consistent management commitment to safety, (2) communication about safety issues between management, supervisors and the workforce, and (3) involvement of employees in safety matters.

The second element in corporate commitment is a process to motivate managers and supervisors to become actively involved in occupational safety and health promotion and activities. Many companies have a safety and health review as part of a manager's annual performance rating and for determining pay increases. Some companies have a policy that managers can be discharged for poor work unit safety performance, or if a serious accident occurs. Other companies provide rewards and prizes for work units and managers that have exemplary safety performance. The important point is that corporate policies and actions have to get the attention of company managers and supervisors that occupational safety and health are very important, and that good performance will be rewarded while poor performance will be punished.

The current era (2000-2008) has seen very risky behavior by managers worldwide in stock market funds, mortgage and finance banking, and in insurance investments that have led to a major collapse of many investment funds, banks and insurance companies.

Yet in the wake of this disaster it is astounding that many of the managers that made very risky and poor decisions received huge bonuses even though the results were poor. Such a reward structure encourages managers to take risks that can lead to unfavorable outcomes. This type of risk management reward process is not what we want to have as a motivational tool for managers in the arena of occupational safety and health. We want managers to be rewarded for reducing the risk of accidents, injuries and illnesses, and for the support they provide to employees to be involved in occupational safety and health efforts.

The third element of corporate commitment and responsibility is the promotion of good communications among all levels of the organization to ensure a knowledgeable workforce. The flow of information must be bi-directional, that is upward as well as downward. One approach for dealing with safety communications is to establish communication networks. These are formal structures to ensure that information gets to the people who need to know the message(s) in a timely way. These networks are designed to control the amount of information flow to guard against information overload, misinformation, or a lack of needed information. Such networks have to be tailored to the specific needs of an organization. They are vital for hazard awareness and general health and safety information. For instance, in a multi-shift plant, information on a critical hazardous condition can be passed from shift to shift so that workers can be alerted to the hazard. Without a communication network, this vital information may not get to all affected workers and an avoidable exposure or accident could occur. This is especially important in work settings where changes can occur very rapidly and, therefore, working conditions may produce new hazards that every worker should be aware of as soon as possible.

The fourth element of corporate commitment is providing the resources necessary to support occupational safety and health efforts. This could include expertise in safety and health participating in facility design, the purchasing of equipment, materials and supplies, training for managers, supervisors and employees, and in carrying out safety and health program activities. At the center of corporate commitment is a structured program of hazard detection, evaluation, analysis and control. This is a visible demonstration to managers, supervisors and employees that safety and health are important and need to be taken seriously. In addition, it is important to recognize that occupational safety and health issues need to be considered whenever changes in technologies and production methods are implemented.

A critical element of corporate commitment is the use of metrics to evaluate the successes and failures of safety and health efforts. Various measurements have been used such as property damage costs, injury costs, insurance premiums, injury frequency rates, employee lost days from work, and production costs of downtime due to accidents and illnesses. The purpose of the metrics is to provide assessment of progress and to pinpoint areas in need of attention. Such metrics are best used at an aggregate level that provides a sufficient number of exposed employees that will allow for reasonable trend analysis. These metrics are seldom useful for detecting trends at the individual department or supervisor level.

Metrics at the department or supervisor level could include the extent of employee training achieved, the number of serious hazards identified and resolved, the number of employee safety contacts, and/or the number of safety meetings in a given period of time.

It has been suggested that the development of Total Quality Management approaches may produce some positive results with regard to occupational safety and health [17]. Power and Fallon [18] have proposed TQM as a framework for integration of health and safety activities with other functions. They argue that the practice of safety management should include the following TQM principles: management commitment to occupational safety and health objectives, plans and policies; development of a health and safety culture; employee involvement in safety activities, such as risk assessment and training of new employees; measurement and monitoring of health and safety performance; and continuous improvement.

K.U. Smith [19] and T.J. Smith [20] have proposed a model for integrating ergonomics, safety and quality based on behavioral cybernetics theory. From a behavioral cybernetics perspective, participatory ergonomics and safety and quality management are effective because they enable workers to control sensory feedback from job-related decisions or working conditions that affect them, and in turn to generate sensory feedback for the control and benefit of other workers. Worker involvement in decision-making, worker control over the production process, and job enrichment enhance the overall level of worker self-control. Use of workers as resource specialists and emphasis on skill development can benefit the integration of ergonomics, safety management, and quality management of the organization. This should lead to quicker discovery and identification of hazards, as well as improved mechanisms for communicating hazard-related information that can be used to improve work systems and processes.

3 The Human Factor

At the center of the work system is the employee who carries out job tasks under the direction of the organization (policies, managers, resources, rewards). There are many theories and concepts that address how employee behavior creates risks for accidents and injuries. Some focus on the characteristics of an employee or the workforce and how these characteristics can lead to risky employee behavior. Others focus on the misfits between the employee and the workplace that lead to employee errors (See Smith and Carayon, 2003 for a discussion of some of these theories). KU Smith [19] proposed that the employee was a critical point of control of hazards, and that this role was much more important in promoting occupational safety and health than the concerns about unsafe acts of employees. He proposed a series of 'behavioral safety codes' that can lead to improved employee behavior and enhanced safety and health.

The employee is the point of interaction with the hazards (physical, chemical, radiation, biological, behavioral) that produce injuries. S/he is the point where energy or toxins are released that can damage property or persons. How the employee interacts with the technology, materials and environment in carrying out tasks affects the risk potential of work activities. Smith and Carayon [3] showed how the nature of this interaction could lead to errors that produce accidents, and that the design of tasks, technology, management and environmental factors often play a significant role in causing employee errors and unsafe behaviors.

Companies can take actions to enhance occupational safety and health promotion among employees. The first action is to provide opportunities for employees to be active in managing the risks of their own work tasks. Employees can be empowered to identify hazards and report them to supervisors. Many hazards are "transient" in that they come and go depending on the circumstances of the tasks, technology and environment. Encouraging employees to immediately report significant hazards to supervisors can lead to quick resolution of the risk. This supposes that supervisors and employees have an open communication channel, good relations and respect for each other. The greater the employee participation and open communication afforded by the company culture, then the greater the probability that employee hazard awareness and hazard reporting will occur; this will then lead to actual changes in work systems and processes that can either eliminate hazards or reduce their potential impact. This process is similar to a participatory ergonomics process in which employees are involved in the redesign of some element of their work systems [21].

A second action is to provide ongoing training for employees in hazard awareness and recognition. Cohen and Colligan [22] found that safety and health training was effective in reducing employee risk. Hazard knowledge is a strong tool that leads to early detection and resolution of risks. Training also keeps employees aware of the need to be alert to hazards, and to behave in ways that reduce rather than increase risk. Several safety and health standards require periodic employee training to keep their knowledge and skills in hazard recognition and avoidance current and at the front of their awareness. Beyond these requirements companies can provide additional training to further reinforce the need for employees to be alert, aware and knowledgeable on how to respond to hazards.

Many theories of accident causation have defined employee unsafe acts or behaviors as the major factor in the cause of accidents. Other theories define human error or employee unintentional or intentional behavior as a primary cause of accidents. Still other theories have proposed that system design flaws and improper management lead to human error that causes accidents. At the heart of all of these theories is the belief that improper employee behavior, whatever its cause, is central to accident causation. If this belief is conceded, then it makes sense to take actions that promote proper employee behavior when confronted with risks or hazards. The probability of proper behavior is increased under the following conditions: (1) employees recognize the risk and know what to do when confronted with the risk, (2) employees have the knowledge, skills and capacity to act properly when confronted with risks, (3) employees are motivated to respond properly to the risks, and (4) action is taken by management (or employees) to control the risks.

A large number of the hazards in the workplace are produced by the interaction between employees and their tools and environment. Some of these hazards cannot be completely controlled through hazard inspection and engineering controls. An ancillary way they can be controlled is by increasing employee recognition of the hazards and by proper and safe employee behavior when confronted with the hazards. Such behavior may be the use of safe work procedures to ensure that hazards will not occur, taking an evasive action to avoid a hazard when the hazard does occur, or informing supervision of the hazards so that appropriate action can be taken. There are very few hazard control efforts that are not in some way dependent on the proper behavior of employees. But, increasing employees' awareness of hazards is meaningless if employees do not behave in a proper and safe way by using their hazard awareness and knowledge.

Conard [23] defined work practices as employee behaviors that can be simple or complex, which are related to reducing a hazardous situation in occupational activities. There are a series of steps that can be used in developing and implementing work practices for eliminating occupational hazards: (a) the definition of hazardous work practices; (b) the definition of new work practices to reduce the hazards; (c) training employees in the desired work practices; (d) testing the new work practices in the job setting; (e) installing the new work practices using motivators; (f) monitoring the effectiveness of the new work practices; (g) redefining the new work practices as needed; and (h) maintaining proper employee habits regarding work practices. Hopkins, Conard and Smith [24] demonstrated the efficacy of this approach for decreasing risky workplace behavior and increasing proper work practices that reduced employee exposures to hazardous chemicals.

To reiterate, proper employee behavior has as its foundation a corporate culture that promotes and rewards the proper behavior, well trained and knowledgeable employees, supervision and management that responds to employee identification of risks, and work systems and processes that promote safe behaviors. In essence the best way to get proper employee behavior is to make it part of the corporate safety and health culture.

4 Task Factors

Work task design is a significant consideration for controlling safety hazards, and management is responsible to ensure proper task design [1-4]. The demands of a work activity and the way in which work is conducted can influence the probability of an exposure to a hazard or an accident. In addition, the influence of the work activity on employee attention, satisfaction, and motivation can affect behavior patterns that increase exposure and accident risk. Task design has to be based on considerations that will enhance worker attention and motivation. Work task considerations can be broken into the physical requirements, mental requirements, and psychological considerations. The physical requirements influence the amount of energy expenditure necessary to carry out a task. Excessive physical requirements can lead to fatigue, both physiological and mental, which can reduce worker capabilities to recognize and respond to workplace hazards. Mental overload and underload can take employee attention away from risks while doing tasks. The use of work design principles to meet the physical, mental and psychological needs of employees will lead to better employee hazard awareness and safer behavior.

Other task considerations include the pace or rate of work, the amount of repetition in task activities, and work pressure due to production demands [1]. Task activities, that are highly repetitive and paced by machinery rather than employee paced, tend to be stressful. Such conditions diminish an employee's attention to hazards and his/her capability to recognize and respond to a hazard. Tasks with relatively low workload and energy expenditure can be very hazardous due to boredom that leads to employee inattention to hazards [1].

Psychological task content considerations, such as satisfaction with job tasks, the amount of control over the work process, participation in decision making, the ability to use knowledge and skills, the amount of esteem associated with the job and the ability to identify with the end products of the task activity can influence employee attention and motivation [1-2]. They also can cause job stress [1]. Job stress can affect employee ability to attend to, recognize, and respond to hazards, as well as the motivation needed to be concerned with personal health and safety considerations. Negative influences can bring about emotional disturbances that limit the employee's capabilities and motivation to respond.

Scientific work design principles can be applied for developing tasks that have proper content to eliminate overload and underload, and will enhance the employee's physical and mental state [1-3]. Work tasks should be under the control of the employee and repetition should be avoided if possible [3]. This latter requirement is sometimes hard to achieve. When work tasks have to be repetitious then providing the worker with some control over the pacing of the task reduces stress associated with such repetition. Employee concentration and attention can be enhanced by providing frequent breaks from the repetitious activity to do alternate tasks or take a rest [3, 6, 9].

Training employees about proper work procedures provides direction that will help employees avoid hazards or to more effectively deal with hazards. The basis of good instruction and training is the job analysis which provides detailed information on the job tasks, environment, tools, and materials used. The job analysis will identify high risk situations. Based on verification of the information in the job analysis, a set of instructions on how to avoid hazardous situations can be developed. The implementation of such instructions as employee behavior will be covered in the next section under training and safe behavior improvement.

5 Technology and Materials Factors

The relationship between the controls of a machine and the subsequent action of that machine dictates the level of skill necessary to perform a task. The action of the controls and the subsequent reaction of the machinery must be compatible with basic human perceptual/motor patterns [6, 9, 19]. If there is incompatibility, then significant interference with performance can occur which may lead to improper responses that can cause errors and accidents [3]. The adequacy of feedback about the reaction of the machine to the control action affects the performance efficiency that can be achieved, and the potential for an operational error. Equipment must conform to principles of proper engineering and human factors design so that the controls that activate the machine, the displays that provide feedback of machine action, and the safeguards to protect workers from the action of the machine are compliant with worker skills and expectations. The action of the machine must be compliant with the action of the controls in temporal, spatial and force characteristics.

The hazard characteristics of materials will affect exposure and risk [4, 6, 9]. More hazardous materials inherently have a greater probability of adverse safety and health outcomes. Sometimes employees will be more careful when using materials that they know have a high hazard potential. But this can only be true when employees are knowledgeable of the materials' hazard level and they know how to respond to the risks posed.

Ensuring that machines are designed properly and that employees are aware of the risks of the materials they work with is the responsibility of management. These issues are part of a comprehensive and effective safety and health program; see discussion above on organizational considerations.

6 The Work Environment

The work environment can expose employees to materials, chemicals, radiation, biological agents and physical agents that can cause harm or injury if the exposure exceeds safe limits [4, 6, 9]. Such exposures vary widely from industry to industry, from job to job, and from task to task. Hazard exposures in the work environment influence the probability for an accident, injury or illness, and the extent of exposure often determines the seriousness of an injury. The hazard potential of different environmental factors can be evaluated using various federal, state and local codes and standards for worker protection, and limits established by scientific and professional groups. A comprehensive safety and health program can be very effective in defining and controlling workplace hazard exposures. Providing a proper work environment that is free of hazards, has adequate sensory requirements, and permits smooth work flow is the responsibility of management. Ensuring that the work environment remains clean and uncluttered is an important issue for good safety performance [10, 11].

A formalized approach to hazard control often includes an inspection system to define workplace hazards, accident investigations, record keeping, a preventive maintenance program, a machine guarding program, review of new purchases to ensure compliance with safety guidelines, materials safety data sheets, and good housekeeping requirements [4, 6, 9]. The effectiveness of specific aspects of such a formalized hazard control approach has been debated [10, 11], but it is clear that structured programs are a good idea [4, 6, 9, 11]. Cohen [10] indicated that more frequent informal inspections may be more effective than more formalized approaches. This may be because the informal programs often involve workers in defining the hazards. However, the significance of formalized hazard control programs is that they establish the groundwork for other programs such as work practice improvement and training. In essence, they are the foundation for other safety approaches.

7 Conclusions

The Balance Theory was created as an attempt to develop a more realistic approach to the design of the work system. It provides an integrated, holistic approach to identifying elements of the work system, as well as a set of principles for the design or redesign of work systems. Consistent with an integrated approach that bridges various areas (job/organizational design, job stress, and human factors and ergonomics), the outcomes of interest of the 'Balance Theory' are diverse and include job satisfaction and stress, and worker health, safety and well-being [7]. The broader work system model encompasses psychosocial, cognitive and physical aspects of work that can create psychosocial, cognitive and/or physical demands and loads on the individual. For instance, the tasks performed by the individual have psychosocial dimensions such as control over work pace, cognitive dimensions such as information overload, and physical dimensions such as repetitiveness. These psychosocial, cognitive and physical loads created by the work system interact with each other and have various impacts on the individual's ability to respond appropriately to risk.

The core principles of work system design of the 'Balance Theory' are:

1. to eliminate negative aspects of each work system model. This requires knowledge in the areas of job/organizational design, job stress, and human factors and ergonomics.
2. to balance the work system. Because it may not be possible or practical to eliminate all negative aspects of the work system, the entire work system needs to be balanced so that the overall impact on the individual is high performance, low job stress, good health, and high safety and well-being. The balance can be achieved by identifying aspects of the work system that can be used to compensate for the negative aspects. Another method for achieving the balance is overall system balance where there are sufficient significant positive aspects that balance out for the negative aspects of work [7, 8].

Carayon and Smith [5] and Carayon [8] have described an expansion of the 'balanced work system' and proposed the 'balanced organization'. The organization is conceptualized as being a collection of work systems that are interconnected; the elements of the organization include: people, strategy, structure, rewards and processes. The work system model can also be expanded to describe phenomena at the team level: a team is comprised of individuals who perform tasks using tools and technologies; the work of the team occurs in a physical environment and is influenced by various organizational factors. This expanded model provides an improved concept for promoting safety, health and wellbeing at the workplace.

References

1. Smith, M.J., Carayon-Sainfort, P.: A balance theory of job design and for stress reduction. International Journal of Industrial Ergonomics 4, 67–79 (1989)
2. Smith, M.J., Carayon, P.: New technology, automation, and work organization: Stress problems and improved technology implementation strategies. The International Journal of Human Factors in Manufacturing 5(1), 99–116 (1995)
3. Smith, M.J., Carayon, P.: Examining the Entire Work System to Better Understand Human Error in Occupational Accidents. In: Proceedings of Human Error in Occupational Safety Symposium, Peachtree City, GA, March 13-14, 2003, pp. 33–53. American Society of Safety Engineers, Des Plains (2003)
4. Smith, M.J., Carayon, P.: Controlling Occupational Safety and Health Hazards. In: Tetrick, L.E., Quick, J.C. (eds.) Handbook of Occupational Health Psychology. American Psychological Association, Washington (in press, 2009)
5. Carayon, P., Smith, M.J.: Work organization and ergonomics. Applied Ergonomics 31, 649–662 (2000)
6. Smith, M.J., Karsh, B.-T., Carayon, P., Conway, F.T.: Controlling Occupational Safety and Health Hazards. In: Quick, J.C., Tetrick, L.E. (eds.) Handbook of Occupational Health Psychology, pp. 35–68. American Psychological Association, Washington (2003)
7. Carayon, P.: Human factors of complex sociotechnical systems. Applied Ergonomics 37, 525–535 (2006)

8. Carayon, P.: The balance theory and work systems model — twenty years later. International Journal of Human-Computer Interaction (in press, 2009)
9. Smith, M.J., Carayon, P., Karsh, B.-T.: Design for Occupational Safety and Health. In: Salvendy, G. (ed.) Handbook of Industrial Engineering: Technology and Operations Management, pp. 1156–1191. John Wiley and Sons, New York (2001)
10. Cohen, A.: Factors in successful occupational safety programs. Journal of Safety Research 9, 168–178 (1977)
11. Smith, M.J., Cohen, H.H., Cohen, A., Cleveland, R.: Characteristics of successful safety programs. Journal of Safety Research 10, 5–15 (1978)
12. Cleveland, R., Cohen, H., Smith, M.J., Cohen, A.: Safety Program Practices in Record-Holding Plants, U.S. Dept. of Health, Education, and Welfare Publication No (NIOSH), pp. 79–136. Government Printing Office, Washington (1979)
13. Cohen, H.H., Cleveland, R.J.: Safety program practices in record-holding plants. In: Professional Safety (March 1983)
14. Zohar, D.: Safety climate in industrial organizations: Theoretical and applied implications. Applied Psychology 65, 96–102 (1980)
15. Zohar, D.: A group-level model of safety climate: Testing the effect of group climate on micro-accidents in manufacturing jobs. Applied Psychology 85, 587–596 (2000)
16. Zimolong, B.M., Elke, G.: Occupational Health and Safety Management. In: Salvendy, G. (ed.) Handbook of Human Factors and Ergonomics, 3rd edn., pp. 673–707. John Wiley & Sons, Inc., Hoboken (2006)
17. Zink, K.: Human Factors and Business Excellence. In: Axelsson, J., Bergman, B., Eklund, J. (eds.) Proceedings of the International Conference on TQM and Human Factors-Towards Successful Integration, vol. 1, pp. 9–27. Centre for Studies of Humans, Technology and Organization, Linkoping, Sweden (1999)
18. Power, F.P., Fallon, E.F.: Integrating Occupational Health and Safety Activities with Total Quality Management. In: Axelsson, J., Bergman, B., Eklund, J. (eds.) Proceedings of the International Conference on TQM and Human Factors-Towards Successful Integration, vol. 1, pp. 445–450. Centre for Studies of Humans, Technology and Organization, Linkoping, Sweden (1999)
19. Smith, K.U.: Performance Safety Codes and Standards for Industry: The Cybernetic Basis of the Systems Approach to Accident Prevention. In: Widner, J.T. (ed.) Selected Readings in Safety. Academy Press, Macon (1973)
20. Smith, T.J.: Synergism of ergonomics, safety and quality – A behavioral cybernetic analysis. International Journal of Occupational Safety and Ergonomics 5(2), 247–278 (1999)
21. Wilson, J.R., Haines, H.M.: Participatory ergonomics. In: Salvendy, G. (ed.) Handbook of Human Factors and Ergonomics, pp. 490–513. John Wiley & Sons, New York (1997)
22. Cohen, A., Colligan, M.J.: Assessing Occupational Safety and Health Training: A literature Review. National Institute for Occupational Safety and Health, Cincinnati (1998)
23. Conard, R.: Employee Work Practices. National Institute for Occupational Safety and Health, Cincinnati (1983)
24. Hopkins, B.L., Conard, R.J., Smith, M.J.: Effective and reliable behavioral control technology. American Industrial Hygiene Association Journal 47(12), 785–791 (1986)

Varying the Office Work Posture between Standing, Half-Standing and Sitting Results in Less Discomfort

Peter Vink[1,2], Ineke Konijn[3], Ben Jongejan[4], and Monique Berger[4]

[1] TNO Work and Employment, Polarisavenue 151, 2130 AS Hoofddorp, the Netherlands
[2] Delft University of Technology, Industrial Design Engineering, the Netherlands
[3] Ergoshop, the Netherlands
[4] Human Kinetic Technology, The Hague University, the Netherlands
peter.vink@tno.nl

Abstract. In this study 10 subjects worked two weeks in their rather new normal work station and two weeks in another work station. These VDU workers were trained and received a table making standing work possible. They also received a chair making half sitting possible. The effects on experienced variation in posture and discomfort were studied. It appeared that most of the time people work in the normal sitting situation (69% in the new and 90% in the old work station). Sometimes the half sitting and standing posture was used in the new situation. This new situation had a significant lower discomfort in the back, neck and shoulder region compared with the old situation.

Keywords: variation in posture, VDU work, sitting, discomfort, standing work.

1 Introduction

In a large part of Scandinavia sit-stand tables are used, which could give more variation in postures [1]. Also, in the Netherlands sit-stand tables are introduced [2]. One of the assumed advantages of these tables is that they contribute to a better health and more comfort. Other effects, like the positive effects on communication have been shown before [3]. It is easier to walk to colleagues when you are starting from a standing position and another advantage is that standing makes it easier for two persons to look at the same VDU screen. Some health effects of sit-standing tables have also been studied before. Aaras et.al. [4] showed for instance with EMG recordings that performing VDU work standing reduced the activity of the m. trapezius significantly compared with sitting VDU work. Vellinga [2] showed that in 84% of the subjects the well being was improved.

However, there is still skepticism on the sit-stand table in the field. The question is whether it will be used or whether it has any effect, especially as the impression is that people do not use the standing position often. This is also affirmed by the study of Vellinga [2] who showed that half of the user group only stood 15 minutes a day and 10% never did use the standing option.

A new possibility is recently introduced by a new seat where a half standing position is possible. It is in between sitting and standing (see fig. 1). However, there is also skepticism among experts and end-users, whether this middle posture will be used.

B.-T. Karsh (Ed.): Ergonomics and Health Aspects, HCII 2009, LNCS 5624, pp. 115–120, 2009.
© Springer-Verlag Berlin Heidelberg 2009

The opinion that variation in posture is important is not so much under debate [5]. It's important not to look only at the ideal posture, but also at the ideal variation in posture. Knowledge is coming available about ideal "work-rest" schemes for keeping the musculoskeletal system in optimal condition. To keep the human body fit, a seat should in fact warn us, when we are sitting too long in one position [5]. The fact that variation is preferable is supported by the epidemiological review of Nordin [6], where she found that sitting in a "restricted posture" is a risk for back complaints. It is also affirmed by scientific experiments. For instance, Dieen et al. [7] found that the length of the human body increased significantly more after sitting in a chair that made people move compared with people sitting in a fixed chair. These movements were imposed by dynamics in chairs making movement of the seat and backrest and seat possible.

The literature also clearly shows that training is an important element if we want the office furniture to be used in the correct way [8]. Therefore, in this study the subjects will be trained in how to use the furniture as well.

Nevertheless, the skepticism on the sit-stand seat in combination with a half sitting position is there. Some evidence on the effects could be helpful to reduce the skepticism. Therefore, this study was done. The question asked by skeptic persons is whether people use the standing and half sitting position of this furniture. It's also the question whether office workers in the Netherlands like it and whether effects on discomfort can be shown. Therefore a pilot study was done with three research questions:

1. Do end-users really use the half standing and standing position?
2. Do these differences have effects on discomfort?
3. What is the general opinion on these extra possibilities of furniture?

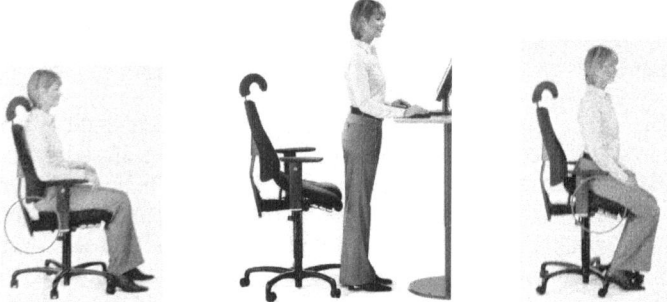

Fig. 1. The three positions possible in using the new furniture: normal sitting (left), standing (middle) and half sitting (right). To prevent gliding off the seat in half sitting the middle of the seat is lifted upwards as is shown in the middle picture.

2 Methods

Ten subjects (6 male, 4 female doing VDU work for more than 6 hours per day, mean age 38,1 year (20-60 years), mean length 1.77 m (1.65-2.00 m) with no diseases were asked to participate in the field-test. Five subjects first received an instruction, a new height adjustable table and the special chair. After a week getting used to this new workstation, recordings were made during a week (incl. Local Postural Discomfort).

During these 5 successive working days subjects had to complete 4 times each day a short questionnaire and a long one at the end of the week. The other five subjects served as a control and followed the same research protocol, but worked at their old workstation. The third and the fourth week these control subjects were "treated" and the others served as controls. The table height was "programmed" at three positions (normal sitting, half sitting and standing) and adjusted to the size of the subjects and in the instruction the corresponding seat heights were shown. By pressing one button the desk adjusted it self to preferred height.

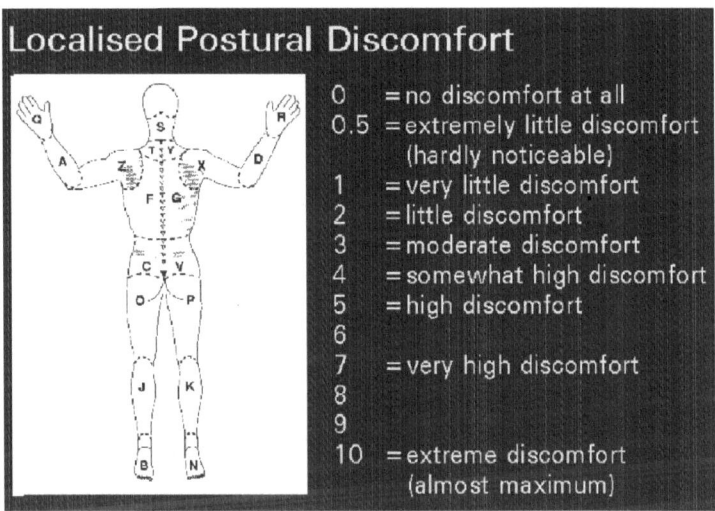

Fig. 2. A method often used in discomfort research: local postural discomfort (LPD). Subjects are asked to score discomfort (from 0-10) in the body map (left). This LPD map of the body shows the separate regions where a discomfort score can be given on a 0–10 scale.

In this project we also used the Local postural discomfort questionnaire (=LPD) developed by Grinten and Smitt [9] (see fig. 2). Recently, a three year follow up longitudinal study showed that a LPD score of 2 or more in the neck region is a predictor for neck pain [10]. A peak score of 2 or more increases the relative risk with 2.56 (n=1001, p<.05). In the back region the relative risk increases with 1.79 [10]. In our study we first teach the subjects the scale by giving them one kg in their hand with their arm elevated 90° and give a score from 0-10 every 10 seconds for the shoulder region. Then we asked subjects to put this score in a body map (see fig. 2). During the experiment we asked the subjects to give this score four times a day in the region where they felt discomfort: before the working day (we subtract these values from the other scores), at coffee break, lunch break and at the end of the day. The scores are normalized per person by dividing it through the highest score of that subject. A two sided t-test for paired comparison (p<0.05) was done for the score at the end of the day of all situations of one subject in the control and treated situation for each region and for clusters. Also, the average pattern of LPD during the day was recorded in both control and treated situation.

In the other daily questions subjects were asked several questions regarding their experience and health and to estimate their movement on a 9-point scale (which was also t-tested).

3   Results

The results show that all subjects adjust their table once in a while. Six subjects use the half standing position each day and three the standing position each day. Subjects were asked to estimate their movement on a 9-point scale each day. In the new situation the score was 5.9 and in the old 2.5 averaged over all days and all subjects, which was significant (p=.000, t-test for paired comparison).

Table 1. Local Postural Discomfort at the end of the day in the new and old situation *=significant

end of the day LPD score	old situation	new situation	p-value
total LPD	0.58 (sd 1.29)	0.26 (sd 0.77)	0.000 *
cluster upper back	0.40 (sd 0.97)	0.05 (sd 0.30)	0.002 *
cluster arms/hands	0.17 (sd 0.69)	0.18 (sd 0.76)	0.828
cluster neck-shoulders	1.23 (sd 1.79)	0.44 (sd 0.96	0.000 *
cluster low back	1.06 (sd 1.59)	0.49 (sd 0.96)	0.004 *
cluster hip/leg	0.27 (sd 0.77)	0.16 (sd 0.57)	0.106
cluster ankle/feet	0.06 (sd 0.38)	0.21 (sd 0.61)	0.109

Table 2. Self reported postures in percentage of the day averaged over all 10 subjects and 5 days. The cell under half sitting in the control situation is empty as this was not possible.

	sitting	half sitting	standing	walking
control	90%		0%	10%
treated	69%	13%	8%	10%

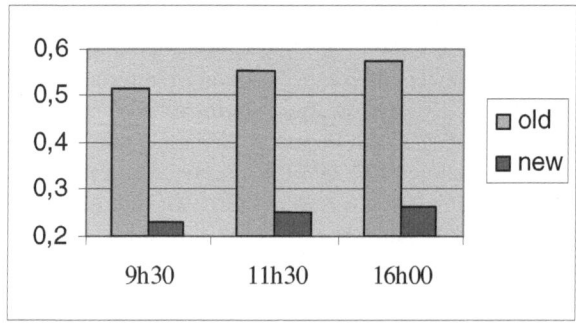

Fig. 3. Discomfort of the total body of all subjects over the day

The discomfort was significantly reduced in the back, neck and shoulder region (see table 1). During the day the discomfort increases, this is both in the old and new situation. The largest effect is shown in the beginning (see fig. 3). If we ask subjects to the percentage of time the subjects were in various postures and we take the mean (see table 2), the time experienced in the sitting posture reduces. If we ask the subjects to their preference after having felt the two conditions for two weeks all subjects preferred their new workstation.

4 Discussion

Regarding the first research question: "do end-users really use the half standing and standing position?", the results indicate that the variation in postures increases (see table 2). Of course it is only the self reported variation in posture and not objectively measured and the quality of these results could be discussed. 13% half sitting is approximately one hour a day and 8% standing is only 2/3 of an hour per day. These values correspond with data of Vellinga (2001) in the sense that users only work standing for a small part of the day. Nevertheless, in our study this variation has a significant effect on discomfort reduction.

The second research question "does adding the standing and half sitting position have an effect on discomfort?" can be answered positively. The discomfort changes in the areas where these effects are to be expected: back and neck/shoulders. This reduction is also of importance because it reduces the chance of musculoskeletal complaints on the long run [10].

The third research question is also answered positively as all subjects prefer the new furniture, while they were already sitting on rather good furniture.

Of course an important disadvantage of this study is the fact that the effects could only be studied of the combination of interventions: a new seat making also half sitting possible, a new table making half sitting and standing possible and the training. Also, Robertson et al. [8] showed that this combination has many effects. The disadvantage is that it is now difficult to distinguish the contribution of the different elements to the effect. Also, this study is only using the opinion of the end user and no other measurements were done supporting the findings. Also, only short term effects are studied. In fact a long-term effect study with more precise movement recordings is needed to show the effects in a better way.

5 Conclusion

This study shows that the new furniture enabling more working postures in combination with training has significant effects on discomfort and there is an indication that people move more. They all prefer the new work stations. More in depth studies are needed with more precise movement recordings and long term effects to show the effects precisely.

Acknowledgement

The authors would like to thank Mr J.P. Builtjes of the Ergoshop for supporting this research financially and by letting us use their products.

References

1. Stranden, E.: Dynamic leg volume changes when sitting in a locked and free floating tilt office chair. Ergonomics 43(3), 421–433 (2000)
2. Vellinga, R.: Researching sit-stand tables (in Dutch). Witteveen Project-Inrichtingen, Ouderkerk aan de Amstel (2001)
3. Miedema, M.: The effect of standing tables in an insurance company (in Dutch). TNO, Hoofddorp (2001)
4. Aaras, A.E.S., Fostervold, K.I., Ro, O., Thoresen, M., Larsen, S.: Postural load during VDU work: a comparison between various work postures. Ergonomics 40(11), 1255–1268 (1997)
5. Vink, P.: Comfort and Design: Principles and Good Practice. CRC Press, Boca Raton (2005)
6. Nordin, M.: Zusammenhang zwischen Sitzen und arbeitsbedingten Rückenschmerzen. In: Wilke, H.J. (ed.) Ergomechanics, pp. 10–35. Shaker Verlag, Aachen (2004)
7. van Dieën, J.H., de Looze, M.P., Hermans, V.: Effects of dynamic office chairs on trunk kinematics, trunk extensor EMG and spinal shrinkage. Ergonomics 44, 739–750 (2001)
8. Robertson, M., Amick, B.C., DeRango, K., Rooney, T., Bazzanid, L., Harrist, R., Moore, H.: The effects of an office ergonomics training and chair intervention on worker knowledge, behavior and musculoskeletal risk. Applied Ergonomics 40, 124–135 (2009)
9. van der Grinten, M.P., Smitt, P.: Development of a practical method for measuring body part discomfort. Industrial Ergonomics and Safety IV, 311–318 (1992)
10. Hamberg-van Reenen, H.: Physical capacity and work related musculoskeletal symptoms. PhD thesis Vrije Universiteit, Amsterdam (2008)

A Person-Centered Measurement System for Quantification of Physical Activity and Energy Expenditure at Workplaces

Britta Weber[1], Ingo Hermanns[1], Rolf Ellegast[1], and Jens Kleinert[2]

[1] Institute for Occupational Health and Safety of the German Social Accident Insurance (BGIA), Dept. Ergonomics, Alte Heerstr. 111, 53754 Sankt Augustin, Germany
[2] Institute of Psychology of the German Sport University Cologne, Dept. Health Research, Am Sportpark Müngersdorf 6, 50933 Köln, Germany
Britta.Weber@dguv.de, Ingo.Hermanns@dguv.de,
Rolf.Ellegast@dguv.de, Kleinert@dshs-koeln.de

Abstract. Accurate quantification of physical activity (PA) and energy expenditure (EE) is a basic prerequisite to evaluate activity promoting measures. A novel approach for determining EE by a person-centered measurement system which operates with motion sensors is presented. The new EE prediction model combines information on the type and intensity of PA as well as personal characteristics. For model calibration eight subjects performed standardized office and locomotion tasks while wearing the measurement system and an indirect calorimeter simultaneously. Via multiple regression analyses different EE prediction equations for sitting, standing, walking, climbing downstairs and climbing upstairs are developed. Model fit statistics revealed good results (adjusted $R^2 = 0.51 - 0.90$). The developed model seems promising for precise EE prediction during the investigated activities.

Keywords: physical activity, inactivity, office tasks, energy expenditure, prediction equation, motion sensors, CUELA Activity System, MetaMax 3B.

1 Introduction

Work with computers means a heavy burden on the employees' well-being: Continuous sitting, inadequate static postures and strong focus on screen and keyboard hardly allow physical activity (PA). Static work tasks and lack of PA constitute a serious health hazard which can be reduced by preventive strategies that promote PA and the variation between sitting, standing and moving at workplaces. To evaluate such measures, a method which provides objective, reliable and detailed information on PA in field studies is required.

Motion sensors are currently seen as the most suitable practice for long-term activity monitoring [4, 6, 11]. In case of adequate data processing, they provide information on type, intensity, duration and frequency of the performed activities as well as estimation of the energy expenditure (EE). Particularly in the context of inactivity, EE – which is often disproportionate to energy intake – has an increased significance. There are basically two approaches in determining EE by means of motion sensors:

B.-T. Karsh (Ed.): Ergonomics and Health Aspects, HCII 2009, LNCS 5624, pp. 121–130, 2009.

1. *Estimation of EE via the intensity of PA (PAI, physical activity intensity):* This approach is based on the assumption that the intensity of human movement is related linearly with activity induced EE. As far as thirty years ago it was discovered that during walking the integrated sums of the accelerations measured on the body are proportional to EE [7]. Today's devices designed for recording PAI and EE are also based on this assumption (e.g. Caltrac, MTI Actigraph or RT3 Activity Recorder). Movement intensity is usually recorded by a single uni- or triaxial accelerometer placed on the hip (as rough representation of the body's centre of mass). The procedure used to determine PAI is always the same: first of all, the raw acceleration signals are high-pass filtered and afterwards the absolute values are subsequently averaged in different ways. The so calculated PAI values are either internally converted into EE or they are displayed as "activity counts" and have to be processed further externally. Both, the internal and the external calculations are based on calibration studies with indirect calorimetry, in which equations for the conversion of activity counts into EE were ascertained via linear regression methods. In many cases, the prediction models include personal characteristics like age, sex, and/or body size.

   Validation studies yielded very heterogenous results. The estimations can be used to distinguish between different levels of activity. However, the precise prediction of EE according to this approach seems difficult [4, 5, 6 ,11]. This may be due to the inability of one hip mounted sensor to reflect the energy cost of arm activities or walking upstairs. Additionally, the relationship between PAI and EE depends highly on the type of activity. Prediction equations which are, for example, developed only on the basis of locomotion activities (e.g. walking and running at different speeds), tend to underestimate the energy cost of everyday activities like household or office tasks [10, 11]. Therefore, it is concluded, covering all possible activities with just one equation seems unlikely, and alternative strategies are needed to obtain more precise estimations of EE which are valid for a broad range of activities [10].

2. *Estimation of EE via the type of PA:* A different approach is pursued by the measurement system IDEEA (Intelligent Device for Energy Expenditure and Activity). By means of five movement sensors, which are placed at the sternum, at both thighs and under both feet, different activities, like sitting, standing, lying, walking, climbing stairs or running, are detected automatically. The IDEEA software contains equations for the determination of EE for the identifiable activities as well as for resting metabolic rate. These equations are taken from especially conducted measurements as well as large databases [1, 2]. As the IDEEA system records accurately type, onset, duration and frequency of PA [15], a more differentiated estimate of EE compared to the first approach can be expected.

   Validated against direct and indirect calorimetry, a high overall accuracy has been shown [14]. Anyhow, there were overestimations and underestimation up to 10%. The authors explain the overestimation of the IDEEA with the fact, that some of the subjects had a high fitness level which is ignored in the prediction equations. The underestimations probably arise because activities of the upper limbs are disregarded again. Furthermore, additional movements during static postures (e.g. fidgeting during sitting) are not considered.

The test protocol for validation against indirect calorimetry solely consisted of static body postures as well as walking and running on a treadmill; everyday activities were not investigated. The main difficulty of this approach is that, even if more sensors were applied, it would not be possible to detect all conceivable activities to consult the respective exact equation for EE determination.

In order to solve the described problems, we developed a new EE prediction model which combines the two presented approaches: The model considers the type of activity as well as PAI. Additionally, personal characteristics are taken into account. For model calibration, we conducted a study in which the required activity information was determined by the multi-sensor CUELA Activity System (computer-assisted recording and long-term analysis of physical activity) and a portable gas exchange analyzer (MetaMax 3B) provided the criterion measure of EE.

2 Methods

2.1 Subjects

Eight subjects (4 females, 4 males) participated in this calibration study. The participants were free from known cardiovascular and metabolic disorders. The physical characteristics are given in Table 1. Besides sex, age and BMI, the activity level was assessed as supposed determinants of EE [12]. The activity level was rated by the subjects themselves on a five-stage scale (1 = inactive, 2 = low, 3 = moderate, 4 = high and 5 = very high) [3]. The sample represents a wide range of physical characteristics: age between 23 and 48 years, BMI between 20.1 and 31.2 kg/m^2 and activity level between 1 and 5.

Table 1. Characteristics of the sample

	Female (n = 4)		Male (n = 4)		Total (n = 8)			
	Mean	SD	Mean	SD	Mean	SD	Min	Max
Age (years)	29.5	8.7	39.3	8.5	34.4	8.7	23	48
BMI (kg/m^2)	25.6	5.3	25.9	5.0	25.7	4.7	20.1	31.2
Activity level [1…5]	3.3	2.1	2.5	1.0	2.9	1.6	1	5

2.2 Activity Protocol

Each subject performed a standardized activity protocol. Sequence and duration of the activities are listed in Table 2. For the protocol we selected activities which occur typically at office workplaces. Furthermore, we considered to have at least two different intensity levels in each activity category. The protocol included office tasks during sitting (sitting quietly, typing, filing) and during standing (standing quietly, filing, sorting files in an office cabinet), walking at different speeds (4, 5 and 6 km/h) as well as going downstairs and upstairs ('slow' and 'medium' speed). In order to standardize the speed during walking and climbing stairs, subjects were accompanied by a person who set the pace with the aid of a clock and distance markers. The complete procedure took about 40 minutes.

Table 2. Activity protocol

Nr.	Activity	Duration [min]	Explanatory notes
1	Sitting 1	5	Sitting quietly
2	Sitting 2	3	Typing
3	Sitting 3	4	Filing
4	Standing 1	2	Standing quietly
5	Standing 2	4	Filing
6	Standing 3	2	Sorting files in a cabinet
7	Walking 1	3	4 km/h
8	Walking 2	3	5 km/h
9	Walking 3	3	6 km/h
10	Downstairs 1	1	Slow speed
11	Downstairs 2	1	Medium speed
12	Upstairs 1	1	Slow speed
13	Upstairs 2	1	Medium speed
Total duration (net)		33	
Total duration		**~40**	**(incl. change of location)**

2.3 Measurements

During the whole activity protocol, subjects were monitored simultaneously by the MetaMax 3B and the CUELA Activity System (see Fig. 1). Additionally, video recordings were conducted for documentation purposes.

Criterion Measure of EE (MetaMax 3B). Indirect calorimetry is considered the most accurate method for free-living assessment of physical activity EE [8] and is, therefore, adequate for application in calibration studies. In the present study, the portable indirect calorimeter MetaMax 3B (CORTEX Biophysik, Leipzig, Germany) was used for metabolic gas exchange analyses and subsequent determination of EE.

The portable MetaMax 3B operates with a volume sensor which is integrated into a mask as well as oxygen and carbon dioxide sensors which are integrated in a chest

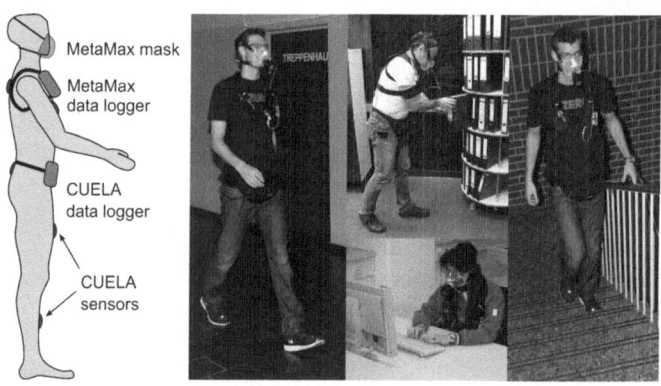

Fig. 1. Measurement instrumentation during activity protocol

worn data logger (see Fig. 1). The system performs gas analysis via breath-by-breath method and yields different outcome measures of EE. In order to allow EE estimates to be independent of body size we use the metabolic equivalent (MET) as expression of EE. METs represent the ratio of working metabolic rate to the resting metabolic rate. One MET is defined as 1 kcal/kg/hour and is roughly equivalent to the energy cost of sitting quietly.

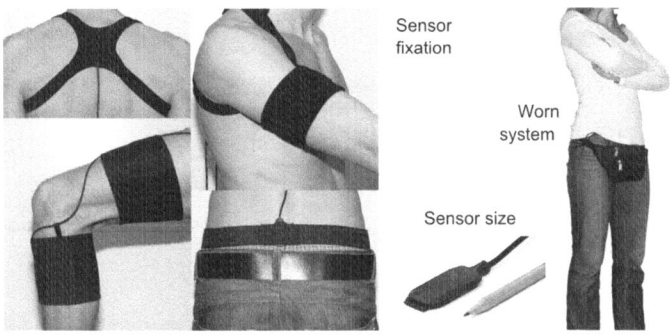

Fig. 2. Measurement setup of the CUELA Activity System

Quantification of PA (CUELA Activity System). The CUELA Activity System is developed by the Institute for Occupational Health and Safety of the German Social Accident Insurance (BGIA) in order to provide differentiated movement data [9]. The system operates with a total of seven miniaturized sensors, each consisting of a triaxial acceleration sensor and an uniaxial gyroscope. The sensors are attached to the back at level of thoracic spine and lumbar spine, both upper and lower legs and the upper arm of the dominant arm (see Fig. 2.). Elastic and breathable straps are used to fix the sensors under the clothing. Over the closing only a hip belt with the data logger is visible.

The sensor signals are stored on a flash card and subsequently imported into the associated analysis software on the PC. For the development of the EE prediction model the following analysis functions are relevant:

- The sensor data is used to determine body angles and postures. Via pattern recognition algorithms the software detects automatically which activity is performed at any given time. The identifiable activities are sitting, standing, lying, kneeling, crouching, walking, running, cycling and climbing upstairs and downstairs.
- The acceleration signals are used to determine PAI values according to the approach of the one-sensor devices. PAI for each body segment fitted by a sensor is calculated as follows: To cover all directions of movement the vector magnitude of the 3D acceleration vector (x, y, z) at time t is determined:

$$\text{VM}_{\text{Segment}_t} = \sqrt{x_t^2 + y_t^2 + z_t^2} \tag{1}$$

Subsequent high-pass filtering removes the constant signal portions, so that only the alternating portion – i.e., the signal representing actually movement – remains. To obtain the current movement intensity a moving root mean square is calculated for the high-pass filtered vector magnitudes (VMfilt) across $T = 150$ readings (equivalent to $3\,s$ at the adopted sampling rate of $50\,Hz$):

$$PAI_{Segment_t} = \sqrt{\frac{1}{T} \int_{t-\frac{T}{2}}^{t+\frac{T}{2}} VMfilt_{Segment_t}^2 (t)dt} \qquad (2)$$

The segment activities determined in this way are combined to calculate whole body PAI (PAI_{total}). According to the distribution of segment masses assumed in bio-mechanical models e.g. [13] the PAI values are merged using the following factors:

$$\begin{aligned}
PAI_{total} = \quad & 0.4 \cdot (\,0.5 \quad PAI_{thoracic\ spine} + 0.5 \quad \cdot PAI_{lumbar\ spine}) \\
+ \ & 2 \ \cdot 0.2 \cdot (\,0.65 \quad PAI_{upper\ leg} \quad + 0.35 \cdot PAI_{lower\ leg} \quad) \qquad (3) \\
+ \ & 0.2 \cdot \qquad PAI_{upper\ arm}
\end{aligned}$$

2.4 Data Analysis

In order to synchronize the data streams the MET values quantified by MetaMax 3B (MET_{MMX}) were imported into the CUELA software. For the accurate identification of the activities from the protocol the recorded videos were also synchronized with the measurement data.

The first part of developing an EE prediction model was to determine MET values according to the type of activity detected by CUELA. These METs are obtained from well-researched databases [1, 2]. As the CUELA System can only identify base activity categories like 'sitting' or 'walking' and not for example 'sitting and sorting files', we call them MET_{Basis}. Therefore, differences between measured and base METs are expected.

The second part of the model was then to examine these differences ($MET_{Diff} = MET_{MMX} - MET_{Basis}$) to correct the MET_{Basis} values appropriately. Following the assumption that differences are on the one hand due to the variety in movement intensity within one base activity category (i.e. identical MET_{Basis} value), scatter plots were drawn to analyze the relationship between MET_{Diff} and PAI_{total} at group level. On the other hand discrepancies may be caused by personal conditions; hence, differences between group and individual MET_{Diff}-PAI_{total} relationships were examined with respect to BMI, age, gender and activity level using scatter plots (all plots not shown).

Multiple regression analyses for the prediction of the MET_{Basis} correction were calculated. For this purpose activities from the protocol were investigated separately. The last 30 % of each activity interval were taken for examination, assuming that a steady state has been reached therein. PAI_{total} and MET_{Diff} were averaged for every activity. Regressions were calculated for each base activity category (sitting, standing, walking, walking downstairs and walking upstairs) whereas MET_{Diff} was the dependent variable and PAI_{total}, BMI, age, activity level and gender were the indepen-dent variables. For the analysis gender was dummy-coded (male = 1; female = 2) and the activity level were converted into scores according to Jurca et al. [3].

3   Results

Base MET values referring to the protocol are given in Table 3. During all performed activities differences between looked-up METs (MET_{Basis}) and measured METs (MET_{MMX}) were found. The mean differences over all subjects and intensity levels within one category are presented in Table 3. The absolute values of the mean differences were the lowest for sitting (0.32 METs) and the highest for climbing upstairs (2.09 METs), whereas the highest relative mean differences occurred during standing (61 %) and the lowest during walking (14 %).

Table 3. Differences between looked-up and measured METs

	MET_{Basis}	$MET_{Diff} = MET_{MMX} - MET_{Basis}$				
		Mean	SD	Mean in %	Min	Max
Sitting	1.0	0.32	0.25	31.64	-0.11	0.71
Standing	1.2	0.73	0.74	61.20	-0.25	2.12
Walking	3.5	0.49	0.70	14.04	-0.87	1.91
Downstairs	3.0	0.69	0.63	23.08	-0.76	1.74
Upstairs	8.0	-2.09	2.04	-26.07	-4.89	1.10

Values are in METs (1 MET = 1 kcal/kg/h), except for Mean in %; MET_{Basis}, looked-up base METs; MET_{MMX}, METs measured by MetaMax 3B.

MET_{Diff} values increased with raising intensity within one base activity category. Scatter plots (not shown) demonstrated strong linear relationships between these differences and PAI_{total}. Linear relationships were also found for the differences between group and individual MET_{Diff}-PAI_{total} relations and the personal characteristics. Multiple linear regression analyses with PAI_{total} (PAI), BMI, activity level (Act), age and gender (G) as predictors yielded the following correction terms for sitting, standing, walking and climbing stairs:

$$Corr_{Sitting} = 0.994 + 48.438 \cdot PAI - 0.032 \cdot BMI - 0.030 \cdot Act - 0.004 \cdot Age - 0.158 \cdot G \qquad (4)$$

$$Corr_{Standing} = 1.513 + 31.416 \cdot PAI - 0.029 \cdot BMI - 0.032 \cdot Act - 0.009 \cdot Age - 0.370 \cdot G \qquad (5)$$

$$Corr_{Walking} = -0.984 + 8.870 \cdot PAI - 0.03 \cdot BMI - 0.049 \cdot Act - 0.018 \cdot Age - 0.238 \cdot G \qquad (6)$$

$$Corr_{Downstairs} = 1.266 + 4.786 \cdot PAI - 0.096 \cdot BMI - 0.310 \cdot Act + 0.006 \cdot Age + 0.228 \cdot G \qquad (7)$$

$$Corr_{Upstairs} = 8.064 + 32.429 \cdot PAI - 0.206 \cdot BMI - 0.315 \cdot Act + 0.040 \cdot Age + 1.076 \cdot G \qquad (8)$$

Standard error of estimate (SEE) and adjusted multiple determination coefficients (adj. R^2) of the correction models as well as the standardized coefficients (beta coefficients) of all predictors are given in Table 4. SEE was the lowest for the correction term for sitting (0.08 METs) and the highest for climbing upstairs (1.37 METs). Compared to the standard deviation of the respective dependent variables (see Table 3) all SEE values are considerably lower. The linear combinations of the adopted predictors explain between 83 and 90 % of the variance of the dependent variable during sitting, standing and walking and slightly more than half of the variance during walking upstairs and downstairs. The prediction models for MET_{Basis} correction were highly significant ($p \leq 0.001$) for sitting, standing and walking and significant for the stair climbing correction terms ($p \leq 0.05$).

In order to show the importance of each predictor within one model standardized beta coefficients are presented here. For all activity categories except for walking downstairs PAI_{total} has the clearly highest influence on the correction term. For walking downstairs the absolute beta coefficient of BMI is somewhat higher than the value for PAI_{total}. Except for age and sex during climbing stairs, the person related variables have a negative sign. Among these predictors BMI is of highest importance for sitting and climbing downstairs and upstairs. For standing gender shows the largest absolute beta and for walking the highest impact is found for age.

For all activities beta coefficients for PAI_{total} are significant. Further significant beta coefficients are found for BMI (for sitting and walking downstairs) and gender (only for sitting).

Table 4. Model fit statistics and standardized coefficients of the base MET correction terms

Correction term for	SEE (METs)	Adj. R²	Standardized coefficients (beta)				
			PAI_{total}	BMI	Act	Age	G
Sitting	0.08	0.90**	0.79**	-0.53**	-0.13	-0.15	-0.32*
Standing	0.30	0.83**	0.93**	-0.17	-0.05	-0.11	-0.26
Walking	0.24	0.88**	0.95**	-0.19	-0.06	-0.24	-0.17
Downstairs	0.44	0.51*	0.54*	-0.65*	-0.54	0.08	0.19
Upstairs	1.37	0.55*	0.83**	-0.43	-0.17	0.16	0.27

* $p \leq 0.05$; ** $p \leq 0.001$; Adj. R², adjusted multiple determination coefficient; SEE, standard error of estimate; PAI_{total}, whole body physical activity intensity; Act, activity level; G, gender.

4 Discussion

The presented approach for EE estimation by means of motion sensors combines the existing methods and addresses their problems at the same time: Using the automatic activity recognition of the CUELA Activity System, it was possible to develop a branched model with different EE prediction equations for the respective activity categories. This proceeding seems inevitable since precise prediction of EE with just one equation for all activities is not possible [10]. As the system can not detect all imaginable human activities, additional movements, for example during sitting or standing, are involved by regarding PAI values of different body regions. PAI of upper and lower legs and trunk as well as the dominant arm are integrated into whole body PAI. Thus, more differentiated information on movement intensity than just PAI measured at hip level is considered. Underestimations of the previous approaches referring to this might be solved. In addition, the integration of BMI, age, sex and activity level may possibly further reduce estimation errors.

The first part of the developed model (consulting look-up tables for EE determination) corresponds to the IDEEA approach. As expected, the looked-up METs (MET$_{Basis}$) differed from the measured METs (MET$_{MMX}$) during all performed activities. The discovered positive linear relationships between these differences (MET$_{Diff}$) and PAI$_{total}$ reconfirmed the approach of estimating EE by PAI: growing energy demand due to increasing movement intensity can be predicted to a large extent by whole body PAI. In order to get a more precise prediction for correcting MET$_{Base}$, multiple regression analyses with supplementary consideration of personal characteristics were conducted. Regarding the small sample size typically a method for step-wise selection of variables would be suitable. Since we used predictors which are well known as EE determinants they were entered into the regression analyses via inclusion method.

Checking the model fit revealed statistical significance for each correction equation. Adjusted R² was lower for the models of walking downstairs and upstairs. This might be due to the experimental protocol: for climbing stairs only two different intensity levels were included and, therefore, less data points are provided for these activities.

With regard to the non standardized regression coefficients it can be stated that, the higher the relative differences between base METs and measured METs are, the larger the coefficients for PAI$_{total}$ tend to be. Beta coefficients for PAI$_{total}$ showed significance for all correction terms and, thus, prove the high importance of PAI on the variance in EE. Negative signs of the regression coefficients of the individual variables agree with known effects of personal characteristics on EE: the correction term is smaller, i.e. EE per kg body weight is lower, (1) for persons who have a higher BMI, (2) for physically more active persons, (3) for older persons and (4) for women. Solely for the climbing upstairs and downstairs correction terms the coefficients for sex and age are positive. However, these coefficients are each of very low impact on the whole equation. Considering the standardized coefficients for the personal characteristics only few of them were significant. This is likely caused by the small sample size and should be investigated again with more subjects.

Anyhow, it can be concluded that combining the information on type of activity, movement's intensity (PAI) and a person's characteristica may improve estimation of EE by motion sensors. By integrating the determined regression models into an EE prediction model linked to the CUELA Activity System, this device seems promising for accurate analysis of PA and EE for a broad range of applications, for example the activity assessment of computer workers in the context of quantification of inactivity and evaluation of PA promotion measures. Currently, we are analyzing data of a validation study, in which the resulting EE prediction model is tested against indirect calorimetry for an independent sample. Once being evaluated, the CUELA Activity System might overcome limitations of methods used to measure PA and EE. The system will, for instance, be more valid than questionnaires or one-sensor systems and more practicable than indirect calorimetry.

References

1. Ainsworth, B.E., Haskell, W.L., Leon, A.S., Jacobs, D.R., Montoye, H.J., Sallis, J.F., Paffenbarger, R.S.: Compendium of physical activities: classification of ener-gy costs of human physical activities. Med. Sci. Sports Exerc. 25, 71–80 (1993)

2. Ainsworth, B.E., Haskell, W.L., Whitt, M.C., Irwin, M.L., Swartz, A.M., Strath, S.J., O'Brien, W.L., Bassett, D.R., Schmitz, K.H., Emplaincourt, P.O., Jacobs, D.R., Leon, A.S.: Compendium of physical activities: an update of activity codes and MET intensities. Med. Sci. Sports. Exerc. 32(Suppl.), 498–516 (2000)

3. Jurca, R., Jackson, A.S., LaMonte, M.J., Morrow, J.R., Blair, S.N., Wareham, N.J., Haskell, W.L., Van Mechelen, W., Church, T.S., Jakicic, J.M., Laukkanen, R.: Assessing cardiorespiratory fitness without performing exercise testing. Am. J. Prev. Med. 29, 185–193 (2005)

4. Mathie, M.J., Coster, A.C.F., Lovell, N.H., Celler, B.G.: Accelerometry: providing an integrated, practical method for long-term, ambulatory monitoring of human movement. Physiol. Measurement 25(review), R1–R20 (2004)

5. Montoye, H.J., Kemper, H.C.G., Saris, W.H.M., Washburn, R.A.: Measuring physical activity and energy expenditure. Human Kinetics, Champaign (1996)

6. Plasqui, G., Westerterp, K.R.: Physical activity assessment with accelerometers: an evaluation against doubly labeled water. Obesity 15, 237–239 (2007)

7. Reswick, J.B., Perry, J., Antonelli, D.: Preliminary evaluation of the vertical acceleration gait analyzer (VAGA). In: Proceedings of the 6th Annual Symposium on External Control of Human Extremities, pp. 305–314 (1978)

8. Starling, R.D.: Use of doubly labeled water and indirect calorimetry to assess physical activity. In: Welk, G.J. (ed.) Physical Activity Assessments for Health-Related Research. Human Kinetics, Champaign (2002)

9. Weber, B., Wiemeyer, J., Hermanns, I., Ellegast, R.P.: Assessment of everyday physical activity: Development and evaluation of an accelerometry-based measuring system. Int. J. Comp. Sci. Sport 6, 4–20 (2007)

10. Welk, G.J.: Principles of design and analyses for the calibration of accelerometry-based activity monitors. Med. Sci. Sports. Exerc. 37(Suppl.), 501–511 (2005)

11. Welk, G.J.: Use of Accelerometry-Based Activity Monitors for the Assessment of Physical Activity. In: Welk, G.J. (ed.) Physical Activity Assessments for Health-Related Research. Human Kinetics, Champaign (2002)

12. Wilmore, J.H., Costill, D.L., Kenney, W.L.: Physiology of Sport and Exercise, 4th edn. Human Kinetics, Champaign (2008)

13. Winter, D.A.: Biomechanics and Motor Control of Human Movement. Wiley, New York (1990)

14. Zhang, K., Pi-Sunyer, F.X., Boozer, C.N.: Improving energy expenditure estimation for physical activity. Med. Sci. Sports. Exerc. 36, 883–889 (2004)

15. Zhang, K., Werner, P., Sun, M., Pi-Sunyer, F.X., Boozer, C.N.: Measurement of Human Daily Physical Activity. Obesity Res. 11, 3–40 (2003)

Management of Work Site Health-Promotion Programs: A Review

Bernhard Zimolong and Gabriele Elke

Ruhr University Bochum, Department of Work- and Organizational Psychology,
Universitaetsstr. 150, 44780 Bochum, Germany
Bernhard.Zimolong@rub.de, ge@auo.psy.rub.de

Abstract. The review starts with the assessment of needs for health promotion, particularly drawing upon the aging of the workforce in Europe and U.S. Basic intervention models for work site health promotion programs (WHP) are outlined. Recent findings of WHP outcomes underscore the requirement to integrate health promotion into the management system of the organization. Based on the framework of healthy work organization and of Health Management Systems the research project INOPE is described. The objective is the development, implementation, evaluation and transfer of a holistic health management system within the German tax administration.

Keywords: Review, occupational health promotion, healthy work organization, health and safety management, tax administration.

1   Need for Health Promotion

The aging of the population in Europe, United States and throughout the world is a challenge for many organizations. The baby boomer generation of 78 million, born between the years of 1946 and 1964, is the largest birth cohort in U.S. history and is rapidly moving into the older age groups. The proportion of the U.S. population in the 65 and older age group has grown from 4.0% at the turn of the century to 8.1% in the 1950s and to 12.4% in 2000. Predictions suggest that by 2030 it could reach a level as high as 20.0% [14].

A significant numbers of older age groups retire, the influx of younger replacement workers will be insufficient to replace those leaving. Several industrial sectors are projecting that a majority of their current workforces will retire within the next 2 decades (e.g. teachers, hospital workers, roofers) raising concerns about the loss of skilled workers along with institutional knowledge und experience. In addition, the movement of large numbers of older workers into retirement will put substantial pressures on social security, pension funding systems, and medicare financing. Public policies will almost certainly need to evolve to encourage workers to stay on the job longer [13].

There appears to be a discontinuity in the trend for advanced retirement of older workers, either by choice or force, and their expressed desires to remain actively engaged. The willingness of the 55-years-and-older group to continue working into the

B.-T. Karsh (Ed.): Ergonomics and Health Aspects, HCII 2009, LNCS 5624, pp. 131–140, 2009.
© Springer-Verlag Berlin Heidelberg 2009

future or to delay retirement is a multidimensional decision [11]. Factors relevant to the person's decision to retire or to continue working include the individual's health status, financial considerations (e.g., retirement income, savings, pensions, and social security payments), job satisfaction, work environment, and social support. In contrast, poor health, involuntary retirement, and changes in marital status (e.g. widowhood or divorce) have negative impacts on retirement attitudes.

Although managing one's physical and mental health requires a high degree of personal responsibility in maintaining a healthy lifestyle and positive attitudes, supports within the workplace (e.g., programs and policies) are essential in maximizing health and productivity. Work Site Health-Promotion Programs (WHP) have emerged as a priority topic among those initiatives.

WHP are initiatives directed at improving the health and well-being of workers and, in some cases, their relatives. They include programs designed to prevent the occurrence of disease or the progression of disease from its early unrecognized stage to one that's more severe. At their core, WHP support primary, secondary, and tertiary prevention efforts [7].

The main driving force behind employers' growing interest in providing WHP services to their workers is undoubtedly rapidly rising health care costs. Employers' health care costs, primarily focused on sickness care, are increasing exponentially with no immediate attenuation in sight. The most recent worksite health promotion survey in Germany in 2004 reports that 20% of the enterprises from a representative panel of 16,000 implemented some form of health promotion activities. Most frequently mentioned were analyses of status of employee's illness, and surveys on health and sickness status (9%), followed by health education (6%), health circles (6%) and other activities (5%) (www.iab.de). If structural, e.g., management and environmental activities as well as individually focused health activities are simultaneously considered, less than 10% of the enterprises make use of an holistic approach.

A recent National Worksite Health Promotion Survey (2004) from the U.S. documents that only 6.9% of employers provide all five elements considered key components of a comprehensive program: (a) health education, (b) links to related employee services, (c) supportive physical and social environments for health improvement, (d) integration of health promotion into the organization's culture, and (e) employee screenings with adequate treatment and follow up [12].

2 Basic Intervention Models

WHP cover a wide range of health promoting activities. The selection and implementation of these activities may be associated with the underlying assumptions about the passive or active roles of individuals within a system or a setting. [16]. According to the passive or individual model, the setting is seen as a neutral and passive environment that simply offers access to populations and favorable circumstances to undertake a range of individually focused health promotion activities, e.g., using media, health counseling and developing personal skills for health. From an active model perspective, the problem still rests within the individual, i.e., the need to change specific health behaviors like smoking or stress managing, however, the nature of solution is broadened to incorporate structural elements of the setting in which the individual lives. The setting is thus seen as an independent and controllable system, which has the potential to contribute to the shaping of individual behavior. Various elements of a health promotion system such as policy development, physical and social environment, information and communication, and skills development are thus set up to deal with specific health problems (smoking cessation, physical activity, dietary fat consumption).

Based on an assumption that over-arching systems are the product of a multitude of processes or individual actions, health promotion in the psychosocial model is mainly seen as the product of psychosocial factors. Organizational communication, mechanism of representation and participation within the setting, and training and development of setting's staff are considered as general representation of health promoting activities. This approach suggests activity that focuses on the ability to strengthen collective participation and action, and that is synonymous with the broad tradition of community development and, in particular, the bottom up approach [16].

The structural model tends to bring about direct and significant changes in setting structure and developing culture which in turn will have significant impacts on the behavior of groups and individuals. The potential for profound and sustainable change comes from relatively powerful agents within the system and, as such, the emphasis tends to be more on broad setting's policies and strategies, with the focus on the direct actions of senior management. This approach includes actions as identifying relevant policy attributes, considering factors that may enhance or inhibit policy change; assessing change options, planning the political process of achieving the necessary legislative, regulatory, financial, organizational or educational changes. In case of work organizations, changes generally deal with the way work processes are structured and managed, such as job design, scheduling, management and leadership, information and communication, and policies and procedures.

These models portray health promotion activities in a rather stereotypical way. There may be significant variability within each model and also a considerable overlap and interaction between them. For example, the psychosocial model and the structural model are often seen to be complementary. However, without top level commitment and at the same time without a strong participatory health development process from bottom-up the entire health promotion process is doomed to failure [21]. As well as overlap, health promoters may use a choice of models at the same time to tackle specific problems within the organization, where progress in one area facilitates progress in another.

3 Recent Findings of WHP Outcomes

Worksite health promotion programs range from single component to multicomponent programs, facing the multicausal causation of several disorders. In an early review on multicomponent WHP and their impact on employee health and productivity, Heaney and Goetzel [10] examined 47 peer-reviewed studies over a 20-year period. They reported that WHP varied widely in terms of their comprehensiveness, intensity, and duration. Consequently, the measurable impact of these programs varied significantly because different intervention and evaluation methods were employed. Despite the variability in programs and study designs, the authors concluded that there was "indicative to acceptable" evidence supporting the effectiveness of multicomponent WHP in achieving long-term behavior change and risk reduction among workers.

Aldana [1] performed a comprehensive literature review of the financial impact of health-promotion programming on health care costs. In his analysis, the average Return Of Investment (ROI) of seven studies reporting costs and benefits was $3.48 for every dollar expended. In the same review, Aldana reported the impact of work site programs on absenteeism. All 14 absenteeism studies reviewed found reductions in employee absenteeism, regardless of the research design applied. In a more recent review of economic outcomes, summarizing results from 56 qualifying financial impact studies conducted over the past two decades, Chapman [4] concluded that participants in work site programs have 25%–30% lower medical and absenteeism costs compared with nonparticipants, over an average study period of 3.6 years.

A recent review of workplace-based health-promotion and disease-prevention programs was reported by the Community Preventive Services Task Force in 2007 [15]. The Task Force examined the literature for worksite programs of 50 studies which qualified for inclusion in the review. Studies include an assessment of health risks with feedback, delivered verbally or in writing, followed by health education or other health-improvement interventions. Additional health-promotion interventions incorporated counseling and coaching of at-risk employees, invitations to group health education classes, and support sessions aimed at encouraging or assisting employees in their efforts to adopt healthy behaviors. Interventions with an environmental or ecological focus cover enhancing access to physical activity programs (exercise facilities or time-off for exercise), providing healthy food choices in cafeterias, and enacting policies that support a healthier work site environment (such as a smoke-free workplace). In most cases, WHP interventions provided at the work site were offered free of charge to encourage participation.

The outcomes included a range of health behaviors, physiologic measurements, and productivity indicators linked to changes in health status. Most of the changes in these outcomes were small when measured at an individual level. For example, the review found strong evidence of WHP effectiveness in reducing tobacco use among participants (with a median reduction in prevalence rates of 1.5 percentage points), dietary fat consumption as measured by self-report (median reduction in risk prevalence of 5.4 percentage points), high blood pressure (median prevalence risk reduction of 4.5 percentage points), total serum cholesterol levels (median prevalence reduction of 6.6 percentage points), the number of days absent from work for the reason of illness or disability (median reduction of 1.2 days per year), and improvements in other general measures of worker productivity.

Aside from changes in health risks, the review reported additional benefits associated with work site programs. These include increasing worker awareness of health topics; increasing detection of certain diseases, or risk for disease at an earlier stage; referral to medical professionals for employees at high risk for disease; and creation of need-specific health promotion programs based on the analysis of aggregate results.

4 Healthy Work Organization

Although there has been considerable discussion of healthy work organization, there have been relatively few attempts to develop or test actual models of healthy work organization. DeJoy and colleagues [5], [18] are representatives of some of the work on this topic. The following working definition of healthy work organization guided their model development and test: 'A healthy organization is one characterized by intentional, systematic, and collaborative efforts to maximize employee well-being and productivity by providing well-designed and meaningful jobs, a supportive so-cial–organizational environment, and accessible and equitable opportunities for career and work–life enhancement' [18].

The model, which was successfully tested using structural equation modeling, in-cludes three rather distinct domains of work life: Job design emphasizes employees' individual perceptions of their immediate work tasks; organizational climate empha-sizes the social and interpersonal aspects of the work situation, while job future con-centrates on job security, equity, and career developments.

Zimolong & Elke [20] performed a longitudinal study in the chemical industry to identify key practices and systems of healthy work organizations, particularly on OHS management systems that are allied to organization's OHS performance. A total of 18 plants participated, with a size ranging from 200 to 1,500 employees. Research topics were best practices, processes and structures in OHS-related planning and design of work systems, in human resource management, in information and communication management, and in cultural aspects. Other topics addressed the control strategies of the human resource subsystems such as guiding, training, and incentive systems, and the kind of substitutes companies have developed to maintain an efficient control loop. The OHS performance level of companies was measured by the frequency of injury days and ill-health related lost work days.

Companies with world leading excellent records in OHS integrate their general achievement systems based on MbO, appraisal-, reward-, and career development systems with the OHS function. They mainly rely on strong leadership responsibility in OHS, on appraisal, and on reward systems that are combined to a holistic human resource management system. These systems do not only include indicators of busi-ness performance, they also address OHS indicators and performance. OHS culture serves as substitute for managerial influence and fosters internalized member com-mitment. Specific contribution of the OHS culture addresses the development of health resources of employees towards self-sustained health consciousness, commit-ment and activities. The traditional approach to managing people focuses on selection, training, performance appraisal, and compensation for individuals in specific jobs. When tall organizations become flatter and/or are restructured around teamwork, different forms of team autonomy and OHS responsibilities are emerging. Selection, performance appraisal, and reward policies are the most likely candidates for change. Contingent pay and peer pressure generated by teams are emerging as substitutes for both managerial influence and internalized member commitment.

From reviews of benchmarking and best-practice studies the following system ele-ments of holistic health programs are described repeatedly as effective WHP practices [8], [22]: (a) integrating WHP into the organization's central operations; (b) addressing individual, environmental, policy, and cultural factors; (c) development of a healthy organizational culture, (d) targeting several health issues simultaneously; (e) imple-mentation of health-screenings, (f) tailoring programs to address specific needs of the population (e.g., provision of a menu-approach), (g) effectively communicating; (h) attaining high participation rates; (i) networking with local and regional healthcare providers and institutions; (j) evaluation and continuous improvement of the program.

The challenge is how to implement those best WHP practices within the work organization to unfold the effects. Basically two approaches are feasible: the organization acquires menu-based health services from health vendors (surface acting) or the organization decides for a sustainable solution and adopts some kind of a health management system (deep action). In this paper we will pursue the management approach.

5 Health and Safety Management

Occupational health and safety has not been recognized by academics as a managerial and organizational research domain [6]. Less than 1% of organizational research published in top journals has focused on occupational safety, a situation that has not changed for more than two decades [2]. Contrary to the academic neglect, safety management has been practiced worldwide successfully by a great number of enterprises for decades. Policies, strategies, procedures and practices of excellent enterprises have been reviewed by business consultants, safety practitioners and academics [3], [19], [23].

Management as a function comprises all processes and functions resulting from the division of labor in an organization such as planning, organizing, leading and controlling. In most organizations more or less formalized management systems serve to structure, develop, and direct business processes. Systems differ with respect to branches, nature of business, company size, and human factors such as culture and policy. As firms grow in size management systems gain complexity and become difficult to use, thus resulting in domain-specific systems such as management of health, safety, environmental resources, quality or personnel. Since Health, Safety and Environmental (HSE) management have a number of over lapses and are actually practiced by the same people in an integrated manner, companies are moving towards integrated HSE management systems as a subsystem of the business/operations management.

OHS management can be understood as a domain-specific management system within a broader risk management domain. Many of the features of OHS management are indistinguishable from the sound management practices advocated by proponents of quality and business excellence. This is reflected in standards usually based on ISO 9000, e.g. BS 7750 and the ISO 14000 series, and in legislative developments in many countries. The British environmental standard BS 7750 and EMAS contributed to the development of the ISO 14000 series 'Environmental Management Systems' standards. Initiatives to launch an international standard for 'Occupational Health and Safety' (OHS) management systems have been delayed. In many countries, national guidelines give guidance on OHS management systems.

The safety management principles of the ISO standards and of the standard textbooks on safety management seem to suggest that science and industry have reasonable models of how safe and reliable organizations work. However, this is not the case. Hale and Baram [9] conducted a thorough literature review on OHS management and revealed a number of lines of research and isolated studies which seem to have few links with each other. They concluded that literature on OHS can be characterized, at least until the 1980s, as accumulated experience of common sense and as general management principles applied to the specific field of health and safety. The management approach of the ISO standards are based on generic management principles which are derived from different theoretical and organizational perspectives. The elements of the systems are considered to present 'best practices' of successful enterprises. They are designed to be used by organizations of all sizes and regardless of the nature of their activities.

From the research on best practices in OHS management and based on findings from literature a holistic framework of OHS management has been proposed [23]. The domain-specific management system must be integrated into the processes of an organization to assure a sustainable effect. OHS activities have to be incorporated into the daily routines of managers, supervisors and employees, and OHS standards and processes into the life cycle of products, services and work systems. Best practices of Human Resource Management (HRM) support long term commitment and involvement of employees to OHS. The system elements to be managed are risk control and health promotion systems. Key elements of the systems are human resources management, management of information and communication, (re)design of work and technology, and development of an OHS supporting culture. Generic management activities include those of the management control loops of the ISO-standards. The health and safety risks associated with the life cycle of systems, products and services are managed by risk assessment in each of the phases of the life cycle and by continuous risk performance measurements as part of the information and communication management.

6 Research Project INOPE

The objective of the ongoing research project INOPE[1] is the development, implementation, evaluation and transfer of a holistic health management framework within the German tax administration. The German fiscal authority operates 645 local tax offices in all federal states of Germany. The tax administration of North Rhine-Westphalia operates 137 local tax offices counting approximately 30,000 employees. The project INOPE proceeds in nine local tax offices of the tax administration Rhineland, tax offices volunteered to participate in the pilot project. They were chosen according to geographical characteristics and transaction volumes. The tax administration Rhineland employs 15,800 women and men, the nine pilot tax offices cover 2,136 people. Each tax office employs between 138 and 380 employees organized in 10-15 functional units.

The organizational change process followed the dual approach of the structural and psychosocial model drawing on top level commitment and from bottom up on strong participatory support of employees, members of employee committees, and health and safety representatives. Starting point was an update of previous and ongoing work site health activities and programs at the level of the local tax offices, an assessment of their outcomes, a health survey, and the participatory implementation of steering committees in each of the tax offices. Their responsibility was to plan, coordinate, evaluate and improve health promotion activities. Participants of the local steering committees

[1] INOPE (Health promotion and prevention supported by Integrated Network, Organizational, and Personnel development) is a project funded by the German Federal Ministry of Education and Research (BMBF, www.inope.de)

were the senior and deputy manager, first-level managers, employees, members of the local employee committee, and health and safety representatives. Taken together, 8 -12 members joined the local committee. The president of the tax administration Rhineland chaired the central steering committee of the 9 tax offices. This committee incorporated all senior managers of the tax offices, central health and safety representatives, members of the central employee committee and the scientific consultants.

Key elements of the management framework to be implemented incorporated processes (structures) and activities of human resource management, e.g., leadership accountability for OHS objectives linked with appraisal and reward systems, top- down and bottom-up health goal settings and negotiations, setting up of monitoring and feedback systems, promoting of OHS responsibility of self-managed teams and individuals, and training systems linked to managers' and subordinates' needs. Additionally, peer pressure with respect to health activities and positive health attitudes generated by work teams served as supplement for both managerial influence and internalized member commitment.

Managerial tasks in the information and communication domain included the establishment of top-down and bottom-up information and communication channels and platforms on health issues, installation of a web-based communication platform, and the start-off of internal communication processes promoted by incentives and personal communication ownerships. Management of job and work design emphasized the allocation of accountability to first line managers and teams. This was linked to an ongoing monitoring and improvement loop with the focus on physical (ergonomic) as well as psychosocial aspects of work place environment. Teams (health circles) developed work process improvements and were encouraged to adjust characteristics of their computer software.

The implementation and continuing improvement of the generic OHS management system was supplemented by health surveys, specifically tailored health interventions (for example, 'Healthy back' program, see Schwennen and Zimolong in this symposium), and ongoing menu offers including physical and psychosocial activities at the local tax offices. A notable part of the offers resulted from networking with local and regional healthcare providers and institutions.

The 'Healthy back' program offered an assessment of health risks with feedback, delivered verbally and written, followed by tailored risk group health education and specific back health-improvement interventions. Health-promotion interventions incorporated counseling and coaching of employees, invitations to group health education and active training classes, and support activities via telephone aimed at encouraging or assisting employees in their efforts to adopt healthy behaviors. Interventions with an environmental focus covered enhancing access to physical activity programs (exercise facilities, time-off for exercise, set-up of training classes such as Nordic Walking), providing healthy food choices in cafeterias, and enacting policies that support a healthier work site environment (such as a smoke-free workplace). In most cases, WHP interventions provided at the work site were offered free of charge to encourage participation.

Comprehensive outcomes from the ongoing research project will be presented at the conference.

References

1. Aldana, S.G.: Financial impact of health promotion programs: A comprehensive review of the literature. Am. J. Health Promot. 15, 296–320 (2001)
2. Barling, J., Loughlin, C., Kelloway, E.K.: Development and test of a model linking safety-specific transformational leadership and occupational safety. Journal of Applied Psychology 87(3), 488–496 (2002)
3. Bird, F.E.J., Germain, L.E.: Practical loss control leadership. In: The conservation of people, property, process, and profits. Institute Publishing, Loganville (1987)
4. Chapman, L.S.: Meta-evaluation of worksite health promotion economic return studies: 2005 update. Am. J. Health Promot. 19, 1–11 (2005)
5. DeJoy, D.M., Southern, D.J.: An integrative perspective on worksite health promotion. J. Occup. Med. 35, 1221–1230 (1993)
6. Fahlbruch, B., Wilpert, B.: System safety - an emerging field for I/O psychology. In: Cooper, C.L., Robertson, I.v.T. (eds.) International review of industrial and organizational psychology, pp. 55–93. John Wiley & Sons Ltd, West Sussex (1999)
7. Goetzel, R.Z., Ozminkowski, R.J.: The health and cost benefits of work site health-promotion programs. Annu. Rev. Public Health 29, 303–323 (2008)
8. Goetzel, R.Z., Shechter, D., Ozminkowski, R.J., Marmet, P.F., Tabrizi, M.J.: Promising practices in employer's health and productivity management efforts: Findings from a benchmarking study. J. Occup. Environ. Med. 49, 111–130 (2007)
9. Hale, A., Baram, M. (eds.): Safety management and the challenge of organizational change. Elsevier, Oxford (1998)
10. Heaney, C., Goetzel, R.Z.: A review of health-related outcomes of multi-component worksite health promotion programs. Am. J. Health Promot. 11, 290–307 (1998)
11. Karpansalo, M., Kauhanen, J., Lakka, T.A., et al.: Depression and early retirement: Prospective population based study in middle aged men. Journal Epidemiol Community Health 59, 70–74 (2005)
12. Linnan, L., Bowling, M., Lindsay, G., Childress, J., Blakey, C., et al.: Results of the 2004 National Worksite Health Promotion Survey. Am. J. Public Health. 98, 1503–1509 (2008)
13. Musich, S., McDonald, T., Chapman, L.S.: Health promotion strategies for the "Boomer" generation: Wellness for the mature worker. American Journal of Health Promotion (23), The Art of Health Promotion 23, 1–9 (2009)
14. Social Security Administration (2000), Actuarial publications, http://www.ssa.gov/OACT/TR
15. Task Force Comm. Prev. Serv., Proceedings of the Task Force Meeting: Worksite Reviews (2007)
16. Whitelaw, S., Baxendale, A., Bryce, C., Machardy, L., Young, I., Witney, E.: Settings based health promotion: A review. Health Promotion International 16, 339–352 (2001)
17. Wilson, M., Holman, P., Hammock, A.: A comprehensive review of the effects of worksite health promotion on health related outcomes. Am. J. Health Promot. 10, 429–435 (1996)
18. Wilson, M.G., DeJoy, D.M., Vandenberg, R.J., Richardson, H.A., McGrath, A.L.: Work characteristics and employee health and well-being: Test of a model of healthy work organization. Journal of Occupational and Organizational Psychology 77, 565–588 (2004)
19. Zimolong, B., Elke, G.: Risk Management. In: Karwowski, W. (ed.) International Encyclopedia of Ergonomics and Human Factors, pp. 1327–1333. Taylor & Francis, London (2001b)

20. Zimolong, B., Elke, G.: Die erfolgreichen Strategien und Praktiken der Unternehmen (The successful strategies and practices of enterprises). In: Zimolong, B. (Hrsg.) Management des Arbeits- und Gesundheitsschutzes - Die erfolgreichen Strategien der Unternehmen (Health and safety management- The successful strategies of enterprises), pp. 235–268. Gabler, Wiesbaden (2001a)
21. Zimolong, B., Elke, G.: Occupational health and safety management. In: Salvendy, G. (ed.) Handbook of Human Factors and Ergonomics, pp. 673–707. Wiley, New York (2006)
22. Zimolong, B., Elke, G., Bierhoff, H.W.: Den Rücken stärken. In: Grundlagen und Programme der betrieblichen Gesundheitsförderung. Hogrefe, Göttingen (2008)
23. Zimolong, B., Elke, G., Trimpop, R.: Gesundheitsmanagement (Health management). In: Zimolong, B., Konradt, U. (eds.) Enzyklopädie der Psychologie (Encyclopedia of Psychology): Band 2 Ingenieurpsychologie (Engeneering Psychology), pp. 633–668. Hogrefe, Göttingen (2006)

Part II

New Trends in Ergonomics

Development of Portable Robotic Operation Terminals to Achieve Increased Safety and Usability and a Study on the Effectiveness of Wireless Terminals

Hidetoshi Fukui, Satoshi Yonejima, Masatake Yamano, Masao Dohi,
Tomonori Nishiki, Mariko Yamada, and Toshihiro Fujita

IDEC Corporation, 1-7-31 Nishimiyahara, Yodogawa-ku, Osaka, 532-8550 Japan
{hifukui,syonejima,myamano,mdohi,nishikit,mayamada,
fujitat}@idec.co.jp

Abstract. In factory automation (FA) industry, it is essential for the working environment using industrial robots to be provided with measures that assure operator's safety and good usability of machines. We have studied the operator's safety and usability of portable robotic operation terminals, and have developed the standardized terminals for one-hand operation suitable to many types of applications. The find`ings and knowledge we obtained through the development materialized recently as the new two-hand portable robotic operation terminal which is designed ergonomically. In this paper, we report on the new operation terminal which provides excellent operational safety and usability, and also a study on the effectiveness of wireless terminals for improving the usability of entire system.

Keywords: Teach pendant, enabling switch, robot, HMI environment, wireless, safety, usability.

1 Introduction

In factory automation (FA) industry utilizing industrial robots, it is widely recognized that the environment where operators and machines interact must be assured of high level safety for operators, at the same time as improving the system productivity.

As figure 1 shows, there are many situations in the working environments where operators and robots interact directly in manual operations, such as system start-up, teaching, process-changeover, error repair, and maintenance. In manual operations where operators need to work in close proximity to a robot, the operator needs to use a portable robotic operation terminal (hereinafter referred to as teach pendant). Because the operator is required to work in a hazardous area, the teach pendant has to be designed so that the safety of operators can be ensured. The requirements of teach pendant and enabling device, which must be used on teach pendants, are described by many international standards as shown in Table 1 [1-5].

B.-T. Karsh (Ed.): Ergonomics and Health Aspects, HCII 2009, LNCS 5624, pp. 143–152, 2009.

Table 1. International Standards for Teach Pendant and Enabling Device

Standards	Requirement
ISO 12100-1 (2003) Safety of machinery - Basic concepts, general principles for design -- Part 1: Basic terminology, methodology	3.26.2 enabling device
ISO 12100-2 (2003) Safety of machinery - Basic concepts, general principles for design -- Part 2: Technical principles	4.11.9 Control mode for setting, teaching, process changeover, fault-finding, cleaning or maintenance
ISO 10218-1 (2006) Robots for industrial environments – Safety requirements – Part 1: Robot	5.8.3 Enabling device
IEC 60204-1 (2005) Safety of Machinery – Electrical Equipment of Machines	10.9 Enabling control device
IEC 60947-5-8 (2006) Control circuit devices and switching elements – Three-position enabling switches	2.1 Enabling device 2.2 Three-position enabling switch
ANSI/RIA ISO 10218-1 (2007) Robots for Industrial Environment – Safety Requirements, Part 1 - Robot	5.8.3 Enabling device
ANSI/RIA R15.06 (1999) for Industrial Robots and Robot Systems Safety Requirements	4.7.3 Enabling device
NFPA79 (2007) Electrical Standard for Industrial Machinery	9.2.5.7 Enabling control
ANSI B11.19 (2003) Performance Criteria for Safeguarding American National Standard for Machine Tools	12.3 Enabling devices
CAN/CSA Z434-03 (2003) Industrial Robots and Robot Systems - General Safety Requirements	4.7.4 Enabling Device
SEMI S2-0706 (2006) Environmental, Health, and Safety Guideline for Semiconductor Manufacturing Equipment	20.4 Industrial Robot and Industrial Robot Systems
UL 1740 (1998) Robots and Robotic Equipment	41.5 Teach pendant

The enabling switch of enabling device enables robot operation when pressed and turned on, and disables robot operation when turned off. The enabling switch is designed to turn off by unintentional action of the operator when the robot moves unexpectedly. There are two-position and three-position enabling switches, and three-position type is the preferred choice for the use in enabling device due to the following reasons.

Two-position enabling switch turns on when pressed, and turns off when released. Three-position enabling switch similarly turns on when pressed and turns off when released, but it also turns off when pressed tightly by the panicked operator. Therefore in emergency, three-position enabling switch turns off either when released or pressed tightly. On the other hand, two-position enabling switch turns off only when released.

According to the experiment by National Institute of Occupational Safety and Health, Japan, operators cannot act calmly when facing with an imminent danger. ANSI/RIA R15.06 also describes that "Tests have shown that human reaction to an emergency may be to release an object, or hold on tighter, thus compressing an enabling device. Design and installation of the enabling device should consider the

Operator
Robot
Teach Pendant

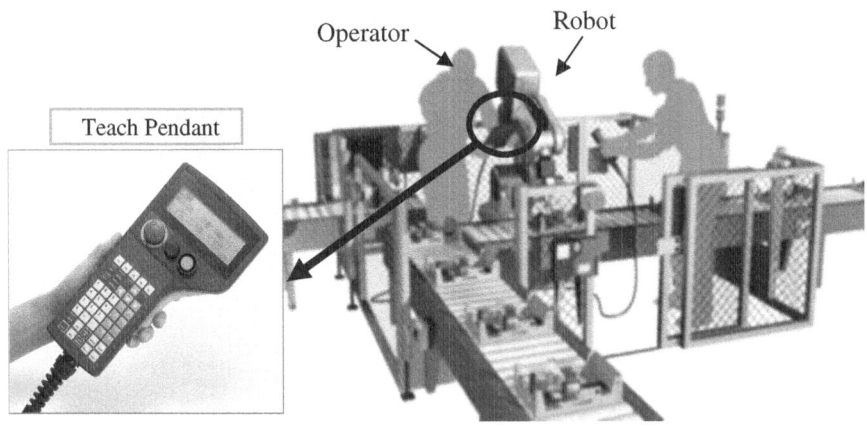

Fig. 1. Operators and robot in working area

ergonomics issues of sustained activation." Therefore when designing a teach pendant, we must consider two types of situation: a panicked operator releases the enabling switch, and the operator holds on to the switch tightly.

Figure 2 shows how the safety of operators is different when using two-position enabling switch and three-position enabling switch. In the figure, an operator uses a grip switch in (A) and a teach pendant in (B). The safety of operator when using the two-position enabling switch is shown in (C), and three-position enabling switch in (D).

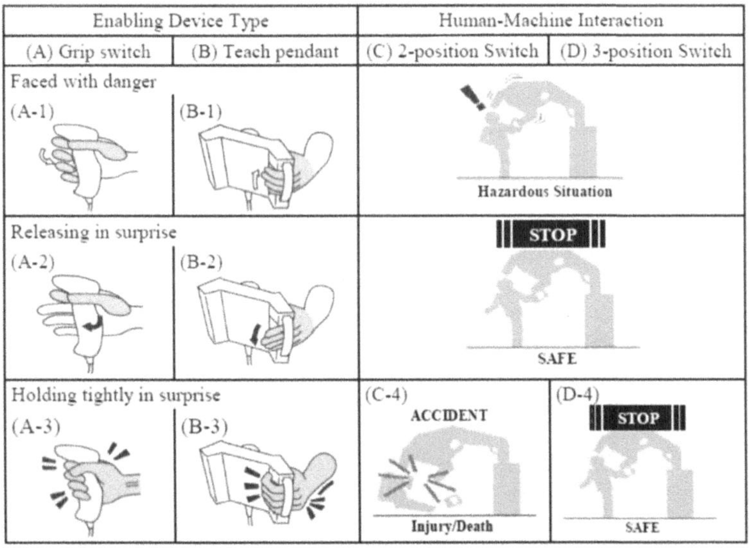

Enabling Device Type
Human-Machine Interaction
(A) Grip switch
(B) Teach pendant
(C) 2-position Switch
(D) 3-position Switch
Faced with danger
(A-1)
(B-1)
Hazardous Situation
Releasing in surprise
(A-2)
(B-2)
STOP
SAFE
Holding tightly in surprise
(A-3)
(B-3)
(C-4)
ACCIDENT
Injury/Death
(D-4)
STOP
SAFE

Fig. 2. Comparison of 2-position and 3-position enabling switches

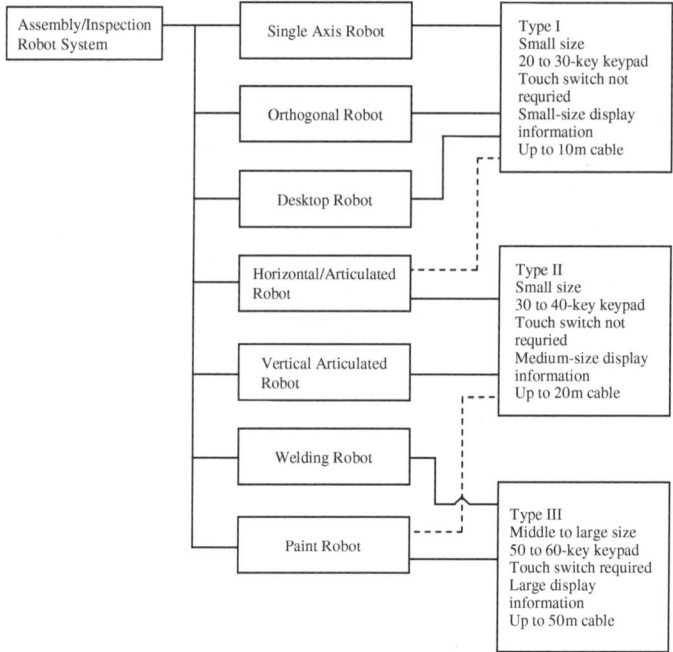

Fig. 3. Three types of teach pendants

As shown in the figure, both two- and three-position enabling switches disable machine operation when released (A-2, B-2). When grasped tightly (A-3, B-3), however, two-position switch keeps activating robot motion, causing possible danger or death to the operator (C-4). On the other hand, three-position enabling switch disables robot motion even when held tightly, assuring operator's safety (D-4).

Therefore, three-position enabling switch is superior to two-position enabling switch, and the requirements of operational performance characteristics are specified in IEC 60947-5-8: Low-voltage switchgear and controlgear – Part 5-8: Control circuit devices and switching elements – Three-position enabling switches. We have long been engaged in the research and development of safety products such as enabling switch and emergency stop switch from the viewpoint of operational safety [6-11].

2 Standardized Teach Pendant for Improved Usability

Pendants are used by holding in a hand, therefore good usability is necessary to minimize stress and to ensure comfort operation for users. Therefore teach pendants must provide users with both operational safety and usability based on ergonomics [12, 13]. Conventionally, each machine manufacturer has developed teach pendant individually with their own design, because specifications required for a teach pendant varies with different types of applications where the pendant is used. Because

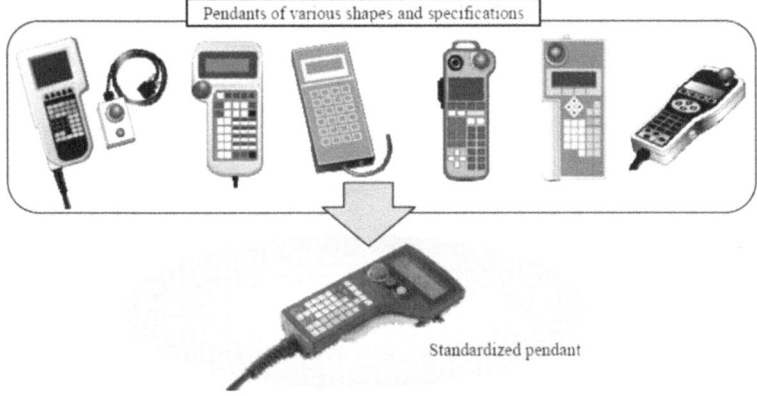

Fig. 4. Standardization of teach pendants

there have been no specific guidelines available for the required components of teach pendant, the pendants designed by machine manufacturers were hardly the optimal choice as a Human Machine Interface (HMI), and there were problems such as lack of safety components, un-ergonomic and inflexible component layout, shape, and size, resulting in bad usability and stressful operation.

To solve these problems, we have studied various teach pendants and requirements for teach pendant used in FA industry, and categorized them in types I, II, and III as shown in figure 3. Based on the research, we have developed the standardized teach pendant that can be used for many types of robots and machines shown in figure 4. Figure 5 shows the HG1H teach pendant we developed for Type I requirement of 20 to 30-key keypad and small display information, and the HG1T teach pendant for Type II requirement of 30 to 40-key keypad and medium-size display information. These pendants were designed not only with good appearance, but also with excellent usability. The enabling switch, which operator needs to keep pressing in enabling position during teaching, is arranged where the palm of the operator is placed invariably when holding a teach pendant. The design makes it possible for the operator to continue teaching operation for a long time almost without realizing it. The shape and position of enabling

	In left hand	In right hand
HG1H teach pendant for Type I requirement	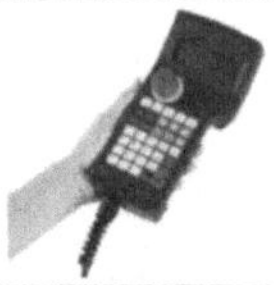	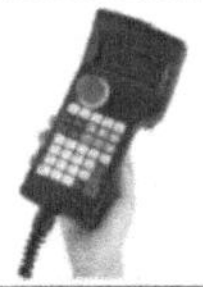
HG1T teach pendant for Type II requirement	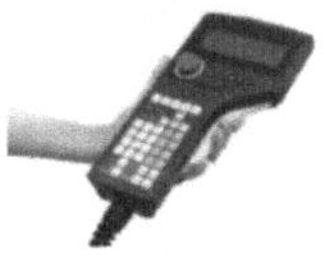	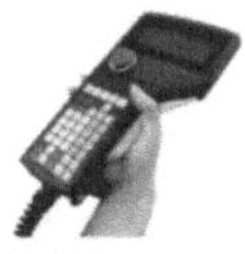

Fig. 5. HG1H and HG1T teach pendants for type I and II requirements

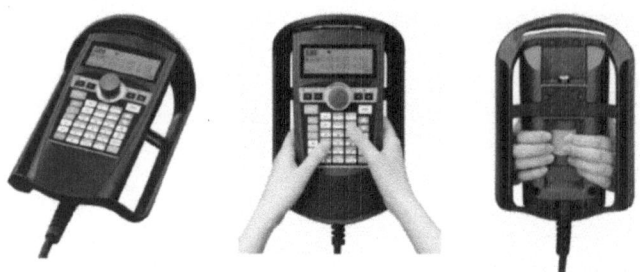

Fig. 6. HG1U Two-hand teach pendant

switch are designed with ergonomic considerations so that it turns off without failure when the panicked operator in emergency releases or holds on to the teach pendant tightly. The enabling switch can also be used easily in either right or left hand [12, 13].

3   Two-Hand Teach Pendant of Excellent Usability

In addition to one-hand teach pendant, some robot-teaching applications require a teach pendant which can be held and operated by both right and left hands. The HG1U two-hand teach pendant shown in figure 6 was developed to meet the new demand.

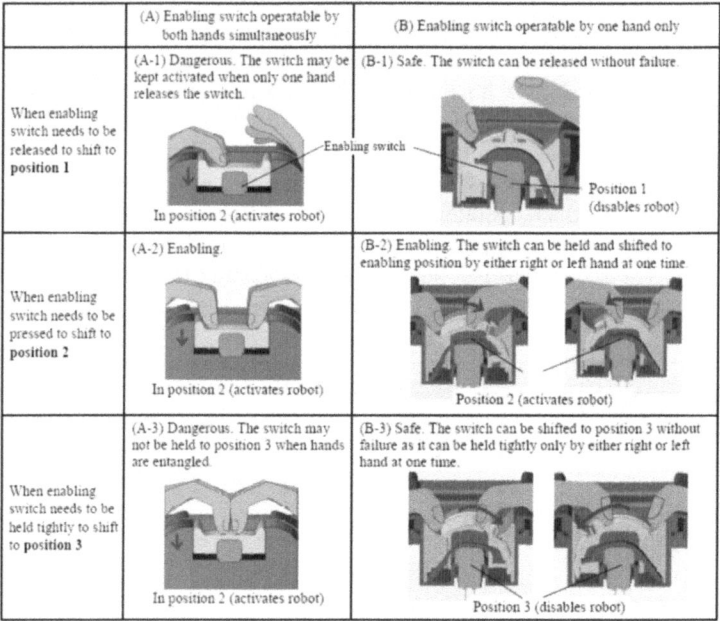

(A) Operatable by both hands simultaneously (B) Operatable by one hand only

Fig. 7. Enabling switch type comparison

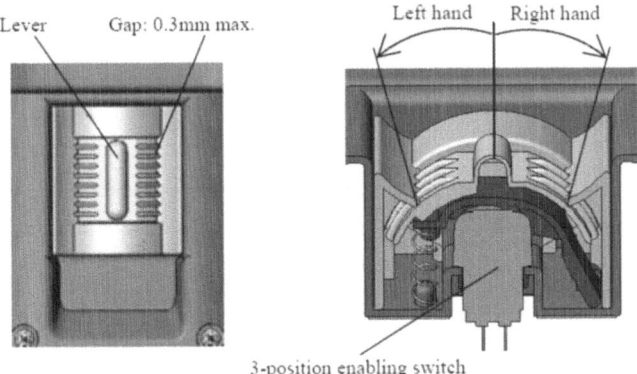

Fig. 8. Enabling switch structure for HG1U teach pendant

Special attention is required when designing the 3-position enabling switches for two-hand teach pendants, because both right and left hands are always in contact with the enabling switch. The switch has to be designed to allow only either right or left hand to operate the switch at one time, otherwise there is a possibility that the switch cannot shift to disabling positions properly when it is supposed to be released or held tightly, as illustrated in (A-1) and (A-3).

The usability problems mentioned above are eliminated in the structure shown in figure 8, which can be operated by one hand only at a time. In this structure, the enabling switch shifts to enabling position only when the lever is held lightly by either right or left hand and pulled to the side as shown in (B-2), and it can be released without failure when needed, as shown in (B-1) and (B-3). The lever's shape, height, width and length are designed with ergonomic considerations to ensure good usability. The lever and the housing have comb-shaped features and have a 0.3mm gap in between, to prevent the entry of foreign objects and trapping of fingers.

In addition to enabling switch, the design of two-hand teach pendant has also achieved excellent usability with the following characteristics.

1. Easy to hold: The operator needs to be able to hold a teach pendant for a long time without developing fatigue. The protector installed around the teach pendant touches the back of the hands lightly, making it possible for the operator to keep holding the pendant comfortably without stress.
2. Easy to operate: The operator needs to be able to press the keys easily while holding the teach pendant. The keys are arranged in positions where the thumb of right and left hands can approach easily.
3. Robustness: The operator might drop the teach pendant accidentally. The teach pendant withstands free-fall from 1.5m without damage.

As explained above, we have developed the standardized two-hand teach pendant that provides excellent operational safety and usability that ensures comfortable and stress-free operation.

Table 2. Comparison of wireless and wired teach pendants

		Wireless	Wired
Usability	Portability	★ ★ ★	★ ★
	Maintenance ease (battery/cable change)	★ ★	★
	Operating duration	★	★ ★ ★
Flexibility	System layout	★ ★ ★	★ ★
	Multiple hosts	★ ★ ★	★
	Mobile hosts	★ ★ ★	★
	Resistance against obstacles in communication (radiowave absorber, EMC)	★	★ ★ ★
Cost		★	★ ★

★ ★ ★ : Excellent   ★ ★ : Good   ★ : Acceptable

4   A Study on Wireless Teach Pendant for Large Robot Systems

Because large systems such as welding robot and paint robot handle information of large volume, they require large-size teach pendant equipped with many keys. The more display information and optional functions must be processed, the thicker and heavier the cable becomes. Also, large systems necessitate operators to move around in wider area, requiring longer cables and resulting in lower portability of teach pendants. There is a growing demand for wireless teach pendants.

Wireless teach pendant is effective not only in large systems but also in systems using multiple and mobile hosts such as service robots. Table 2 shows the comparison of wireless and wired teach pendants.

As the table shows, wireless teach pendants have the following advantages in usability.

- God portability. Can be used anywhere without a concern of distortion/toppling over/stepping on the cable.
- No cable replacement.
- Good flexibility. Responds to layout change quickly.
- Hosts can be changed easily by re-login.
- Can be used with mobile hosts such as service robot by remote connection.

There are also challenges for achieving practical usage of wireless teach pendant as follows.

- Because safety signals from enabling switch and emergency stop switch are sent wirelessly, reliable communication and fast response speed are required for safety.
- Stable communication for preventing robots from stopping every time when a communicational error occurs.
- Small and energy-efficient design.
- Proper communication distance according to system size.

As the project entrusted by the Ministry of Economy, Trade and Industry, Japan, we have been engaged in the "Development Project of Next-generation Intelligent Robot Technology." The purpose of the project is to realize efficient teaching,

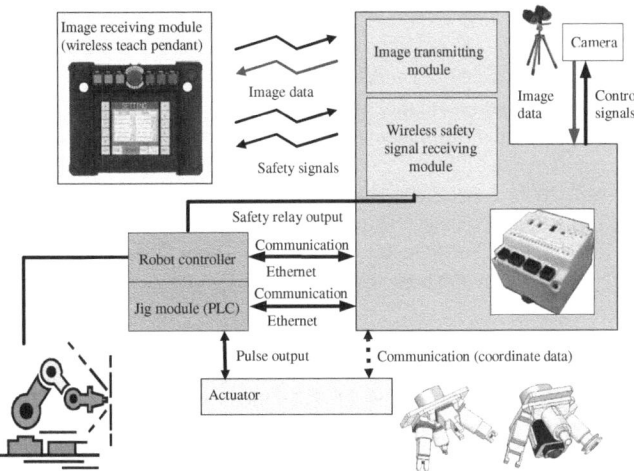

Fig. 9. Next-generation robot system using the wireless teach pendant under development

improved productivity, and good usability in workplaces using robot systems. The effort to realize efficient teaching includes the study of teach pendants that can handle a camera's image data, which requires wireless system as shown in figure 9. As explained, we have been making efforts to establish reliable and stable wireless communication for achieving the practical use of wireless teach pendants of excellent safety and usability.

5 Conclusion

For the purpose of standardizing teach pendants, we have developed one-hand small teach pendants for small robots and also two-hand small teach pendants with enabling switch of innovative structure. We have also studied the effectiveness of using wireless teach pendants used in large robot systems. We will continue working on wireless communication technology of both safety and good usability, in order to develop the standardized wireless teach pendant in applications not only of large robot systems but also small robot systems. We will also continue making efforts for the goal of establishing the optimum HMI environment that assures stress-free and comfortable working environment for operators.

Acknowledgement

The authors would like to thank the Ministry of Economy, Trade and Industry and the New Energy and Industrial Technology Development Organization (NEDO) for their invaluable support, advice, and trust in the Development Project of Next-generation Intelligent Robot Technology.

References

1. ISO12100-1, -2: 2003, Safety of machinery-Basic concepts, general principles for design-Part 1: Basic terminology, methodology-Part 2: Technical principles and specifications
2. IEC 60204-1: 2005, Safety of machinery-Electrical equipment of industrial machines, Part 1: General requirements (2005)
3. IEC 60947-5-8: 2006, Low-votage switchgear and controlgear – Part 5-8: Control circuit devices and switching elements – Three-position enabling switches (2006)
4. ANSI/RIA R15.06:1999, for Industrial Robots and Robot System-Safety Requirements
5. SEMI S2-0706–Environmental, Health, and Safety Guideline for Semiconductor Manufacturing Equipment
6. Fukui, T., Nobuhiro, M., Sekino, Y., Maeda, I., Matsumoto, A., Fujita, T.: Requirement of Three-position Enabling Switches for Installing in Enabling Devices to Achieve Operational Safety of Robotics and Automation Applications. In: Third Annual IEEE Conference on Automation Science and Engineering (IEEE CASE 2007), Scottsdale, Arizona, USA, pp. 111–116 (2007)
7. Sakai, T., Iwami, T., Fujimoto, M., Fujitani, S., Matsumoto, A., Fujita, T.: Development of New Emergency Stop Switch which Assures Operator's Safety at Its Foreseeable Failure. In: 4th International Conference Safety of Industrial Automated Systems (SIAS 2005), Chicago, IL, USA (2005)
8. Fukui, T., Nobuhiro, M., Matsumoto, A., Fujita, T.: Application of Three-position Grip Switch for Inherent Safety of Machinery. In: 3rd International Conference Safety of Industrial Automated Systems (SIAS 2003), pp. 3.121–3.126. Institut National de Recherche et de Securite, Nancy (2003)
9. Fukui, T., Nobuhiro, M., Sekino, Y., Fujita, T.: Development of Ergonomically Designed 3-position Enabling Switches for Operational Safety and Installation in Universal Industrial Application. In: ISA ETCON (Emerging Technologies Conference) 2002, Chicago, IL, USA ETC02-S003 (2002)
10. Fujita, T.: Importance of Ergonomically Designed 3-position Enabling Devices for Operational Safety of Machinery. In: 2002NRSC (National Robot Safety Conference), Ypsilanti, MI, USA (2002)
11. Sekino, Y., Fukui, T., Sugimoto, N., Fujita, T.: Development and Applications of 3-position Enabling Switches Embodying Operation Safety Based on Ergonomics. In: 2nd International Conference Safety of Industrial Automated Systems (SIAS 2001), Berufsgenossenschaftliches Institut für Arbeitssicherheit (BIA), Bonn, Germany, November 13-15, 2001, pp. 407–408 (2001)
12. Matsumoto, A., Nobuhiro, M., Fukui, T., Fujita, T.: Ergonomics and Usability of Pendant Terminals for Improved Safety. In: 3rd International Conference Safety of Industrial Automated Systems (SIAS 2003), Institut National de Recherche et de Securite, Nancy, France, pp. 3.81–3.86 (2003)
13. Mamiya, M., Nishiki, T., Sugimoto, N., Fujita, T.: Development and Application of Pendant Terminals for Improved Safety. In: 2nd International Conference Safety of Industrial Automated Systems (SIAS 2001), Berufsgenossenschaftliche Institut für Arbeitsschutz (BIA), Bonn, Germany, pp. 403–404 (2001)

Participatory Ergonomics as a Method of Quality Improvement in Maintenance

Małgorzata Jasiulewicz-Kaczmarek

Poznan University of Technology, Faculty of Management Engineering
11 Strzelecka Str., 60-965 Poznan, Poland
malgorzata.jasiulewicz-kaczmarek@put.poznan.pl

Abstract. Modern enterprises are forced to constantly improve ways of management and to introduce changes. One of the changes is a alteration of organizational culture and acceptance of participation of employees in designing and implementing new solutions. Striving for general improvement of system efficiency involves joint design of technical and social systems to achieve the best fitness to goals and requirements of system and its parts possible. Not only technical objects, but also workers and workplaces (work environment) require keeping in good condition. Such approach to maintenance stresses human importance and workers place in systems they work in. It also stresses necessity for not engineers, but also quality and ergonomics experts as well as technical objects users to involve into maintenance actions and processes. The paper presents potential of participatory ergonomics to maintenance quality improvement use.

Keywords: maintenance, participation, participatory ergonomics, stakeholders.

1 Introduction

Improvement is an undertaking striving for gaining extra benefits for both, organization and its customers. Usually in literature on the subject, the term is presented in pro-quality activities context – 'continuous improvement' and most authors associates the term with Japanese methods of effectiveness and efficiency of organization activities for the benefit of internal and external customers improvement. According to the definitions by S. Piersiala and S. Trzcielinski presented in [1], continuous improvement is planned, organized and systematic process of continuous change for the purpose of losses elimination/limitation, as well as productivity and competitiveness improvement, requiring commitment of employees on all the levels of organization structure.

Hence, improvement is solving problems, which are both, discrepancies (differences) between requirements and results (effects), and searching for opportunities/possibilities to improve effectiveness and efficiency of actions and processes [2]. Thus, to improve, the knowledge of processes (or objects analysed) and of methods and tools that can be applied, as well as skills in using them, is necessary.

In contemporary company the maintenance function has become an integral part of the overall profitability of an organization. It has been proven that with no doubt maintenance as support function in businesses is crucial for companies performance and new strategies i.e. lean manufacturing, just-in-time production, total quality control and

B.-T. Karsh (Ed.): Ergonomics and Health Aspects, HCII 2009, LNCS 5624, pp. 153–161, 2009.

six-sigma programs implementation (see: [3], [4], [5], [6], [7]). Thus, improving levels of utility and efficiency of actions and process performer in UR system [8] is necessary. Many organisations tend to adopt the proactive maintenance philosophies such as total productive maintenance (TPM) and reliability-centered maintenance (RCM), since these approaches are committed to long-term improvement of maintenance management. The basic rules of contemporary maintenance concepts/ approaches (TPM, RCM, etc.) include:

- Top managers commitment,
- Team work, active communication and cooperation between all the interested parties (participation),
- Pro-preventive orientation, based on searching for and eliminating potential threats and their causes,
- Trainings and qualifications and skills of employees improvement,
- Joining operators in maintenance actions, delegating responsibilities and powers,
- Methods of work, work environment and safety improvement.

The goal of the paper is to present opportunities and potential benefits from quality of maintenance improvement (from both internal and external perspective) that can be achieved with participatory ergonomics.

2 Participation Aspects

Improving quality and efficiency of actions and processes of maintenance system requires joint (combined) design of technical and social subsystems[1]. Not only technical objects (tools, machines etc.) should be kept 'in shape', condition of work environment and people performing processes – company's employees, is even more important. The approach to maintenance presented above is human-centric, focusing on people and their place in the system analysed. It also stresses the necessity to join experts on quality and ergonomics, and not only engineers, in maintenance improving actions. Safety, satisfaction of employees, quality of professional work and mood (disposition) of employees are positively synergetic in maintenance system, which means that total efficiency of a system is much bigger than a sum of its parts (components).

Contemporary concepts of maintenance management show necessity to join all the process parties and performers in improving actions, they stress importance of participation and team work.

Wenger [9] refers to participation as 'a process of taking part and also to the relations with others that reflect this process'. It is a complex process that includes, for example, doing, talking, thinking, feeling and belonging. Participation involves action, e.g., talking with someone, and connection, e.g., feeling that one takes part.

Participation method is more and more often used in companies to improve ergonomics of work and workplaces – participatory ergonomics. It is an important factor promoting initiatives of employees and high efficiency in implementing actions

---

[1] Maintenance system is socio-technical (social subsystem includes individuals (people) and social groups, organizational culture they create, as well as goals, tasks and organizational strategy, while technical subsystem includes machines, tools and Technologies, as well as actions taken to perform the tasks).

improving work methods, work conditions and risk management (see: [10], [11], [12]). The literature presents numerous definitions of participatory ergonomics (see [13], [14], [15], [16]). The common characteristic is that in a change process, attention is paid explicitly to the role of participants [17]. Participants of improving changes can be divided into two groups: internal stakeholders, including:

- top management, their commitment and role is usually strategy, goals and budget definition (when changes are local and not cost-generating, the top-management role is small),
- middle management, usually regarded as the head of the department where the changes really took place,
- employees, their commitment is crucial for success of the project/ undertaking, They know how the work is done normally and how the improvement works with respect to their typical work. They are necessary when it comes to taking decisions on changing work method or realisation or implementing new organisation because they usually know what is wrong and how to implement changes,
- experts, they are necessary at the stage of problem analysis, solution choice and solution testing,
  and external stakeholders, including:
- facility management, sector organizations, clients and suppliers, they define their requirements, show necessity to implement changes, provide knowledge and skills (f.ex. trainings).

Their role and commitment in particular stages of participatory improving changes design can be different. According to [17] in participatory ergonomic project, ergonomists and employees play an essentials role in the improvement process ('ergonomists (or other experts working on work improvement) are involved, because they add a new realistic vision and employees are involved because of changes in their work—and they may know best what and how to change').

Though the role of ergonomists and employees is indisputable, nowadays the role of facility management, sector organizations, clients and suppliers in initiating improving changes in organizations they cooperate with is more and more often appreciated and stressed in business practice.

3 Maintenance Stakeholders and Their Requirements

Maintenance system is a set of organizational units and relations between them defined by maintenance processes accordingly to technologies accepted and used. Combination of maintenance actions and repeated actions striving for processing inputs into outputs is a maintenance process (ISO/IEC 15288 (2002)). Applying process approach to organize maintenance system actions allows to meet the most important needs of contemporary organization: pro-customer orientation (in maintenance case it is direct orientation on internal client and indirect orientation on external client), changes implementation (improvement) and barriers between departments crossing (maintenance actions are performed not only by maintenance department employees, but also production, supplies an some other department employees) [18].

The ISO 9000:2005 standard defines clients as 'an organisation or a person receiving the product'. The definition by Juran and Blanton [19] is wider, as it defines client as 'anyone who is affected by the product or by the process used to produce the product'. Clients (both internal and external) are also stakeholders (stakeholders – person or group having an interest in the performance or success of an organization (example: customer, owners, people in an organization, suppliers, bankers, unions, partner or society) (ISO 9000:2005). In the following paper, when analyzing an organization as a system (a set of elements and relations between them) the term 'stakeholder' will be used instead of the term 'client' as to improve maintenance quality it is necessary to identify stakeholders interested in maintenance system, as well as relations between them since they are supposed to enable appointing a common, general goal and motivate to active cooperation – participation – striving for the goals appointed achievement.

Maintenance should be analysed in two perspectives:

- internal perspective, in which maintenance system is analysed in reference to meeting obligations towards employees (process performers) and other internal processes of the company (maintenance system in the aspect of processes performed by the company and relations between them – processes aspect)[2],
- external perspective, in which maintenance system is regarded as management system and analysed in reference to meeting obligations towards environment as well as values, methodologies and tools used to perform management functions.

Maintenance internal perspective is a perspective of internal stakeholders while external perspective is a direct perspective of external stakeholders and indirect perspective of internal stakeholders. Taking both perspectives into consideration allows to identify present and future (potential) problems and to choose proper tools supporting their solution, and thanks to stakeholders identification it allows to build responsible and competent teams.

Importance and positive influence of internal perspective of maintenance improving project is widely discussed in literature on the subject, external perspective is taken into consideration only in a small degree.

3.1 Internal Maintenance Perspective

Maintenance exists, because disregarding the branch of a company and products it provides, it has resources (technical objects) which need to be maintained. Maintaining means making the technical object perform tasks and actions defined by their user. Hence, the goal of maintenance is guaranteeing that technical objects fulfill their functions and their performance meets the requirements of their operators. Realization of the goal above mentioned depends mostly on active participation and commitment of the operators (employees) and managers.

As maintenance system works for internal clients, the goal of maintenance should be defined to meet general requirements of internal client and then decomposed to meet specific requirements of maintenance processes and workstations (as presented in Figure 1), where:

$P_1, ..., Pn$ – maintenance processes,
$S_1, ..., Sn$ – workstations.

---

[2] „Internal client's satisfaction provides perfect quality, because if an organisation meets the needs of its clients and enables its internal clients performing their tasks, then the organisation (the net of internal clients) cooperates for clients (internal and external) [20].

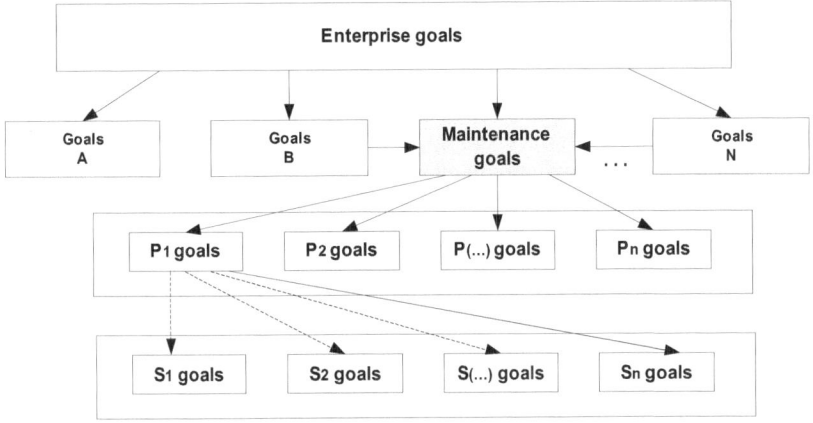

Fig. 1. Maintenance goals structure

Goals identified and presented to the employees, along with necessary resources provided and properly managed, are maintenance tools.

Continuous integration of enterprise management systems is the reason why maintenance systems lost organizational autonomy they had so far and became an element of internal chain of stakeholders: production – quality – maintenance [21] (relation presented in Figure 2).

As the requirements of the internal system's stakeholders are continuously changing, the goals are changing as well. The changes include time, processes realization and working conditions [22]. The concept of "working conditions" consists of two dimensions: "conditions of work," describing the practical conditions under which people work and cope with a specific technical and organizational environment, and "conditions of employment," describing the rules and status under which people are employed and trained.

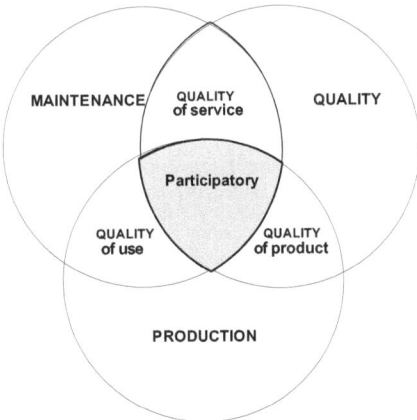

Fig. 2. Maintenance and internal stakeholders

The result of actions improving working conditions is employees' well-being, which includes job satisfaction, motivation, organizational commitment and job involvement. Each well organized, goal-oriented process in which people take part, should provide human well-being as one of its outputs, hence processes are performed by people and their improvement is mostly in exploiting people's capacity and turning from simple communication to interactive communication and commitment – participation (communication is critical to achieving genuine participation). Each of the stakeholders should be aware not only of realization of goals of processes take part in, but also of processes of suppliers and clients, as they are internal stakeholders. Internal quality of services is interpreted with people's attitude to each other and the way they help one another. It is one of the aspects of quality culture of organizations, culture inside organization influences how the services for its employees are performed.

By including internal perspective of maintenance, quality and ergonomics into improving actions better integration of human and systems is provided and the central role of the user in systems design is stressed. A key principle of participatory ergonomics is that workers are the experts in what they do. Therefore, maintenance workers should be involved in the identification and analysis of hazards in the workplace, and the development of solutions that could reduce these hazards.

Work environment plays the main role in preventing discordances and in provoking discordances in maintenance system. The factors provoking maintenance discordances are believed to be: procedures (f. ex. complex, unrealistic, out of date and out of range), equipment (f. ex. Lack of proper equipment, equipment that does not meet requirements), knowledge (f. ex. lack of knowledge, trainings, experience), work organization (f. ex. problems with communication between workers, lack of teamwork), time pressure (f. ex. rush, misdefined maintenance schedules), however designing and realizing trainings can limit the mistakes and failures above mentioned and their consequences as well. To achieve this, it is necessary to build teams and support their work with experts, both internal and external, advice.

An example:

A middle-sized company of mechanical branch employs 123 workers. In the company, two teams were appointed, both including production workers and maintenance workers. There was also safety and hygiene of work expert taking part in both teams' works. For both teams he organized and realized training on workplace hazards and risk connected with their previous routines. The task for the teams was to analyse actions (workplace preparation) as they were realized so far. There were two meetings every week in three months time. After each meeting a report including suggestions for changes and potential benefits was prepared. The outcome of teams work was following:

- Analysis of hazards and potential risks during operations, thanks to which unnecessary actions were identified, operations order was changed and necessary tools were identified, as well as supervision rules,
- Modification of old reports and the way they were filled in, rules of communication process in case of failure existing or potential (expected),
- Responsibilities ranges for operators were developed, as well as instructions for workplaces (for both, operators and maintenance workers).

Result of changes implemented were assessed on the meeting of both teams after six months. According to employees, they believed in possibility to implement changes themselves and they were ready to accept more responsibility. Employees have learned to evaluate the improvements and are able to choose and evaluate the consequence of changes in the workstation and organization. The work and environment limit some possibilities, but the employees have enough control to change the work. They tested various new ways of working and workstations, and could experience how it works. This positive experience could have played a role in the success.

3.2 External Maintenance Perspective

Improving quality of actions and processes in organizations should closely connected with needs and expectations of external stakeholders as the performance of an organization depends upon the interaction between business functions and stakeholders both within and outside of the company. External integration of processes performed by a company becomes the more important, the more important supply chain in which the company takes part in is. Organization's ability to provide clients with products meeting their requirements is as important as product's technical features, and the ability seems to accurate infrastructure and competent, satisfied workers. Organization's stakeholders are, in many cases, integrators of engineering best practices, and they believe sharing knowledge and improving supply chain processes are their duties.

In food branch companies, pharmaceutical companies and automotive industry stakeholders participation is a common standard, and training programmes are oriented, besides from technical issues, also on building proper relations between stakeholders, care for work environment and quality of life at work. Participation of ergonomics and quality are believed to be the basic element of delegating and receiving responsibilities and rights of workers. Consequence in 'managed development' realization is reflected in the following sentence 'my benefit is your benefit' and in the following question 'what can be done to make me happy thanks to your satisfaction?'.

4 Summary

The paper presents two aspects of including participatory ergonomics to maintenance quality improving set of methods. The first aspect is internal perspective of maintenance and its place in he structure of processes performed by a company. The second is the external perspective, in which maintenance system and its improvement is strictly connected to needs and expectations of external stakeholders. Because of growing importance of relations between an organization and its stakeholders (f. ex. in food and pharmaceutical industry), the second perspective seems to be very important. Though initially maintenance seems to be important for stakeholders only indirectly, author's work as an expert in design, implantation and exploitation of pro-quality systems and as an auditors in stakeholders audits has proven that most of discordances and notices is on infrastructure supervision not only in technical, but usually in social aspects. The consequence is increasing commitment of stakeholders in internal processes improvement. Teams of workers, initiated by organization partners, in which experts appointed by organization partners participate in changes implementation, are more and more common. Managers usually do not speak on participatory ergonomics, but they use it. The most important is that thanks to changes implemented in participative way companies build new organizational culture based on awareness of common goals, responsibilities and competences, in which workers feel safe (both physically and psychically) and are appreciated.

References

1. Piersiala, S., Trzcieliński, S.: Maintenance Systems. In: Fertsch, M., Trzcieliński, S. (eds.) Koncepcje zarządzania systemami wytwórczymi, pp. 114–126. Publishing House of Poznan University of Technology (2005)
2. Brilman, J.: Nowoczesne koncepcje zarządzania. PWE, Warszawa (2002)
3. Pun, K.F., Chin, K.S., Chow, M.F., Lau, H.C.W.: An effectiveness-centred approach to maintenance management. Journal of Quality in Maintenance Engineering 8(4), 346–368 (2002)
4. Cua, K.O., McKone, K.E., Schroeder, R.G.: Relationships between implementation of TQM, JIT, and TPM and manufacturing performance. Journal of Operations Management 19(6), 675–694 (2001)
5. Hansson, J., Backlund, F., Lycke, L.: Managing commitment: increasing the odds for successful implemention of TQM, TPM or RCM. International Journal of Quality & Reliability Management 20(9), 993–1008 (2003)
6. McKone, K.E., Schroeder, R.G., Cua, K.O.: Total productive maintenance: a contextual view. Journal of Operations Management 17(2), 123–144 (1999)
7. All-Najar, B.: Cost –Efective & Continous Improvement of Production Process and Company's Business when using Total Quality Maintenace (TQMain). In: International Conference on Maintenance Engineering, ChengDu, China (2006)
8. Murthy, D.N.P.: Strategic maintenance management. Journal of Quality in Maintenance Engineering 8(4), 287–305 (2002)
9. Wenger, E.: Communities of practice: Learning, meaning, and identity. Cambridge University Press, Cambridge (1998)
10. Zalk, D.M.: Grassroots ergonomics: initiating an ergonomics program utilizing participatory techniques. The Annals of Occupational Hygiene 45, 283–289 (2001)
11. Kawakami, T., Kogi, K.: Action-oriented support for occupational safety and health programs in some developing countries in Asia. Int. J. Occup. Safety Ergon. 7, 421–434 (2001)
12. Hignett, S., Wilson, J.R., Morris, W.: Finding ergonomic solutions—participatory approaches. Occup. Med. 55, 200–207 (2005)
13. Wilson, J.R.: Solution ownership in participative work redesign: the case of a crane control room. Int. J. Ind. Ergon. 15, 329–344 (1995)
14. Wilson, J.R., Haines, H.: Participatory ergonomics. In: Salvendy, G. (ed.) Handbook of human factors and ergonomics, 2nd edn., pp. 490–513. Wiley, Chichester (1997)
15. Kuorinka, I.: Tools and means of implementing participatory ergonomics. Int. J. Ind. Ergon. 15, 365–370 (1997)
16. Haines, H., Wilson, J.R., Vink, P., Koningsveld, E.A.P.: Validating a framework for participatory ergonomics. Ergonomics 45, 309–327 (2002)
17. Vink, P., Imada, A.S., Zink, K.J.: Defining stakeholder involvement in participatory design processes. Applied Ergonomics 39, 519–526 (2008)

18. Jasiulewicz-Kaczmarek, M.: "Process approach" in maintenance. In: Fertsch, M., Grzybowska, K., Stachowiak, A. (eds.) Logistyka i zarządzanie produkcją – nowe wyzwania, odlegle granice, pp. 260–270. Publishing House of Poznan University of Technology (2007)
19. Juran, J.M., Blanton, G.A.: Juran's Quality Handbook. McGraw-Hill, New York (1999)
20. Zairi, M.: Managing customer satisfaction: a best practice perspective. The TQM Magazine 12(6), 389–394 (2000)
21. Pawłowski, E., Pawłowski, K., Wachowski, M.: Komputer Aide Maintenance Systems. In: Fertsch, M., Trzcieliński, S. (eds.) Koncepcje zarządzania systemami wytwórczymi, pp. 104–113. Publishing House of Poznan University of Technology (2005)
22. Jasiulewicz-Kaczmarek, M.: Macroergonomic design for improved quality performance in maintenence, Foundations of Control and Management Sciences, vol. 11, pp. 171–183. Publishing House of Poznan University of Technology (2008)

What Is Prospective Ergonomics? A Reflection and a Position on the Future of Ergonomics

Jean-Marc Robert[1] and Eric Brangier[2]

[1] Ecole Polytechnique de Montréal, Dept. of Math & Industrial Engineering – P.O. Box 6079, Station Centre-ville, Montréal, Québec H3C 3A7 Canada
[2] Université Paul Verlaine – Metz. 2LP, Laboratoire Lorrain de Psychologie. Faculté des Sciences Humaines et Arts. BP 30309. Île du Saulcy – 57006 Metz (France).
jean-marc.robert@polymtl.ca, brangier@univ-metz.fr

Abstract. This paper presents a reflection on the future of ergonomics and a clear position for the use of prospective in this discipline. We propose to structure ergonomic activities around corrective, preventive (design) and prospective ergonomics, where the latter looks forward in time to defining human needs and activities so as to create human-centered artifacts that are useful and provide a positive user experience. The place of prospective ergonomics is upstream of projects, before a problem or request is raised by a client, and before projects exist. We describe several characteristics of prospective ergonomics and compare them with those of corrective and preventive ergonomics. We show that prospective ergonomics has major impacts on education and practice, since ergonomists should not only be trained as human factor experts but also as strategists to reflect on the future and as project managers. Prospective ergonomics requires the "intelligence analysis" of a lot of data and experts' opinions, as well as perspicacity, intuition, creativity, motivation and initiative. It represents a huge potential for the advancement and evolution of ergonomics and for the achievement of its full maturity.

Keywords: Corrective ergonomics; Preventive ergonomics; Prospective ergonomics; Design; Human-centered projects.

1 Introduction

In this article we present a reflection on the future of ergonomics and we take a clear position for the use of prospective in this discipline. We reconsider the classification of ergonomic activities in two large categories that are commonly mentioned by authors and that correspond to corrective and preventive ergonomics. We propose to define three categories of activities around corrective, preventive, and prospective. This exercise is not only academic since we believe it may have a major impact on our discipline. Above all, it allows us to emphasize a new type of activity that should be promoted in our field: the prospective. In the new classification, we continue to use corrective ergonomics whose role is clear and consistent among authors. We use preventive ergonomics to cover all design activities that were included so far in what authors called prospective ergonomics, and we add prospective ergonomics with a new content entirely related to prospective.

B.-T. Karsh (Ed.): Ergonomics and Health Aspects, HCII 2009, LNCS 5624, pp. 162–169, 2009.
© Springer-Verlag Berlin Heidelberg 2009

In the earlier classification, there was almost complete overlap between design and prospective. Authors considered that design *is* prospective since one is searching for new ideas, concepts, and solutions that will hopefully lead to the creation of artifacts. We have reservations regarding this position because we consider that such overlap limits the scope of prospective ergonomics by leaving the prospective completely in the shadow. Prospective ergonomics should not be limited to the mining of ideas for projects that have already been decided and that exist somehow, almost always due to others' initiative. This corresponds to what we call the *defined future*. In fact, its scope is much larger than that. It should include the search for projects that have yet not been decided and that do not even exist, and that might come true due to ergonomists' initiative. This corresponds to what we call the *undefined future*. The goal of the restructuring with the addition of prospective ergonomics is to shed light on the challenge of dealing with the future and innovation.

By so doing, while preserving the current assets of ergonomics for correction and prevention (or design), we expand the field of the discipline by pushing the boundaries and discovering a new territory: the prospective. We also enlarge the roles and enrich the tasks of ergonomists by giving them new responsibilities and challenges as strategists and managers. This major change calls for a debate on the validity of doing prospective in ergonomics, and for an analysis of the impacts of this new kind of activity on education and practice. Our hope is that our reflection and position in favour of the prospective will contribute to the advancement and evolution of ergonomics, and to the achievement of its full maturity.

The article is structured as follows: we introduce and define prospective ergonomics, we describe its characteristics and compare them with those of corrective and preventive ergonomics, and we examine its impacts on education and practice.

2 Definition

Prospective is concerned with or related to the future. More precisely, it consists in looking forward in time (as opposed to retrospection) through the "intelligence analysis" of several factors (individual, social, cultural, political, economic, scientific, technological, environmental) whose relative importance depends on each line of business, and of multiple data, experts' opinions, and scenarios of the future ([3,10]). It yields uncertain results because of the difficulty to predict the future. It is used in a variety of areas such as consumption, jobs, technology, energy, financial markets, movement of people, etc. One can adopt four different attitudes and behaviours when facing the evolving future:

- Reactive: opposing the changes to come and trying to slow, stop, or even reverse it;
- Passive: taking no positive or negative actions, yielding to or accepting it;
- Active or proactive: taking positive actions to rapidly adjust and even taking advantage of the change;
- Leading: taking positive actions to initiate, orient, drive and even accelerate the change to come.

Prospective ergonomics is obviously related to the future. The scope it was given by different authors actually corresponds to that of preventive ergonomics, and it is this restricted prospective ergonomics that they compared to corrective ergonomics. M. de Montmollin [6] talks of corrective ergonomics and preventive ergonomics, the former for correcting existing artifacts, and the latter "for systems that do not exist yet in reality; it is ergonomics at the stage of project". He is the only author who uses the term preventive (préventif in French) to designate what others call prospective ergonomics. Laurig [5] associates "corrective ergonomics" with traditional ergonomics and describes it as developing "corrections through scientific studies", whereas "prospective ergonomics" corresponds to a more modern approach that brings a more-forward looking concept of design. Later, Laurig & Vedder [7] asserted that "prospective ergonomics means searching for alternatives in work design which prevent fatigue and exhaustion on the part of the working subject in order to promote human productivity ("… for the benefit of ourselves and others"). Bubb [2] examines the difference in ergonomics between the traditional "a posteriori" design and the modern "a priori" design which uses computer-based human models. This observation leads from an earlier "corrective ergonomics" to a new "prospective ergonomics". Finally, Karwowski [4] compares "retrospective analysis" to "prospective analysis", where the former corresponds to past-oriented activities (e.g., root cause analysis, cognitive task analysis, ethnographic studies) and the latter corresponds to future-oriented activities (e.g., creative thinking, evaluation of consequences). The difference between them is consistent with that made by previous authors between corrective and prospective ergonomics.

On one hand, we agree with the common position of these authors concerning a broad distinction between a past-oriented corrective ergonomics and a future-oriented prospective ergonomics since it is clear enough, it has a high face validity, and it can be useful for identifying these two categories of activities. On the other hand, we are critical, but also constructive, about the position of these authors concerning the content and scope of prospective ergonomics. First, there is an overlap between design and prospective in their definitions of prospective ergonomics since both are basically perceived as looking forward for ideas and concepts. Even though design is future-oriented, it does not have the same scope and it is not concerned with the same activity as prospective. Second, the future is too short-term and the actions are too low level in their definitions of prospective ergonomics. They simply correspond to the use of modern future-oriented design methods that help designers to do their work. A good example of this is the common use of scenarios in human-computer interface design [9]. Third, there is no distinction between existing projects initiated by others where the ergonomist plays the role of a human factor expert, and non-existing projects that will be initiated by the ergonomist and where he/she will play the roles of strategist, manager, and human factor expert. Our critiques are about positions that limit too much the scope of prospective ergonomics. Our standpoint is that it is different from the design activity, it should not be too short-term nor too low level, and it should not be limited to already existing projects and to projects initiated by others. Prospective ergonomics goes far beyond that.

Thus, we propose to have a new classification of activities around corrective, preventive, and prospective ergonomics. In this classification, the content of corrective ergonomics is the same as it was in the definitions and explanations given by the above mentioned authors. The content of preventive ergonomics focuses on design and corresponds to nearly all of what the authors included in prospective ergonomics.

The content of prospective ergonomics is redefined since most design activities were transferred to preventive ergonomics and since the focus is now on prospective. This will be the scope and the niche of prospective ergonomics for the rest of the paper.

3 Prospective Ergonomics

Prospective ergonomics can be defined as the part of ergonomics that attempts to anticipate human needs and activities so as to create new artifacts that will be useful and provide positive user experience. Different criteria can be used to evaluate the user experience, namely well-being, human development, learning, entertainment, pleasure, networking, sense making, performance, satisfaction [8]. Its place is upstream of projects when there is no request or problem brought by a client, and no existing project; it corresponds to the very first step of projects such as can be found in various design disciplines (e.g., industrial design, engineering, computer science, film making).

The anticipation of human needs and activities is based on the analysis of numerous factors and data, and on scenario planning as it is done in prospective. It requires having close contacts with people in their environment in order to be able to observe and interview them and collect data on different aspects of their life.

Prospective ergonomics emphasizes the investigation of the use of artifacts to discover their strengths and flaws, and sources of satisfaction and dissatisfaction that could lead to the improvement of current artifacts or the design of new ones [1]. Furthermore it is human-centered since users should be involved in the anticipation exercise through interviews, observations, surveys, complaints analysis, usability tests, emotions evaluations, satisfaction and performance measurements, etc. Finally, prospective ergonomics requires a sharp sense of observation for ergonomists and a great deal of perspicacity, intuition, creativity, motivation (with an entrepreneurial mindset), and initiative to innovate.

Prospective ergonomic is multidisciplinary since it relies on the theories, models, methods, and tools of human and social sciences (e.g., anthropology, sociology, ethnography, demography, psychology, marketing, epidemiology) to define future human needs and activities, and on those of computer science and engineering to anticipate the evolution and cost of technology that will support future interactive artefacts.

Prospective ergonomics partially overlaps corrective ergonomics and preventive ergonomics, and these two partially overlap, as shown in Figure 1. Design is often required in corrective ergonomics to conceive and develop solutions. Correction is inevitable in preventive ergonomics to change and improve different versions of a design, and prospective may apply to both correction and design. For instance, in a specific project, one looks forward in time to finding other applications of the solution or the design, or other groups of users that could benefit from it. For instance, in a bottom-up process, a problem addressed in corrective ergonomics (e.g., sleepiness of truck drivers that causes accidents) may generate the development of an innovative solution (e.g., head movement recognition system connected to a warning system) that could apply to other groups of people with the same problem (e.g., system controllers).

Prospective ergonomics can operate both in a technology-pull mode and a technology-push mode. The former means that human needs precede, stimulate, and orient

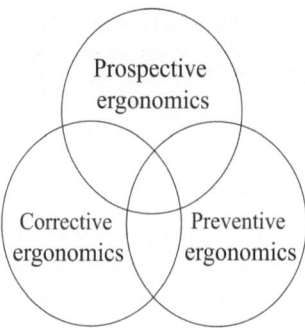

Fig. 1. Interaction between corrective, preventive, and prospective ergonomics

the development of technology, whereas the latter means that technology is available but has not found applications thus far. Considering the increasing number of computer-based interactive artifacts that people will be using in the future, and the importance of technology in innovation, it can be predicted that most projects that will emerge from prospective ergonomics will be strongly influenced by computer technology.

For obvious reasons, projects that will come out of prospective ergonomics will have to go through feasibility tests, cost/benefit analyses, and comparative studies. The projects that will be retained after selection will require financial set-up. The commercial dimension is explicit and brings to the fore the need for ergonomists to have management skills. Despite the unavoidable technical and financial evaluation criteria, since these projects are all concerned with future human activities, they should be guided by positive values that improve the quality of life.

Prospective ergonomics is explicitly associated with innovation. Its middle-term and long-term temporal coverage, high-level actions, as well as the inevitable role of technology may create favorable conditions. Even though corrective and preventive ergonomics can also lead to innovation, they are different on this point because innovation is not their primary goal, and the solution or design they propose is limited to specific projects.

Prospective ergonomics seems ready to be adopted judging from young ergonomists' reactions. In our teaching, we encounter numerous graduate students coming to human factors from different design-oriented disciplines (e.g., industrial design, graphic design, engineering, computer science, architecture, information systems). They end up with multiple competencies in human factors and in design, engineering, computer science, management, and sociology. Some of them, who are both innovative and endowed with an entrepreneurial mindset, want to pursue their design activity in human factors projects. Prospective ergonomics seems natural to them because it offers an opportunity both to innovate and have an impact on others' lifes.

We end this section with Table 1, which presents a comparison of the main characteristics of corrective, preventive and prospective ergonomics. This will help to have an overview of the specificities of each branch of ergonomics.

Table 1. A comparison between Corrective, Preventive, and Prospective Ergonomics

	Corrective Ergonomics	Preventive Ergonomics	Prospective Ergonomics
Temporality:	Past	Present	Future
Nature of work:	Correction	Design	Anticipation
Starting point:	The request of a client (problem to correct)	The request of a client (object to design)	The initiative of the ergonomist (object to create)
Main focus:	The problem to correct	The artifact to design	The needs and activities to define
User sample:	Small	Variable (depending on the project)	Variable (usually large)
Associated disciplines:	Anthropometry Biomechanics Physiology Psychology Engineering Computer science Design	The same + Anthropology Ethnography Sociology Arts	The same as the two previous ones + Management Marketing
Focus of data collection:	Causes of losses such as accidents, incidents, errors, overload, etc.	Users' responses to prototypes and simulations	People's complaints, needs, expectations, and responses to simulations
Status of the human factors:	Recovering factor	Integrating factor	Innovating factor
Nature of the intervention:	Reactive	Active	Anticipatory
Production of wealth:	By reducing or eliminating losses	By optimizing performance and user experience	By creating new products or services
Possibility of revenues:	Low	Medium	High

4   Impacts on Education and Practice

The new scope we give to prospective ergonomics in this paper calls for a revision of current educational programs. It is no longer sufficient to train human factor experts to correct problems and design artifacts. Even though ergonomics remains their main strength, they must also be trained as strategists to look forward in time and be able to initiate projects on their own, and as managers to plan, finance, and make these projects come true. In our opinion, this requires the acquisition of new knowledge in at least five areas: prospective (e.g., strategic planning), innovation, product development, marketing (e.g., of new technology), and management (e.g., financial set-up, project management). The detailed analysis of an enriched educational program in ergonomics requires a broad discussion in the human factor community; however this falls outside the scope of this paper.

The new scope of prospective ergonomics is also expected to have a major impact on ergonomists' tasks since they may choose to become strategists and managers. With prospective ergonomics, ergonomists not only do correction and design for specific projects, but also search for new ones. They not only work on others' projects, but also on their own. They not only react to requests, but are also proactive with their own projects. They not only join design teams and provide human factor expertise, but also solicit expertise. They are not only managed by others, but also manage their own projects. With these new responsibilities, ergonomists will become more versatile and autonomous. These changes in the profession are expected to improve the status and recognition of the profession.

5 Conclusion

Prospective ergonomics provides ergonomists with the opportunity to play a constructive and active role in the definition of the future. It encourages them to be creative, innovative, and inventive, and to initiate and pilot their own human factor projects. It represents a great opportunity to expand the field, acquire new skills in prospective, innovation and management, enlarge their roles and tasks, and improve the status and recognition of the profession. Above all, it allows the discipline to make a giant step in its development and evolution and acquire its full maturity.

Acknowledgment

The authors wish to thank Gracia Gingras for her numerous insightful comments on previous versions of the paper.

References

1. Brangier, E., Bastien, J.-M.-C.: L'analyse de l'activité est elle suffisante et/ou pertinente pour innover dans le domaine des nouvelles technologies? In: Vallery, G., Amalberti, R. (eds.) L'analyse du travail en perspectives: influences et évolutions, pp. 143–156. Octarès, Collection "Entreprise", Travail, Emploi, Toulouse (2006)
2. Bubb, H.: Ergonomic design by means of human models. In: Human Factors and Ergonomic Society Annual meeting Proceedings, Proceedings 6 - Multiple Session Symposia, vol. 51, p. 814. Human Factors and Ergonomic Society (2000)
3. Godet, M., Roubelat, F.: Creating the future: The use and misuse of scenarios. Long Range Planning 29(2), 164–171 (1996)
4. Karwowski, W. (ed.): International Encyclopedia of Ergonomics and Human Factors, 3278 p. CRC Press Inc./ Taylor & Francis (2006)
5. Laurig, W.: Prospective Ergonomics: New Approach to Industrial Ergonomics. In: Karwowski, W. (ed.) Trends in Ergonomics/human Factors III. Elsevier Science Publisher B.V, North-Holland (1986)
6. Montmollin, M.(de): Les systèmes Homme-Machine. PUF, Paris (1967)

7. Laurig, W., Vedder, J.: Overview (section 29.2 on Ergonomics). In: Mager Stellman, J. (ed.) Encyclopaedia of Occupational Health and Safety, 4th edn., vol. 1, p. 29.2. International Labour Office, Geneva (1992)
8. Robert, J.-M.: Vers la plénitude de l'expérience utilisateur. In: Proceedings of IHM 2008. ACM International Conference Proceedings Series, Metz, September 3-5, 2008, pp. 3–10 (2008)
9. Rosson, M.B., Carroll, J.M.: Scenario-based design. In: Jacko, J., Sears, A. (eds.) The human-computer interaction handbook: Fundamentals, Evolving technologies and Emerging applications, LEA, pp. 1–35 (2002)
10. Roubelat, F.: Scenarios to challenge strategic paradigms: Lessons from 2025. Futures 38, 519–527 (2006)

Improving in-Vehicle Display and Control Design for Older Drivers

Jaeheok Ryu[1], Gyohyeon Song[2], Seongil Lee[2], Yoonhyung Cho[1],
Gyouhyung Kyung[1], Hyungkee Kim[1], and Kyungkuk Baek[2]

[1] Package Engineering Team 2, Hyundai-Kia Motors, Korea
[2] System Management Engineering Department, SungKyunKwan University, Korea

Abstract. Guidelines for older driver-friendly automobile interior design have been determined by taking into account older people's physical and cognitive characteristics. Twenty three older people (aged from 54 to 78) and five younger people (from 20 to 29) performed several tasks in actual driving conditions, in which their reaction times and performance errors were recorded. Some design factors were found to be related to older drivers' visibility and controllability. Several design guidelines were proposed in terms of cluster color and font, display location, and HVAC control type. Proposed guidelines are expected to satisfy a wider range of older drivers as these will facilitate automobile interior designs which are fitter to older drivers' visual, cognitive, and manual capabilities.

Keywords: older driver, automobile interior, automotive ergonomics, visibility, controllability.

1 Introduction

With the increase in the average length of life, Korea is expected to enter an advanced age society in a short time. Generally, older people are those who are aged 65 or older according to WTO (World Trade Organization) and UN (United Nations). The aging society is where the proportion of older people among its total population is more than 7%, whereas the advanced age society is where the proportion is more than 14%, and the post-advanced aged society with more than 20% of older people in its population. Korea has already entered the aging society as of the year 2000 when 7.2% of its population aged 65 or older, and recently it has been approaching to an advanced aged society very rapidly. Driving tasks are usually harder for older people due to their decreased physical and cognitive abilities. Hence, the needs and abilities of older drivers should be carefully taken into account when designing automobiles. Studies on older drivers' abilities have been increasing and become vital with the rising number of older drivers involved in car accidents in Europe and North America. Relevant studies led by Toyota, Honda, and Nissan in Japan are more focused on developing welfare vehicles for physically challenged people. Comparatively, studies on older driver-friendly vehicle design in Korea are scarce.

This study attempted to propose automobile interior design guidelines for older drivers in terms of visibility and controllability when interacting with LCD display, cluster gauge, and HVAC (Heating Ventilating, and Air Conditioning) controls.

B.-T. Karsh (Ed.): Ergonomics and Health Aspects, HCII 2009, LNCS 5624, pp. 170–176, 2009.

2 Experiment

2.1 Process

First, this study attempted to find older drivers' characteristics and interior design factors through actual driving tests. Second, simulation tests were performed under various design conditions of LCD display, cluster gauge, HVAC and center fascia controls. Lastly, older driver-friendly automobile interior design guidelines were determined. Experiments involved older drivers and large-size sedans.

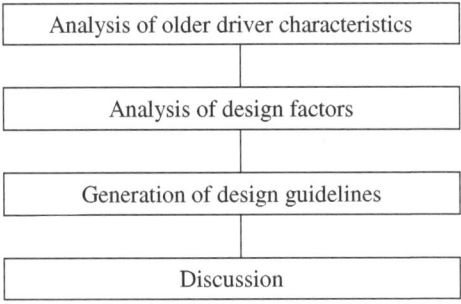

Fig. 1. Research process

2.2 Methods

Analysis of Older Driver Characteristics
Twenty three older drivers (aged from 54 to 78) and five younger drivers (from 20 to 29) performed several tasks and their characteristics and performance data were analyzed. Twenty three older drivers were further classified into two groups, one aged from 54 to 64 and the other aged 65 or older (the latter was referred to as 'the older driver group' in this paper). Experiments consisted of actual driving conditions. Participants performed tasks according to prescribed task scenarios, while driving an experimental vehicle and verbalized their thought using the think aloud method. Their task performance was recorded by 4 pin-hole cameras. Three cameras were mounted

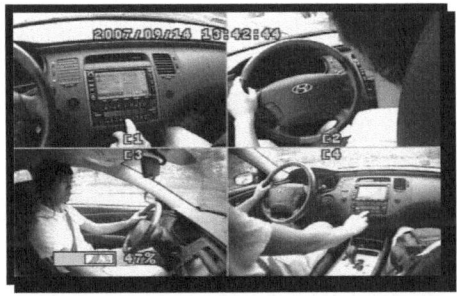

Fig. 2. Recorded actual driving test

at the driver-side center pillar ('B' pillar) for videotaping the cluster gauge area, the passenger-side front pillar ('A' pillar) for recording driver's reaction, and the left side of the passenger headrest for videotaping the center fascia area. The last one was a headset type for driver's visibility. Fourteen specific task scenarios involve interactions with four interior parts (i.e., LCD display, cluster gauge, and HVAC and center fascia controls) to analyze the older drivers' visibility and controllability. Tasks were performed during day and at night, and reaction times and errors of subjects were also recorded.

3 Results

3.1 Performance in Actual Driving

First of all, a task was performed to find interior parts that were strongly related to older drivers' visibility and controllability. With drivers' age advanced, longer reaction times and higher error rates were observed when performing tasks in general. In terms of reaction time, old driver group took longer time than those aged from 54 to 64 (7.65s vs. 4.46s). Older people took 3 times longer than younger people. The older driver group showed a higher error rate than the other two groups. In other words, increased reaction time and error rate were observed with age increasing.

The older driver group also showed the longest reaction time and the highest error rate for functional tasks among three age groups. The results were especially influenced by LCD display, cluster gauge, and HVAC controls.

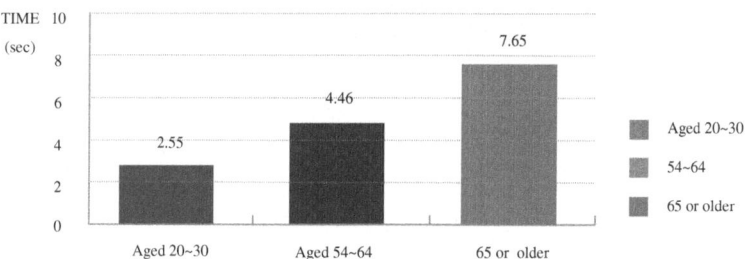

Fig. 3. Task reaction time of three age groups

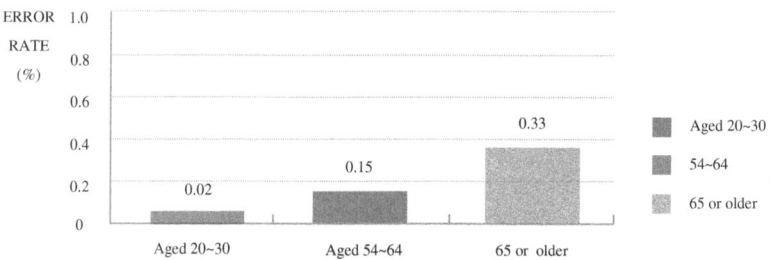

Fig. 4. Task error rate of three age groups

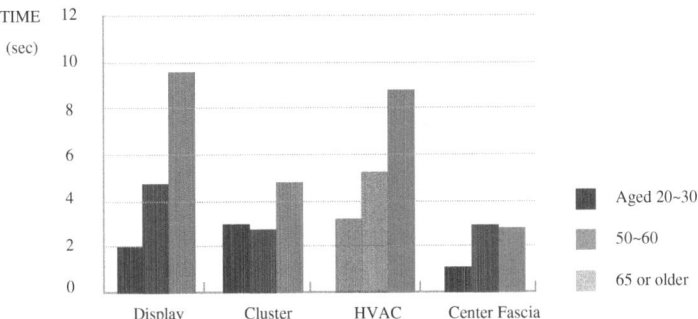

Fig. 5. Task reaction time for function of interior

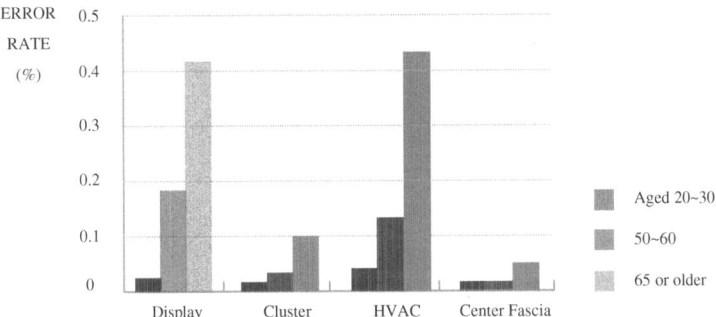

Fig. 6. Task error rate for function of interior

From actual driving tests, differences in driving performance were found according to age and function of automobile interior. Somewhat lower driving performance was observed at night than in daytime.

3.2 Analysis of Relevant Design Factors

From actual driving tests, it was found that LCD display, cluster gauge, and HVAC controls influenced older drivers' visibility and controllability. A further experiment was done in the lab environment to determine appropriate levels of design factor of LCD display, cluster gauge, and HVAC controls. To find levels of design factors, the task performance was measured using actual driving task video in the lab setting. It was made up of twelve task scenarios. Task performance was measured in terms of reaction time, error rate, and additionally subjects' satisfaction index was used.

First, a task involving interactions with an LCD display was performed. Four design factors (the display's lateral angle, vertical slope, height, and degree of protrusion) were manipulated. By changing levels of four factors and attaching touch sensors on the display, reaction time and error rate for each task were measured. Satisfaction level was reported verbally as well as recorded on the questionnaire.

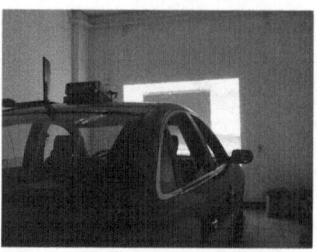

Fig. 7. Simulation test setting

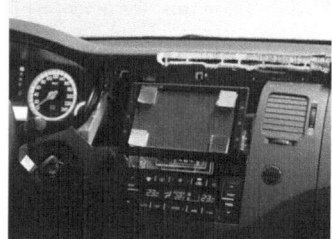

Fig. 8. LCD display test setting

Different task performances were observed between the older driver group and the other two groups when the display's lateral angle was changed. The fastest reaction time and the lowest error rate for the older driver group was when the display was laterally tilted 15 degrees toward the driver, whereas this factor showed little influence on the performance of the remaining groups.

Display slope also led to different task performance between the older driver group and the other groups. The lowest error rate was observed when display slope was set twenty five degrees. When display slope was set fifteen degrees, there was no significant different task performance observed between the older driver group and the other groups, compared to when twenty five degrees were used. However, satisfaction index was a little higher for the older driver group with the display slope of fifteen degrees. Though higher display location was associated with higher satisfaction level, there was little task performance difference between groups. Desirable display height was found to be about 50mm higher than the initial location. There was little significant performance difference in terms of display protrusion level. Only for the older driver group, increased protrusion level led to decreased error rate and increased reaction time.

A second simulation test was performed with HVAC controls. HVAC controls were classified into three types (i.e., mode, dial, and switch types). The mode type had different ventilation direction controls than the switch type; The latter comes with one-switch, one-direction controls, while the former had one-switch, multi-direction controls. LED was added to the mode type HVAC control and traditional color-coding was used for temperature (i.e., Red for increasing temperature, and blue for decreasing temperature). HVAC control type was associated with different performance. A faster reaction time and the lowest error rate were found when using the switch type HVAC control, which was rated most intuitive by the participants.

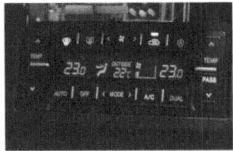 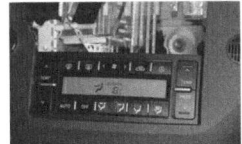 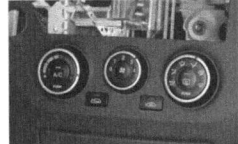

Fig. 9. Three HVAC control types (mode, switch, and dial types)

Lastly, cluster gauge visibility was tested using a total of eight different cluster films that varies by color (4 levels: white, blue, red and orange) and font (2 levels: type A and B). Type B font came from a bestselling large sedan in the USA.

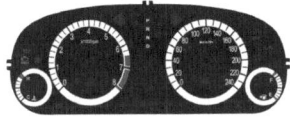 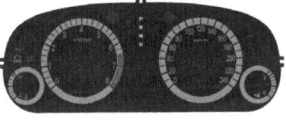

Fig. 10. Examples of cluster prototypes used (white and orange background colors)

Generally, a letter can be designed with a different width, space between letters, thickness, and font type and so on. The letter width and space between letters used for the car B were 3mm and from 0.5 to 1mm, respectively, while those of the car A were 4mm and 0.5mm. Letters of the car A cluster were hence thicker and wider than those of the car B.

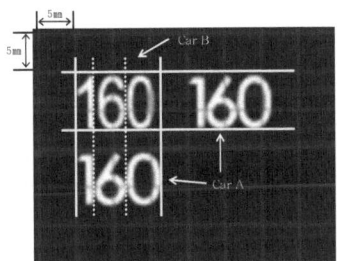

Fig. 11. Comparison of cluster gauge letters

In conclusion, increased reaction time and error rate and decreased satisfaction were observed when the red-colored cluster was used for the older driver group. Increased satisfaction was associated with the white-colored cluster for the older driver group, and with the white-colored and the blue-colored cluster for the other two groups. And in the case of the older driver group, faster reaction time was observed with the car A cluster. Letter thickness and wide space between letters used in the car A cluster seems to be associated with this result. Additionally, some subjects misperceived '6' used in the car B cluster as '8'.

3.3 Design Guidelines

1. LCD display height is recommended to be placed about 50mm higher than considered for the car B, and the display should be slanted in fifteen to twenty five degrees. Visibility and controllability can be further improved when the display could be tilted 15 degrees toward the driver.
2. HVAC controls should be designed using proper switch types which are intuitive the older drivers. Additionally, adding the red and blue color on the switch improves visibility and controllability.
3. In the case of the cluster gauge, white and/or blue color, and letter thickness of 1mm are recommended. Also, the length and width ratio of a letter should be set to 5:7 to improve readability.

4   Conclusion

Several guidelines for older driver-friendly automobile interior design have been determined by taking into account older people's physical and cognitive characteristics. Some design factors related to older drivers were determined through the actual driving test. Design guidelines for LCD display, cluster gauge, and HVAC controls could be proposed through the simulation test. Further study will be needed with more participants. The results from the current study will contribute to increasing the older drivers' safety and convenience, and will help to meet their needs.

References

1. Wickens, C.D., Hollands, J.G.: Engineering Psychology and Human Performance, 3rd edn., p. 573. Prentice Hall, Englewood Cliffs (1999)
2. Wickens, C.D., Gordon, S.E., Yili, L.: An Introduction to Human Factors Engineering, 750 p. Prentice Hall, Englewood Cliffs (1997)
3. Herriotts, P.: Applied Ergonomics 36, 255–262 (2005)
4. Smith, D.: Human factors and aging; an overview of research needs and application opportunities. Human Factors 32(5), 509–526 (1990)
5. Misugi, K., Kanamori, H., Koyama, N., Atsumi, B.: Toyota's Program for Universal Design in Vehicle Development. In: Designing For The 21st Century III, Brazil (December 2004)

Relationship between Emotional State and Pupil Diameter Variability under Various Types of Workload Stress

Kiyomi Sakamoto[1], Shoichi Aoyama[1], Shigeo Asahara[1],
Haruki Mizushina [2], and Hirohiko Kaneko[2]

[1] Corporate R&D Strategy Office, Panasonic Corporation,
3-1-1 Yagumo-naka-machi, Moriguchi City, Osaka 570-8501, Japan
Tel: +81-6-6906-0718, Fax: +81-6-6906-1662
{sakamoto.kiyomi, aoyama.shoichi,
asahara.shigeo}@jp.panasonic.com
[2] Department of Information Processing, Tokyo Institute of Technology,
4259-G2-3, Nagatsuta, Midori-ku,Yokohama-city, Kanagawa, 226-8502 Japan
Tel.: +81-45-924-5292, Fax: +81-45-924-5293
{mizushina,kaneko }@ ip.titech.ac.jp

Abstract. We carried out two experiments to explore the relationship between the frequency characteristic of pupil diameter variability and emotional state under various types of workload. The workload required the subjects to listen to spoken words and categorize them. The difficulty of the task was adjusted by changing the time interval of the stimulus presentation in Experiment 1 (time-based task) and the number of categories in Experiment 2 (cognitive-based task). Pupil diameter was monitored and recorded using an infrared video camera while observers were performing the tasks. In both experiments, a significant correlation was observed between the frequency characteristic of pupil diameter variability and emotional state. Our results indicated the frequency characteristic of pupil diameter variability to be a potentially useful index for evaluating mental stress.

Keywords: Pupil diameter, audio stimuli, psychological state, variability in pupil diameter

1 Introduction

Technological progress in computer and information systems is delivering higher system performance and an increasing range of functions, but on the other hand, their growing complexity causes increased mental stress during use. Further development of these systems will require an easy-to-use human-machine interface (HMI) to be developed. Measurement of mental stress will be an essential element of this process. Current methods of evaluating mental stress depend chiefly on subjective responses, in spite of these responses often showing considerable variation among individuals. Thus, an objective measurement method of mental stress is needed to improve the accuracy and usefulness of evaluations of HMI.

B.-T. Karsh (Ed.): Ergonomics and Health Aspects, HCII 2009, LNCS 5624, pp. 177–185, 2009.
© Springer-Verlag Berlin Heidelberg 2009

Previous studies of objective estimation of users' psychological state have utilized physiological indices, including heart rate (HR) variability, brain waves, and galvanic skin response (GSR). However, wearing the various electrodes and sensors needed for measuring these vital signs may be stressful in itself. One solution to reducing user stress during measurements may be to monitor pupil diameter (PD) using a remote infrared video camera. Pupil diameter is controlled by the autonomic nerve system, as is the heartbeat; and it has been shown that in humans, patterns of change in pupil diameter are closely related to psychological state, especially mental stress. In this study, we explored the relationship between emotional state and pupil diameter variability under various types of workloads using a remote video camera. We also attempted to explore the relationship between heart rate (HR) variability and pupil diameter (PD) variability to confirm the validity of using PD variability as an evaluation index of psychological stress.

2 Experiment 1: Task with Time Pressure

In Experiment 1, pupil diameter (PD) and heart rate (HR) were monitored while the subjects performed the categorizing tasks following the audio stimuli presented at different time intervals. These stimuli induced different levels of psychological stress in the subjects.

2.1 Methods

Subjects: Six adults aged from their 20s to 50s participated in this experiment.

Measurements: The following items were measured as indices of the psychological stress experienced by the subjects: the subjective evaluation of psychological state through interviews, the pupil diameter (PD) as monitored by an infrared video camera, and the heart rate monitored by an electrocardiogram (ECG). Heart rate (HR) variability was obtained from a time series of R-R intervals. In this study, we adopted LF/HF ratios of PD and HR variabilities as indices of frequency characteristics. LF/HF was defined by the power ratio of the low frequency band (LF: 0.04–0.15 Hz) to that of the high frequency band (HF: 0.15–0.5 Hz), calculated by employing FFT analysis [1] [2]. It was assumed that the LF/HF of PD variability might reflect the level of sympathetic nerve activity in the same way as does the LF/HF of HR variability.

Apparatus: Subjects sat in a chair and performed tasks in a dark room. The subjects had to fixate steadily at a point presented on the screen, and their pupil diameter was monitored and recorded by eye movement measurement equipment comprising an infrared video camera (Arrington Research, ViewPoint EyeTracker, Sampling rate 60 Hz). To measure the pupil diameter precisely, the head of the subject was anchored with a head and chin rest. Auditory stimuli were generated by a PC (Apple, MacBook) and presentation software (Cedrus Corporation, SuperLab 4.0) and presented via noise canceling headphones (Bose). Subjects responded to the task using a keyboard (Cedrus Corporation, RB-530 Response Pad).

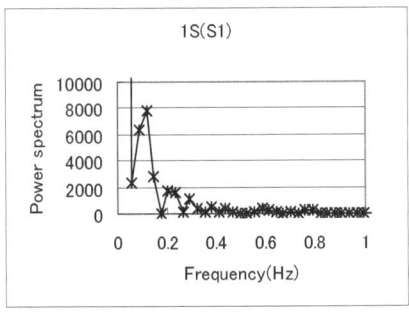

Fig. 1. Power spectrum of LF/HF (PD) at 1 s for S1 (Experiment 1)

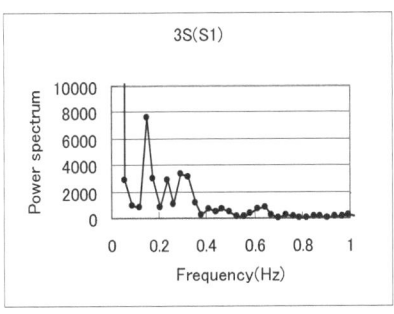

Fig. 2. Power spectrum of LF/HF at 3 s for S1 (Experiment 1)

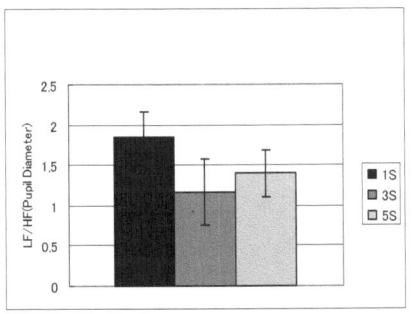

Fig. 3. Power spectrum of LF/HF (PD) at 5 s, for S1 (Experiment 1)

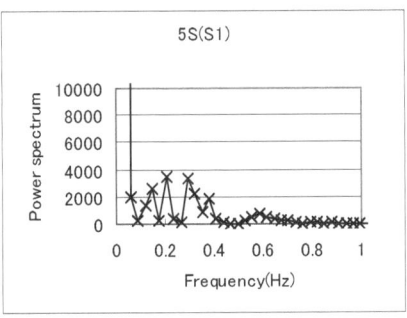

Fig. 4. Average of LF/HF (PD) at 1 s, 3 s and 5 s (Experiment 1)

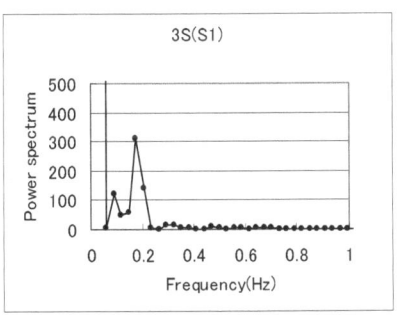

Fig. 5. Power spectrum of LF/HF (HR) at 1 s, for S1 (Experiment 1)

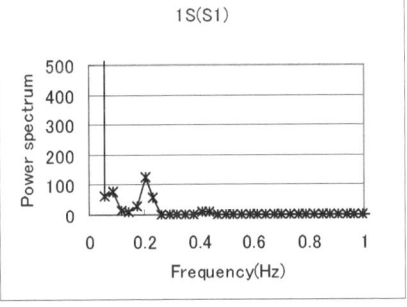

Fig. 6. Power spectrum of LF/HF (HR) at 3 s, for S1 (Experiment 1)

Procedure: The subjects performed the categorizing tasks in response to audio stimuli presented at different time intervals (1, 3 and 5 seconds). Pupil diameter (PD) and heart rate (HR) were monitored throughout the trial. These stimuli induced psychological stress in the subjects. Their task was to answer whether the word presented via the headphones belonged to the specified single category or not. There were 6 categories: Vegetables, Fruit, Fish, Insects, Birds, and Mammals. Each trial lasted about 60

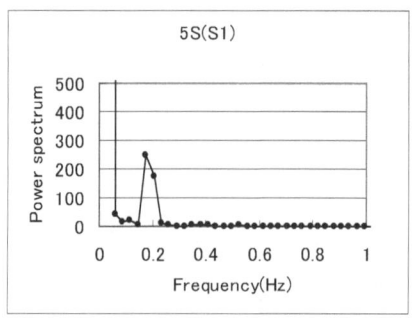

Fig. 7. Power spectrum of LF/HF (HR) on 5 s, for S1 (Experiment 1)

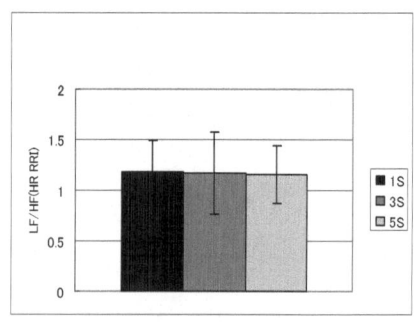

Fig. 8. Average of LF/HF (HR) on 1 s, 3 s and 5 s (Experiment 1)

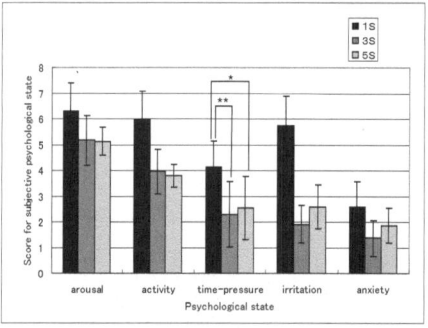

Fig. 9. Score for subjective assessment of psychological state (Experiment 1)

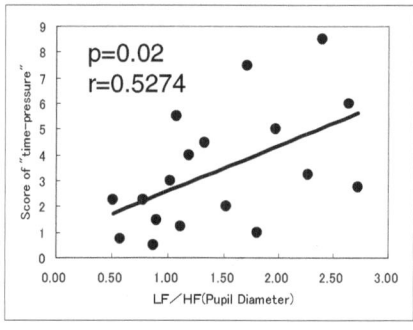

Fig. 10. Correlation between LF/HF (PD) and 'time-pressure' (Experiment 1)

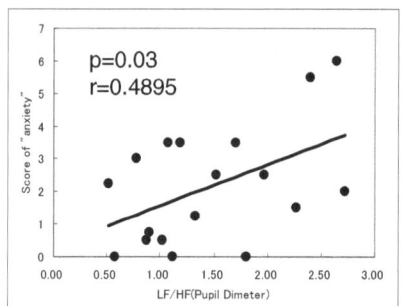

Fig. 11. Correlation between LF/HF (PD) and 'anxiety' (Experiment 1)

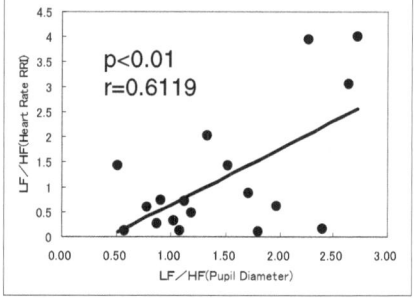

Fig. 12. Correlation between LF/HF (PD) and LF/HF (HR) (Experiment 1)

seconds. During each trial, the time interval between each test word was set at a constant value of 1, 3, or 5 seconds. After each trial, the subject gave a subjective evaluation of their psychological state ('arousal,' 'activity,' 'time-pressure,' 'irritation,' and 'anxiety'), on a score of 0 to 10. The order of the time interval tested was changed for each subject.

2.2 Results

PD variability: Figures 1, 2 and 3 show the power spectrum of PD variability for the conditions of 1 s, 3 s and 5 s for subject S1, respectively. In the case of workload stress for 1 s, the power spectrum of PD variability peaked at around 0.1 Hz (Fig. 1). That for the 3-s condition peaked at around 0.15 Hz (Fig. 2), and that for the 5-s condition peaked at around 0.2 Hz and 0.32 Hz (Fig. 3). The maximum of peak frequency at 5 s shifted to higher frequency than that for 1 s and 3-s conditions. Figure 4 shows the average LF/HF of PD variability across six subjects for each time interval. There was no significant difference in the LF/HFs.

HR variability: Figures 5, 6 and 7 show the power spectrum of HR variability for the conditions of 1 s, 3 s and 5 s respectively for subject S1. In the case of workload stress at 1 s, power spectrum of heart rate variability peaked at around 0.08 and 0.2 Hz (Fig. 5). That for the 3-s and 5-s conditions peaked at around 0.2 Hz (Fig. 6) and around 0.20 Hz (Fig. 7), respectively. Figure 8 shows the average LF/HF of HR variability across six subjects for the 1-s, 3-s and 5-s time intervals. There was no significant difference in the LF/HFs. This is probably due to the large individual differences.

Subjective evaluation of psychological state: Figure 9 shows the average scores of subjective evaluation of psychological state across eight subjects. The horizontal axis indicates the psychological state items, and the vertical axis indicates the score. For all the items, the scores tended to be higher for the 1-s condition. The score for 'time-pressure' for the 1-s condition was significantly higher than that for 3 s ($p < 0.01$) and also higher than that for 5 s ($p < 0.05$).

Correlation among LF/HF of PD variability, LF/HF of HR variability and Subjective evaluation of psychological state: A significant correlation was observed between the LF/HF of PD variability and the score for 'time-pressure' ($p = 0.02$, $r = 0.5273$) (Fig. 10) and between the LF/HF of PD variability and the score for 'anxiety' ($p = 0.03$, $r = 0.4895$) (Fig. 11). Moreover, a significant correlation was observed between the LF/HF of PD variability and that of HR variability ($p < 0.01$, $r = 0.6119$) (Fig. 12).

3 Experiment 2: Task with Cognitive Load

In Experiment 2, pupil diameter (PD) and heart rate (HR) were monitored while the subjects performed categorizing tasks in response to audio stimuli with varying specified numbers of categories. These stimuli induced different levels of cognitive stress in the subject.

3.1 Methods

Subjects: Six adults aged from their 20s to their 50s participated in this experiment. All the subjects had taken part in Experiment 1.

Measurements: Subjective evaluation of psychological state through interviews, pupil diameter (PD) monitored by infrared video camera and heart rate (HR) monitored by electrocardiogram (ECG), as in Experiment 1. All the apparatus used in this experiment was the same as in Experiment 1. The LF/HF of PD variability and that of HR variability were also calculated in the same way as in Experiment 1.

Procedure: The subjects performed the categorizing task in response to audio stimuli. The time interval was set at a constant 2 seconds in all trials. Each trial lasted about 70 seconds. The number of categories to which the word might belong was set at 1 (level 1: 1L), 2 (level 2: 2L), 3 (level 3: 3L) or 4 (level 4: 4L). Increasing the number of categories raised the level of cognitive-task difficulty. We used the same categories for the task as in Experiment 1: Vegetables, Fruit, Fish, Insects, Birds, and Mammals. After each trial, the subjects made a subjective evaluation of their psychological states ('arousal,' 'activity,' 'time-pressure,' 'irritation,' 'anxiety'), on a score of 0 to 10. The order of cognitive load levels was changed for each subject.

3.2 Results

PD variability: Figure 13, 14, 15 and 16 show power spectra of PD variability for the conditions of 1L, 2L, 3L and 4L for subject S1. In the case of a workload level of 1L, the power spectrum of PD variability showed a peak value around 0.18 Hz (Fig. 13). In the case of a workload level of 2L or 3L, the peak frequency was around 0.15 Hz (Fig. 14, Fig. 15). For a workload level of 4L, the peak frequency was around 0.08 Hz (Fig. 16). The peak frequency of power spectrum of PD variability tended to shift to a lower frequency on increasing the level of cognitive load. There was no significant difference in the average LF/HF of PD variability across the six subjects during the present task with different levels of cognitive load. (Fig. 17).

HR variability: There was no significant difference in the average LF/HF of HR variability across the six subjects for different conditions of cognitive load (1L, 2L 3L and 4L) (Fig. 18). However, the LF/HF of HR variability showed wide variation among subjects.

Subjective evaluation of psychological state: Figure 19 shows the average scores of subjective evaluations of psychological state across eight subjects. The horizontal axis indicates the items of psychological state, and the vertical axis indicates the score. For all items except 'time pressure,' the scores increased as the level of cognitive workload increased.

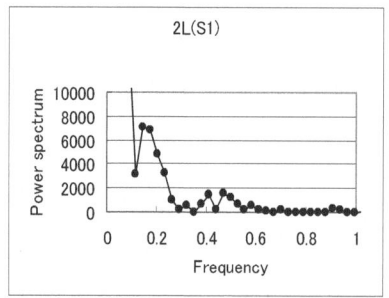
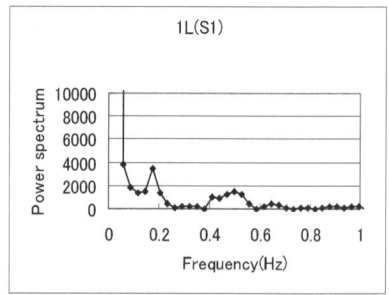
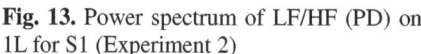

Fig. 13. Power spectrum of LF/HF (PD) on 1L for S1 (Experiment 2)

Fig. 14. Power spectrum of LF/HF (PD) on 2L for S1 (Experiment 2)

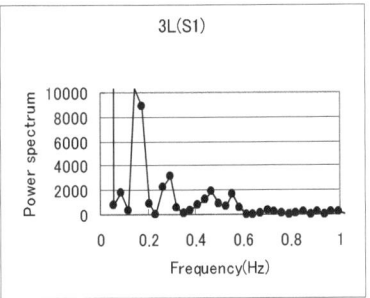

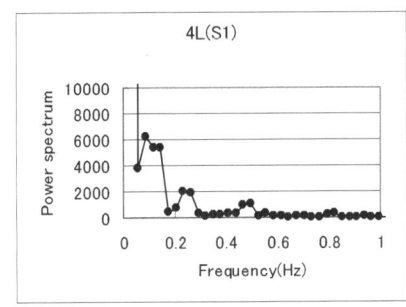

Fig. 15. Power spectrum of LF/HF (PD) on 3L for S1 (Experiment 2)

Fig. 16. Power spectrum of LF/HF (PD) on 4L for S1 (Experiment 2)

Correlation among LF/HF of PD variability, LF/HF of HR variability and Subjective evaluation of psychological state: There were no significant correlations observed between the LF/HF of PD variability and each of the other two measured indices (the subjective score of psychological states and the LF/HF of HR variability). According to our previous study [4], it is possible that the optimum frequency bands for defining LF/HF of PD and HR variability depend on the kind of task. For calculating the LF/HF shown in Fig. 17, we used 0.04–0.15 Hz for the low frequency band (LF) and 0.15–0.5 Hz for the high frequency band (HF) as in Experiment 1. Here, we recalculated the LF/HF of PD and HR variability using adjusted bands as follows:

Definition A: (LF: 0.08–0.18 Hz, HF: 0.18–0.5 Hz)
Definition B: (LF: 0.08-0.20 Hz, HF: 0.20-0.5 Hz)
Definition C: (LF: 0.10-0.20 Hz, HF: 0.20-0.5 Hz)

As a result of adjusting the bands for defining LF/HF, a significant correlation was observed between the LF/HF of PD variability using Definition A and the subjective score of 'arousal' ($p = 0.02$, $r = 0.4857$) (Fig. 20). A significant correlation was also observed between the LF/HF of PD variability using Definition A and the LF/HF of HR variability using Definition C ($p = 0.04$, $r = 0.4166$). Similarly, a pattern of correlation was observed between the LF/HF of PD variability using Definition A and the LF/HF of HR variability using Definition A ($p < 0.1$, $r = 0.3642$).

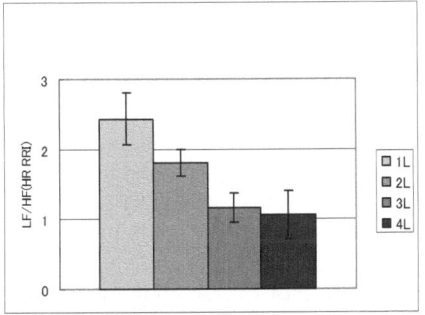

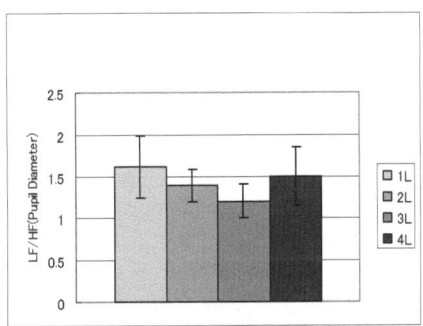

Fig. 17. Average of LF/HF (PD) on 1L, 2L, 3L and 4L (Experiment 2)

Fig. 18. Average of LF/HF (HR) on 1L, 2L, 3L and 4L (Experiment 2)

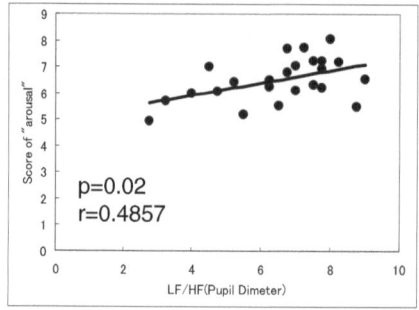
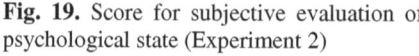
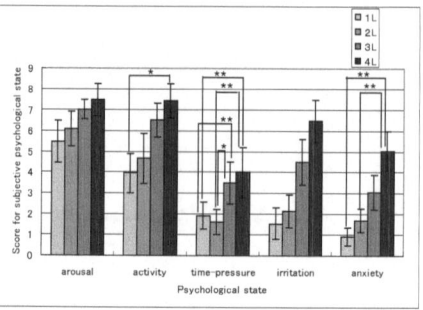

Fig. 19. Score for subjective evaluation of psychological state (Experiment 2)

Fig. 20. Correlation between LF/HF (PD) and 'arousal' (Experiment 2)

4 Discussion

The results of Experiment 1 show that subjective responses of 'arousal,' 'activity' and 'time-pressure' increased on increasing the level of the task workload. The shape of the curve for LF/HF of PD variability was U-shaped, bottoming at the workload with the 3-s interval, and significant correlation was observed between LF/HF of PD variability and the score for 'time-pressure' and 'anxiety,' indicating the possibility that high LF/HF value of PD variability at 1 s might reflect the mental stress caused by too high a workload, and high LF/HF value of PD variability at 5 s might reflect the mental stress caused by too little a workload.

Moreover, the maximum peak frequency of power spectrum of PD variability of the 5 s interval condition shifted to a higher frequency than those for 1-s and 3-s intervals. This indicates that the peak frequency of the power spectrum of PD variability value might reflect workload level. In Experiment 1, a significant correlation was also observed between the LF/HF of PD variability and that of HR variability. These results therefore indicate that LF/HF of PD variability is an evaluation index of mental stress, and could be used as a substitute for LF/HF of HR variability when measuring mental stress.

The results of Experiment 2 show that subjective responses of 'arousal', 'activity,' 'irritation' and 'anxiety' increased with increasing the level of cognitive load. These results indicate that the settings of each level of difficulty were appropriate for inducing different degrees of mental stress. However, the curve for LF/HF of PD variability was U-shaped curve and bottomed at 3L, and LF/HF at 1L and 4L (the lowest and highest cognitive task level, respectively) were higher than those for 2L and 3L. These results indicate that higher LF/HF of PD variability at 4L and 1L might be due to the mental stress caused by too high a workload and too low a workload, respectively. It is possible that the optimum task level might be at the lowest point of LF/HF of PD variability.

Moreover, the peak frequency of the power spectrum of PD variability that took maximum value shifted to a lower frequency on increasing the cognitive level. This indicates that the peak frequency of the power spectrum of PD variability that takes a maximum value might reflect workload stress.

The optimum frequency bands for LF/HF of PD variability in which significant correlations with mental stress were observed in Experiment 1 were different from those in

Experiment 2. The optimum bands used in the analysis to indicate stress from the cognitive load as presented in Experiment 2 shifted to a higher frequency than that from the time pressure as presented in Experiment 1. These facts indicate the possibility that the optimum bands for LF/HF of PD and Heart Rate variability may change according to type of task.

5 Conclusions

The results in Experiment 1 and 2 show that subjective responses to psychological states ('arousal', 'activity,' 'time pressure', 'irritation' and 'anxiety') increased on increasing the task workload. Moreover, using the same frequency band as that of heart rate variability (LF/HF), during the task with time pressure in Experiment 1 revealed a significant correlation between the ratio of lower-to higher-frequency components (LF/HF) of PD variability and subjective psychological state. A significant correlation was also observed between LF/HF of PD variability and LF/HF of HR variability in Experiment 1. During the cognitive load task in Experiment 2, a significant correlation was observed between subjective psychological state and LF/HF of PD variability, as calculated from the different frequency band, as that of HR variability.

These results indicate that LF/HF of PD variability is an effective index of mental stress, and could be used as a substitute for LF/HF of HR variability when measuring mental stress.

Acknowledgements

We thank all the subjects who took part in these experiments for their many valuable comments. This work is supported in part by the Collaborative Development of Innovative Seeds of the Japan Science and Technology Agency.

References

1. Ishibashi, K., Kitamura, S., Kozaki, T., Yasukouchi, A.: Inhibition of Heart Rate Variability during Sleep in Humans By 6700 K Pre-sleep Light Exposure. Journal of Physiological Anthropology 26(1), 39–43 (2007)
2. Ishibashi, K., Ueda, S., Yasukouchi, A.: Effects of Mental Task on Heart Rate Variability during Graded Head-Up Tilt. Journal of Physiological Anthropology 18(6), 225–231 (1999)
3. Murata, N., Mizushina, H., Sakamoto, K., Kaneko, H.: Investigation of the relationship between workload and pupil diameter during task execution using auditory stimuli. In: Technical Report of IEICE HIP 2007-.55, vol. 107(117), pp. 117–121 (2007)
4. Sakamoto, K., Aoyama, S., Asahara, S., Mizushina, H., Kaneko, H.: Effects of the Task Workload on Pupil Diameter Variability. Correspondences on Human Interface 10(1), 125–130 (2008)

Combined Measurement System
for the Evaluation of Multi Causal Strain

Holger Steiner[1], Dietmar Reinert[1], and Norbert Jung[2]

[1] BGIA - Institute for Occupational Health and Safety of the German Social Accident Insurance, Alte Heerstraße 111, 53757 Sankt Augustin, Germany
[2] University of Applied Sciences Bonn-Rhein-Sieg,
Grantham-Allee 20, 53757 Sankt Augustin, Germany
{mail@holgersteiner.de, dietmar.reinert@dguv.de,
norbert.jung@h-brs.de }

Abstract. This work addresses the problem of measuring psychological strain in humans by the use of physiological data. The aim of the work is the research, development and evaluation of a measurement system for the acquisition of such data from humans and the differentiation of psychological and physical strain with the help of machine learning algorithms. The developed system records and analyzes the ECG, the EMG, as well as the skin conductance, and combines these physiological parameters with the subject's physical activity. The main purpose of this measurement system is to assess both types of strain in employees at their workplaces.

Keywords: multi causal strain, stress, strain, ambulatory monitoring, physiological monitoring, physical activity, decision tree learning, machine learning.

1 Introduction

Strain can have multiple causes and consequences, which might be a risk for the health of employees and result in high costs for health insurance companies (see [9]). Researching the strain employees encounter during their work can help to prevent or reduce the strain, for example by modifying the working environment or tools, leading to safer working conditions for the employees and reduced costs for the insurance companies.

In this context, different types of strain have to be distinguished, as strain can be physical (that is, the body of the subjects is affected directly) or psychological: high mental workload or an emotionally stressful working environment might lead to psychological problems, such as depression, but can also be the cause for physical problems, such as illness or back pain.

To distinguish between the different types of strain and to classify their magnitude and their influence on employees, a complex measurement system is necessary, as different parameters for physical and psychological or emotional strain have to be acquired simultaneously. The research and development of such a measurement system is the aim of this work.

B.-T. Karsh (Ed.): Ergonomics and Health Aspects, HCII 2009, LNCS 5624, pp. 186–194, 2009.
© Springer-Verlag Berlin Heidelberg 2009

1.1 Measurement of Physical Strain

For the measurement of physical strain and physical activity, a well-suited measurement system is available that has been developed at the BGIA Institute for Occupational Health and Safety: the CUELA system ([2]). CUELA is a German abbreviation and stands for *"Computer-unterstützte Erfassung und Langzeit-Analyse von Belastungen des Muskel-Skelett-Systems"*, which can be translated as *"computer-assisted measurement and long-term analysis of strain on the musculoskeletal system"*. The system has been used in a large number of applications since the year 1997, primarily for the assessment of physical strain that employees encounter at their workplaces. The standard CUELA system is a sensor suite that can be worn over the working clothes. It is able to measure physical strain of a subject on the basis of the body posture and movements. It uses mechanical sensors to measure the angles of the thoracic and lumbar spine, the torsion of the back, as well as the angles of the hip and knee joints.

On the basis of the standard CUELA system, a modified measurement system called "CUELA Activity" has been developed in the last two years by Weber (see [12]). It uses accelerometers and gyroscopes to measure the actual body posture and movement instead of the mechanical sensors of the standard CUELA system, thus reducing the weight, size and complexity of the sensor suite significantly. The main purpose of the Activity system is to evaluate the actual activity of a subject in terms of both the type of the performed activity and the speed or intensity of movement.

The data that is measured by the system is recorded by a so-called "datalogger" and analyzed at a later time with a software called WIDAAN (which stands for "Winkel-Daten-Analyse", or "angle data analysis", respectively). WIDAAN runs on Windows computers and allows to display the recorded data in the form of graphs over time, as well as in the form of an animated 3D-skeleton figure. WIDAAN is also able to synchronize the measured data with a video recording. It handles every sensor or calculation result as a "channel", which can be viewed as a chart or graph over the time, and allows to synchronize, mark and edit single or multiple data channels at once ([2], [3]). The design of the WIDAAN software allows to extend it with new data channels or new "plug-in" components for the calculation of strain data easily.

1.2 Measurement of Psychological Strain

It is obvious that psychological strain can not be measured by using physical data alone. Therefore, the main idea of this work is to develop an additional physiological measurement system that can be combined with either one of the already existing CUELA systems. Appropriate physiological parameters and sensors that are suited to acquire these parameters have been researched in the scope of this work.

Compared to the physical activity, physiological parameters represent a more direct way to measure and evaluate the strain of a subject. In general, these parameters measure the reaction of the human body to both physical and psychological strain of any kind. The results that can be achieved by the assessment of these parameters are always subjective to a certain extend, as the subject's personal fitness and individual perception of the stressor have an influence on the physiological parameters (see [6]). The heart rate and the heart rate variability, which are both measured by an electrocardiogram (ECG), the electrodermal activity (skin conductance response, respectively) and the muscle activity in the Trapezius muscle, which is measured by an electromyogram (EMG), have been selected due to their importance for the measurement of strain (compare to [4], [10], [11], [14], [15]).

While the heart rate is strongly correlated with the overall strain of the body, the heart rate variability, which represents the variations of the heart rate from beat to beat, can be used to assess mental strain ([6]). It is typically assessed in terms of the "root mean square of successive differences" (RMSSD) and the standard deviation of the beat-to-beat-intervals (SDRR), which are both measured in milliseconds. In contrast to this, the skin conductance response allows the detection of emotional strain and arousal (see [15]). The skin conductance (that is, the ability of the skin to conduct electricity) is measured in Siemens and depends on the amount of sweat in the sweat glands of the skin. The activity of the Trapezius muscle, which is situated in the shoulder and neck region of the human body, is also known to be an indicator for strain, especially when activity is detected during phases without body movements (compare to [10], [11]).

To provide context data in addition to the physiological parameters, the physical activity, which is measured by the use of either the standard CUELA system or the Activity system, is recorded simultaneously.

2 Methods

2.1 Basic Idea

As previously described, there are several parameters that are of interest for the measurement of both psychological and physical strain. The physical activity can be acquired and analyzed in detail by the use of the CUELA system in its different variants. However, in the scope of this work, only the CUELA Activity system has been used, as it already provides a parameter called "Physical Activity Intensity (PAI)", which is well-suited for this purpose. Therefore, this system is a very good basis for the development of the proposed multi causal strain measurement system. The implementation of microcontroller-based intelligent sensor systems for the acquisition and analysis of the physiological parameters, which can not be acquired by the CUELA system so far, and the integration of these sensor systems into the CUELA system is the basic idea of this work.

2.2 System Concept

The concept for the combined measurement system is shown in figure 1. The first and most important part of the system concept is represented by the physiological sensor systems themselves, which are shown in the upper left corner of the figure. On the hardware side, they consist of the actual sensor for the acquisition of the physiological signal, electrical circuitry and components for the analog signal conditioning, as well as one microcontroller IC-chip. On the software side, several functions are implemented on the microcontroller to deal with all signal processing steps that are applied on the digitalized signal. The developed microcontroller-based sensor systems are able to filter, digitalize and analyze the acquired sensor readings autonomously.

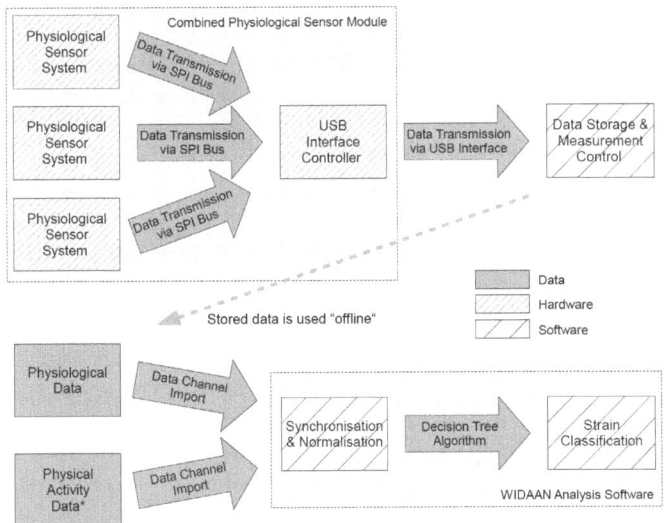

Fig. 1. System concept and data flow chart. *Data* and its flow is shown in dark grey, while *hardware* components are shown in (dashed) light grey and *software* components in (dashed) white.

The physiological sensor systems are combined on one hardware module (represented by the area marked in light grey), together with an USB interface controller. The sensor systems transmit their data to the USB controller by using a SPI bus interface. The USB controller unites the data and transmits it over its USB bus interface to a host device, which stores the data and controls the measurement process by sending control commands back to the physiological sensor systems (via the USB controller). This host device, which is called "datalogger" in conjunction with the CUELA system, can be any personal computer or notebook, as well as a personal digital assistant (PDA) or handheld computer, or even a mobile phone with USB host capabilities and sufficient memory to store the entire measurement data. Therefore, only a software tool that is able to manage the storage of the acquired data and that allows a user to control the measurement system has to be developed in order to implement this component of the system.

From this point on, the data is stored and available for "offline" use, which means that it can be viewed and analyzed after the measurement has been completed. All further components of the system work with this stored data. They are implemented completely in software, which runs on typical computer hardware like a desktop PC or a notebook. The basis for the software implementation is the WIDAAN analysis software of the CUELA system, which provides a graphical user interface to view, edit and analyze the recorded data and to synchronize the different data streams. The stored data from both the physiological and the physical sensor systems is imported into WIDAAN and new data channels are created for each sensor.

Afterwards, a decision tree algorithm is used to classify the data in the course of time with respect to the type and amount of strain that the subject experienced. Again, a new data channel is created in WIDAAN and the results of the algorithm's calculations are stored and graphically represented in this channel. In order to develop appropriate decision rules for the classification of the strain data, a learning algorithm is used on suited learning data. The resulting strain classification method is the final step of the system concept and represents the result of the approach that is proposed in this work.

2.3   Details of the Physiological Measurement System

In the physiological sensor systems, the physiological signals that are acquired by the use of electrodes are "conditioned" before they are digitalized, which means that they are amplified and filtered in order to remove noise and to limit their bandwidth by attenuating frequencies above a certain threshold. This is necessary in order to digitalize the signals correctly: according to the Nyquist-Shannon sampling theorem, the sampling rate, which is applied during the digitalization, has to be more than twice as high as the highest frequency occurring in the signal ([8]). If this theorem is broken, disturbing aliasing effects are the consequence. Therefore, a sampling rate is chosen which is sufficiently high for the respective sensor system.

After the digitalization, an additional digital notch filter is applied on the signal to remove 50Hz and 60Hz noise caused by main power lines. This noise gets easily picked up by the human body and can not be attenuated sufficiently by the analog signal conditioning process, as it is too close to the useful signals' frequency ranges. In the ECG sensor, the resulting signal is analyzed by an algorithm that detects the so-called R-wave, which is the highest peak in the signal. The R-wave marks the exact moment of the heart beat and can therefore be used to calculate the heart rate, as well as the heart rate variability, by measuring the time interval between two successive R-waves. In the skin conductance sensor, the readings are derived in order to gain the skin conductance response. In contrast to this, the readings of the EMG sensor are used without further calculations.

The hardware components of the sensor systems are implemented on one single circuit board, together with an USB controller, which gathers the data from all sensor systems and transmits it to a connected datalogger, as proposed in the system concept. The complete sensor module is powered by the datalogger via the USB connection and small enough to avoid hindering the subject in any way.

2.4   Data Classification

The data that is recorded by the combined measurement system has to be analyzed as a whole in order to evaluate the type and amount of strain that the subject experienced during the measurement. This can be done manually by viewing and evaluating the data in numbers or as a graph, but this approach would be much too time-consuming to be performed for long time measurements or for a series of measurements with different subjects. Therefore, an automatic and autonomously working algorithm is needed that is able to perform this task in less time.

On the basis of the combined measurement system, algorithms for the differentiation between physical and psychological strain have been researched. A machine learning algorithm, which is able to automatically classify new data according to rules that it has learned before, promises to be an optimal solution for the given task. In order to gain training data for the use in such learning algorithms, a number of different strain classes have been specified and for each of these classes, a respective working scenario has been created with the intention to induce the specific amounts of psychological and / or physical strain. These scenarios include parts of both low and high physical and mental workloads, which are induced by a bicycle ergometer and a computer-based math and color recognition test (the so-called Stroop color test) that is based on the dual-task-paradigm (see [13]). Table 1 presents the nine specified strain classes and a description of the respective working scenario.

Table 1. Strain classes and the respective working scenarios for the generation of training data

Strain Class	Description
1 - no strain	Resting phase, also used to determine baseline values for reference. At least ten minutes.
2 - low psychological strain only	Combination of simple mathematical and colour exercises with a fair solving time of 15 seconds.
3 - high psychological strain only	Combination of difficult mathematical and colour exercises with a stronger limited solving time of 10 seconds.
4 - low physical strain only	Cycling with a low workload of approx. 50 Watts.
5 - low physical and low psychological strain	Cycling with low workload and solving of simple mathematical and colour exercises, 15s solving time.
6 - low physical and high psychological strain	Cycling with low workload and solving of difficult mathematical and colour exercises, 10s solving time.
7 - high physical only	Cycling with higher workload of approx. 150 Watts.
8 - high physical and low psychological strain	Cycling with high workload and solving of simple mathematical and colour exercises, 15s solving time.
9 - high physical and high psychological strain	Cycling with high workload and solving of difficult mathematical and colour exercises, 10s solving time.

For the generation of data for the specified strain classes, a respective measurement setup has been developed and performed by several subjects. The resulting data has been analyzed and split up in a training and a test data set. A machine learning algorithm is applied on these data sets in order to find attributes and rules for the reliable classification of the data with respect to type and amount of strain. Due to the given characteristics of the input data (a fixed set of attribute-value pairs with numerical values, possibly containing errors or missing values due to incorrect sensor readings or loss of data), a decision tree learning algorithm was selected for this purpose (see [4], [7]). In decision tree learning, the data is split up by a number of simple decisions that together form a tree: for every data set, decision rules are applied following one path along the edges of the tree until a leave, which represents one of the specified classes, is reached. This type of learning algorithm produces static decision rules for the data classification, which can easily be implemented in the analysis software in order to perform the data classification automatically. The resulting decision rules will classify each of the data sets into exactly one of the previously defined (disjoint) categories.

3 Results

The proposed physiological measurement system has been evaluated in terms of the theoretical and technical implementation of the combined sensor system, as well as by a functional evaluation with respect to the practical use of the system. The results of the evaluation showed that the sensor modules are working correctly and produce good and sufficiently reliable results, even if the subject is in motion.

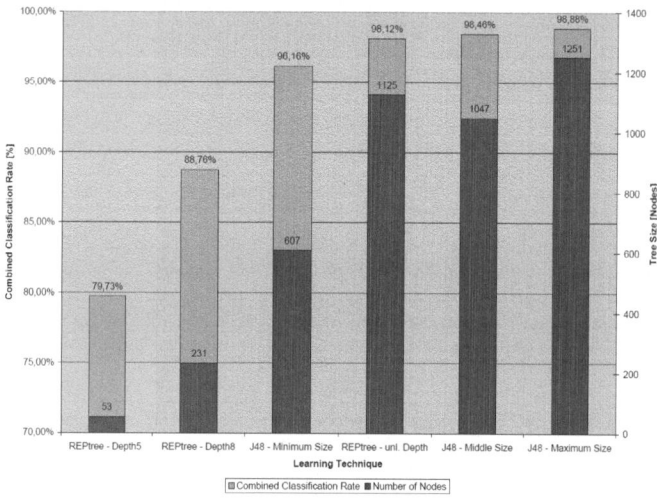

Fig. 2. The performance in terms of the *combined classification rate (left Y-axis)* of different decision tree *learning techniques (X-axis)*, which were applied on the joint data set of two subjects, compared to the respective *tree size (right Y-axis)*

Two data sets from subjects, who performed the specified measurement setup with the nine different working scenarios, were chosen to be used as training data for the learning algorithm. The decision tree learning algorithm delivers a very good performance for the classification of the data of each subject. Correct classification rates of more than 90% can be achieved even by comparably small decision trees with about 50 nodes (or decisions, respectively), which can easily be implemented in an analysis software. By using more complex trees with more than 500 nodes, correct classification rates of up to 98% could be achieved.

In order to find a classification that can be used for both subjects, the data sets were combined and the algorithm was applied on this combined data set. It was found that the correct classification rate is almost identical to the results of the algorithm for just one single data set. Unfortunately, this is achieved by a significant increase of the trees' sizes. However, if the tree's depth is limited to a fixed value (which is possible by modifying the algorithm's parameters), the size of the resulting trees is only moderately increased while still providing a good classification rate. Figure 2 shows the performance of different decision trees on the joint data set compared to their respective sizes.

4 Discussion

This work addressed the problem of measuring both psychological and physical strain in humans, especially in employees at their workplaces, and of differentiating between the types of strain the subject encountered. On the basis of intelligent sensor systems, a combined measurement system for the acquisition of physiological parameters has been designed and implemented. This measurement system can be used in conjunction with the CUELA system in order to acquire both physiological and physical parameters of a subject and all acquired data can easily be combined by the use of a single analysis software.

In order to automatically classify the combined data with respect to the type of strain that the subject encountered, the use of machine learning algorithms has been proposed. Nine different strain classes have been specified and respective strain induction scenarios have been performed by several subjects in order to gain training data with a known combination of strain for the use in the learning algorithm. It was shown that the decision tree learning algorithms deliver a good performance for the classification of the data. However, to achieve reliable classification results for unknown data that has been acquired from a new subject, using a tree that has been learned with the data from only one subject is not sufficient.

A decision tree that was learned with data from two subjects achieved a constantly high correct classification rate for both subjects, which is very promising with regard to a more general applicability of this method. This indicates that in order to find a decision tree, which can be applied successfully to the data of arbitrary subjects, training data from a large number of subjects has to be collected. This requires an additional study and further research in order to find convenient ways of normalizing the data, as well as the design of respective calibration phases that have to be performed by each new subject.

A different approach is to implement a complete decision tree learning algorithm into the data analysis software that learns a new decision tree for every new subject. This would require to extend the calibration phase that has to be performed by each subject, as it has to include all specified strain induction scenarios. Advantages of this approach are that the data does not have to be normalized and that it is not necessary to collect training data from a large number of subjects in advance. Additionally, the results of the classification algorithm might be better, as the distinctive features of each class are based on the specific subject's data only. However, the feasibility of both approaches has to be evaluated in detail in future work.

References

1. Cutmore, T., James, D.A.: Sensors and Sensor Systems for Psychophysiological Monitoring: A Review of Current Trends. Journal of Psychophysiology 21(1), 51–71 (2007)
2. Ellegast, R.-P., Hermanns, I.: Einsatz des Messsystems CUELA zur Erfassung und Bewertung physischer Arbeitsbelastungen. BGIA - Institute for Occupational Health and Safety of the German Social Accident Insurance, Sankt Augustin, (2006)
   http://www.hvbg.de/d/bia/fac/ergonomie/pdf/cuela.pdf
3. Hermanns, I., Post, M.: Das CUELA-Messsystem. Information des Berufsgenossenschaftlichen Instituts für Arbeitsschutz - BGIA, Sankt Augustin (2003),
   http://www.hvbg.de/d/bia/fac/ergonomie/pdf/text1a.pdf
4. Mitchell, T.M.: Machine Learning. McGraw-Hill, Columbus (1997)
5. Myrtek, M., Fichtler, A., Strittmatter, M., Brügner, G.: Stress and Strain of Blue and White Collar Workers During Work and Leisure Time: Results of Psychophysiological and Behavioral Monitoring. Applied Ergonomics 30, 341–351 (1999)
6. Myrtek, M., Foerster, F.: On-Line Measurement of Additional Heart Rate - Methodology and Applications. In: Fahrenberg, J., Myrtek, M. (eds.) Progress in Ambulatory Assessment - Computer-Assisted Psychological and Psychophysiological Methods in Monitoring and Field Studies, pp. 399–414. Hogrefe & Huber Publishers, Göttingen (2001)
7. Russel, S., Norvig, P.: Künstliche Intelligenz. Prentice Hall / Pearson Education, New Jersey (2004)
8. Smith, S.W.: The Scientist and Engineer's Guide to Digital Signal Processing. California Technical Publishing, San Diego (1999)
9. Steiner, H.: Erfassung von physiologischen Daten mit einem Embedded Controller. BGIA - Institute for Occupational Health and Safety of the German Social Accident Insurance / University of Applied Sciences Bonn-Rhein-Sieg, Sankt Augustin (2006)
   http://www.inf.fh-bonn-rhein-sieg.de/data/ informatik/
   fb_informatik/personen/reinert/steiner.pdf
10. Taelman, J., Adriaensen, T., van der Horst, C., Linz, T., Spaepen, A.: Textile Integrated Contactless EMG Sensing for Stress Analysis. In: Engineering in Medicine and Biology Society, EMBS 2007, 29th Annual International Conference of the IEEE, pp. 3966–3969. IEEE Press, New York (2007)
11. Vogt, J., Kastner, M.: Psychophysiological Monitoring of Air Traffic Controllers: Exploration, Simulation, Validation. In: Fahrenberg, J., Myrtek, M. (eds.) Progress in Ambulatory Assessment - Computer-Assisted Psychological and Psychophysiological Methods in Monitoring and Field Studies, pp. 455–476. Hogrefe & Huber Publishers, Göttingen (2001)
12. Weber, B., Hermanns, I., Ellegast, R.P., Kleinert, J.: Assessment Of Physical Activity at Workplaces. In: Bust, P. (ed.) Contemporary Ergonomics. Taylor & Francis, Oxfordshire (2008)
13. Wickens, C.D., Gordon, S.E., Liu, Y.: An Introduction to Human Factors Engineering. Addison Wesley Longman, Harlow (1998)
14. Wilson, G.: In-Flight Psychophysiological Monitoring. In: Fahrenberg, J., Myrtek, M. (eds.) Progress in Ambulatory Assessment - Computer-Assisted Psychological and Psychophysiological Methods in Monitoring and Field Studies, pp. 435–454. Hogrefe & Huber Publishers, Göttingen (2001)
15. Wilhelm, F.H., Pfaltz, M.C., Grossman, P., Roth, W.T.: Distinguishing Emotional From Physical Activation. In: Ambulatory Psychophysiological Monitoring, Rocky Mountain Bioengineering Symposium & International ISA Biomedical Sciences Instrumentation Symposium (2006)

Development of Non-contact Monitoring System of Heart Rate Variability (HRV) - An Approach of Remote Sensing for Ubiquitous Technology -

Satoshi Suzuki[1], Takemi Matsui[1], Shinji Gotoh[1], Yasutaka Mori[1], Bonpei Takase[2], and Masayuki Ishihara[2]

[1] Tokyo Metropolitan University, Asahigaoka 6-6, Hino, Tokyo 191-0065, Japan
[2] National Defense Medical College, Namiki 3-2, Tokorozawa, Saitama 359-8513, Japan
ssuzuki@cc.tmit.ac.jp

Abstract. The aim of this study was to develop a prototype system to monitor cardiac activity using microwave Doppler radar (24.05 GHz frequency, 7 mW output power in average) without making contact with the body and without removing clothing; namely, a completely noncontact, remote monitoring system. In addition, heart rate and changes in heart rate variability (HRV) during simple mental arithmetic and computer input tasks were observed with the prototype system. The experiment was conducted with seven subjects (23.00 ± 0.82 years old). We found that the prototype system captured heart rate and HRV precisely. The strong relationship between the heart rates during tasks (r = 0.963), LF (cross-correlation = 0.76) and LF/HF (cross-correlation = 0.73) of HRV calculated from the microwave radar data and from electrocardiograph (ECG) measurements were confirmed.

Keywords: noncontact monitoring, microwave radar, heart rate variability.

1 Introduction

"Ubiquitous technology" is interpreted in some terms, however, it means essentially that user does not feel the presence of any device and sensing. The sensing technique unnoticeable to the users is one of the important elemental technologies for creating a ubiquitous info-communications environment.

Recently, nonrestrictive and noninvasive sensing techniques to measure vital signs have been actively researched and developed. Examples include using a strain gauge [1], pressure sensors [2], and a piezoelectric polymer called polyvinylidene fluoride film (PVDF) in sensors [3] used to measure heartbeat and respiration from the subject's dorsal body surface. This kind of sensing technique is useful for patients who have suffered heavy burn injuries and serious lacerations, because it avoids having to paste electrodes directly onto the body. Furthermore, patients who should be isolated because of the risk of secondary infection resulting from exposure to toxic chemicals or infectious organisms are treated in an isolator and in such cases a stable remote sensing method is needed to measure vital signs from outside of the isolator.

B.-T. Karsh (Ed.): Ergonomics and Health Aspects, HCII 2009, LNCS 5624, pp. 195–203, 2009.

We have previously reported on a complete noncontact system for monitoring respiratory rate and heart rate using a microwave radar antenna at 1215 MHz to measure the vital signs of casualties inside an isolation unit [4, 5]. In addition, we developed a noncontact method using a ceiling-mounted microwave radar to monitor the respiratory rates of subjects in bed through their bedding [6]. These methods are aimed at detecting motion at extremely minute scales on the body surface caused by cardiac and respiratory motion. The method was originally developed to search for survivors under earthquake rubble [7, 8]. Microwave radar has the following characteristics: (1) microwaves can be transmitted through most objects except metals and water; and (2) it is possible to detect movement of the object from some distance and without actually needing to touch it. If we attempt to use this system for humans, it is possible to observe the motion of the body surface from some distance without removing their clothing.

We have already tried to monitor changes in HRV that are induced by stressful audio stimuli using a noncontact measurement system with a 24 GHz compact microwave radar, which can easily be attached to the rear surface of the back of a chair [9]. The aim of this study was to develop a prototype of the same type of system for cardiac monitoring, using microwave radar without making contact with the body and without removing clothing-namely, a complete noncontact, remote monitoring system. In addition, heart rate and changes in heart rate variability during tasks were measured by utilizing the system.

2 Prototype System

The prototype system for noncontact cardiac monitoring we designed consisted of a microwave Doppler radar antenna (Tau Giken Co., Yokohama, Japan), a device for controlling the power supply to this antenna, and a PC for analyzing the output data from the antenna. The frequency of this microwave radar antenna for cardiac monitoring was 24.05 GHz, with a normal average output power of approximately 7 mW (the maximum output power is under 10 mW). The diffusion angle (θ_d) of the microwave radar antenna is about 40°, the antenna gain is 10 dBi, and the electrical field intensity is 0.7 mW/cm^2. This antenna has approximately the same specifications as that used in our previous research [9].

Damage caused by electromagnetic waves has been discussed in the literature, especially in the case of human applications. At frequencies over 3 GHz, the electrical field intensity limit is 1 mW/cm^2 according to the guidelines for radio waves established by the Telecommunication Bureau of the Ministry of Internal Affairs and Communication in Japan. Also, the 24.05 GHz frequency of our device is within the frequency band for normal use of radio waves as approved by Japanese law.

Before input into a PC for analysis, data were acquired at a sampling frequency of 100 Hz using an A/D converter (USB-6008, National Instruments, Texas, USA). After digitization, the data were analyzed by a system we developed using a Lab-VIEW (National Instruments, Texas, USA). In this analyzing system, in order to reduce noise and select data related to the motion associated with heart rate, a band-pass filter was used for transferring data from the microwave Doppler radar antenna. This filter was set between 0.5 Hz and 2.5 Hz; this setting covers a range of 30 to 150 heartbeats per minute.

3 Experiment

3.1 Experimental Settings

Experiments to measure heart rate and changes in HRV using the prototype system were conducted. At the same time, the ECG was measured by the contact monitoring system using normal electrodes. We compare the results for the ECG with the results acquired by the prototype system.

The subjects were employed seven healthy male subjects (mean age 23.00 ± 0.82 years; range 22–24 years). Each subject wore a 2 mm-thick cotton T-shirt and sat on a chair with mesh back composed of 2 mm-thick polyester plastic (Baron-Chair, Okamura Co., Tokyo, Japan) (see Figure 1). The distance of the antenna of the prototype system to the chair back was 30 mm, and it was placed about 60 mm to the left of the spine at around the level of the fourth intercostal space.

Following a period of 2 minutes' silence for resting, the subjects were asked to perform a simple arithmetic task with pairs of two-digit numbers for a period of 2 minutes. Two-digit numbers in randomly produced pairs were displayed on a personal computer screen. The subject calculated in his head and inputted the answer from the ten-key keyboard within 3 seconds.

The subject rested his right elbow on the armrest of the chair and was directed to keep it there when he inputted the answers using the keyboard. All subjects were right-handed. We did not give the subjects any instructions on breathing, such as holding the breath, and informed consent was obtained from each subject.

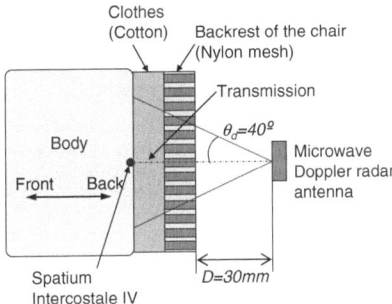

Fig. 1. Setting position of a microwave radar antenna to measured dorsal point of the subject

3.2 Analysis

The output signals from the prototype system and a reference precordial ECG signal from the V_5 position were sampled by the A/D converter with a sampling frequency of 100 Hz. Band-pass filters were used for the prototype system outputs to reduce noise and interference. The band-pass filters were set at between 0.5 Hz and 2.5 Hz; this model band-pass filter covers a range of 30 to 150 heartbeats per minute. After the filtering, power spectra of heartbeat intervals - as low frequency (LF) (0.04 - 0.15 Hz), high frequency (HF) (0.15 - 0.4 Hz), and LF/HF—were calculated to monitor

HRV by using the maximum entropy method (MemCalc software, GMS Co., Tokyo, Japan); this system is normally used for medical research [10, 11].

The intervals of the peaks in amplitude in outputs from the prototype system were assumed to correlate with the R-R interval for the ECG, and HRV was calculated by using peak-to-peak intervals in the output signal of the prototype system. The power spectra of HRV (i.e., LF, HF, and LF/HF) for R-R intervals derived by the ECG were also calculated by using the MemCalc software. Cross-correlations were examined for the LF, HF, and LF/HF derived from our noncontact system and the LF, HF, and LF/HF derived from the contact ECG system. Quantitative data are expressed as mean ± standard deviation (*SD*). sample size was determined to achieve sufficient assurance for the paired t-test for relatively uniform subjects.

4 Results

4.1 Heart Rate

Figure 2 shows sample data for subject S_1 monitored for 5 seconds. Figure 2(A) shows the output signal of the ECG and Figure 2(B) shows the output signal acquired by the prototype system. While small phase shift between R-waves of ECG and the cyclic oscillations acquired by the prototype system was confirmed, however, the repeat cycles of the two systems were nearly identical.

Figure 3(A) shows comparisons between the heart rates determined by the prototype system and those obtained by the reference ECG during the silent period of 2 minutes' rest before the tasks were performed. The horizontal axis indicates the heart rate calculated from the R-R interval in the data derived from the normal ECG. The vertical axis indicates the heart rate estimated by using the data from the prototype system using microwave Doppler radar. A strong positive correlation $(r = 0.954)$ in the two indices was confirmed for all subjects.

Figure 3(B) shows the correlation between heart rates determined by the prototype system and heart rates determined by the normal ECG during the performance of the

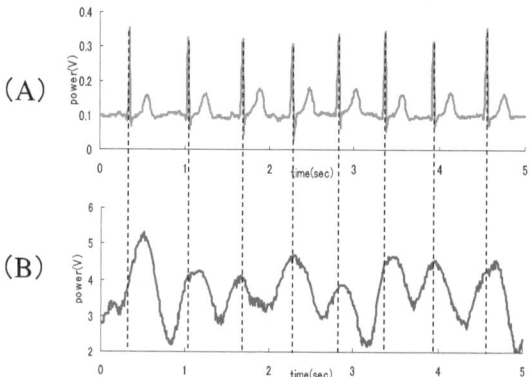

Fig. 2. Sample data for subject S1 monitored by two measurement systems in a 5–second period

arithmetic and computer input task ($r = 0.963$). The high correlation between the heart rates derived by the two systems was confirmed for all subjects irrespective or whether the subjects were performing the task or resting. Therefore, the prototype system measures heart rate stably and independent of the subjects' task.

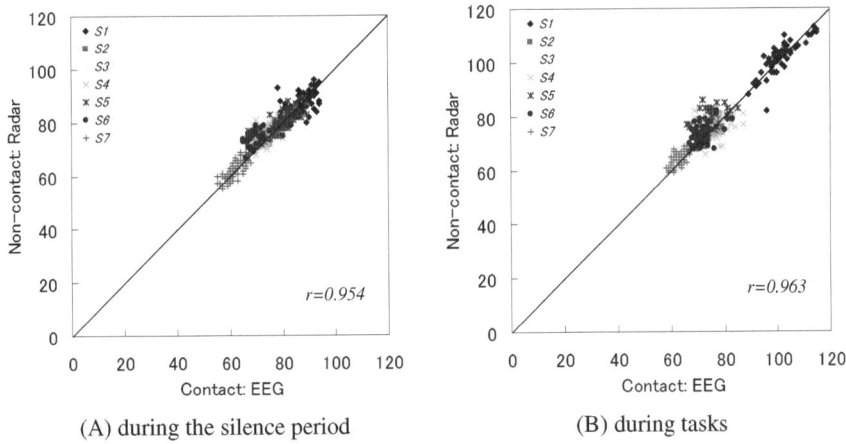

(A) during the silence period

(B) during tasks

Fig. 3. Correlation diagrams for both the noncontact and contact monitoring methods under two conditions of resting and task performance

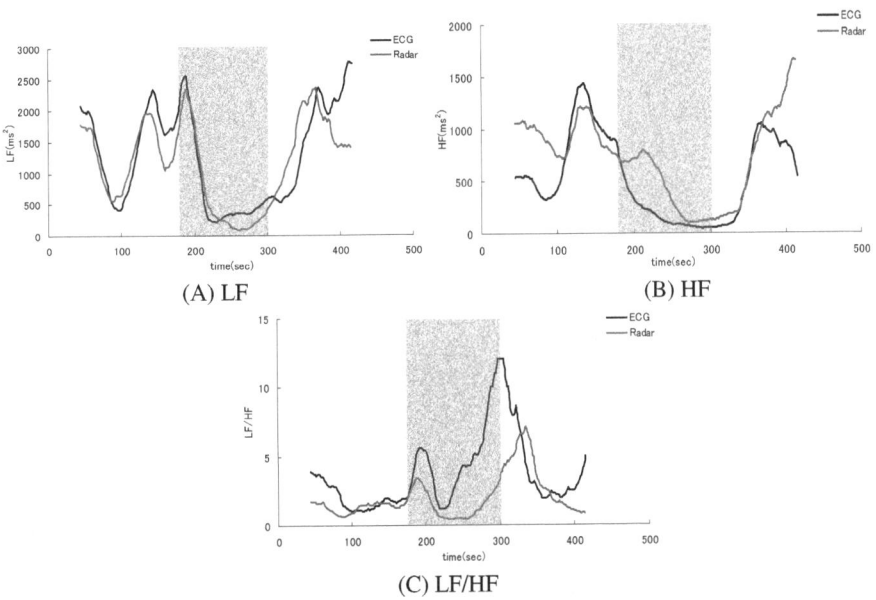

(A) LF

(B) HF

(C) LF/HF

Fig. 4. Sample data for subject S1 showing changes in HRV for the noncontact and contact monitoring systems

4.2 Changes in HRV and Cross-Correlation between the Contact and Noncontact Monitoring Systems

For both the prototype system using microwave radar for noncontact cardiac monitoring and the normal ECG system for contact monitoring as a reference, the HRV parameter LF for subject S_1 reflected mainly sympathetic activation (Figure 4(A)); they both showed a similar change at the 2-minute rest period and during the performance of the task. The HF for the same subject, reflecting parasympathetic activity, did not show any distinctive change during the mental arithmetic and computer input task (Figure 4(B)). The LF/HF for the same subject, reflecting sympathovagal balance, exhibited a peak during the task (Figure 4(C)).

Table 1 shows the results of cross-correlations of HRV for the seven subjects monitored by the noncontact and contact methods during rest and task performance. Maximum cross-correlation values in LF between the noncontact and contact methods averaged 0.76±0.11 for the seven subjects. Maximum cross-correlation values in HF averaged 0.58±0.16 for the seven subjects, and maximum cross-correlation values of LF/HF averaged 0.73±0.15 for the seven subjects.

Table 1. Results of cross-correlation of HRV for seven subjects measured by both the noncontact and contact monitoring systems

Subjects	LF	HF	LF/HF
S_1	0.84	0.68	0.74
S_2	0.75	0.48	0.73
S_3	0.64	0.81	0.76
S_4	0.66	0.57	0.46
S_5	0.95	0.55	0.96
S_6	0.69	0.68	0.70
S_7	0.76	0.30	0.79
Average	*0.76*	*0.58*	*0.73*
SD	*0.11*	*0.16*	*0.15*

5 Discussion

We developed a prototype system using 24 GHz microwave radar for noncontact cardiac monitoring. Compared with other noninvasive measurement methods (i.e., strain gauge [1], pressure sensors [2], and PVDF sensors [3]), our method is completely noncontact and also does not require the removal of clothing. We designed the antenna with relatively small dimensions to obtain high gain with high spatial resolution; the small size also reduces the possibility of signal absorption through the human body, at 24 GHz more than with lower frequencies. In addition, a high gain allows a smaller area to be analyzed. As a result, a small antenna at 24 GHz is easier to integrate into a monitoring system, and is suitable for civil applications.

In order to evaluate the relationship between the intervals detected between peaks in the output signal acquired from the prototype system for noncontact cardiac monitoring and the R-R intervals measured by the ECG, the correlation of heart rates obtained with the two methods was calculated. The results confirmed that peak-to-peak intervals captured by our prototype system are quite similar to the R-R intervals captured by the ECG signal, because the estimated heart rates determined by using the data captured by our prototype system are roughly in accordance with actual measurements. Results confirmed that our microwave system can capture information similar to that obtained with the ECG system.

In addition, the changes in HRV measured by both methods were also similar, although there were some differences in the absolute values. These results mean that our prototype system can capture signals with sufficient accuracy to calculate heart rate and HRV. This success is attributed to improved resolution with the higher-frequency microwave radar. Other research has aimed at capturing heart rate [12, 13, 14]; the frequencies used in those studies were from 1.6 to 2.4 GHz. In order to observe changes in HRV, accurate R-R intervals have to be captured. Our prototype system has a higher-frequency microwave radar antenna with a 24 GHz frequency and has the advantages of higher resolution and noninvasiveness.

However, the signals for some subjects were sometimes distorted during task performance. It is thought that this noise was caused by motions of the upper limbs induced by task performance. We predicted before the experiments that signals would be affected by upper limb motion, because there is some space between the body and the microwave radar antenna, and the device can be affected by other body motions. However, this noise was observed in only some of the data during task performance, and high values of cross-correlation between HRV measured by the noncontact and contact methods during task performance in all subjects were confirmed. Future work should aim to resolve this problem by using filters with appropriate settings or by interpolation.

At the start of this research, we thought that the sympathetic nervous activation related to task performance could be shown - namely, by LF and/or LF/HF increases or HF decreases. The results confirmed that LF/HF increased in many subjects; however, the trend of decreasing LF was confirmed for many subjects. It is thought the task difficulty and the 3-second interval set for each trial were not appropriate. It will be necessary to set a time limit or time pressure for each trial in future experiments.

6   Conclusion

We describe here a novel prototype system using microwave radar for noncontact cardiac monitoring that requires neither direct contact with the body nor the removal of clothing. We monitored changes in HRV during task performance with the system in efforts to monitor human autonomic activation induced by task performance.

The antenna of our prototype system is relatively small and can easily be attached to office furniture in the workplace (i.e., to a chair back or chair arm). This means that the device is suitable for civil applications at a low cost. We will examine actual use in office settings in the future.

The device is sensitive to other body motions since there is a space between the body and the microwave radar antenna. The signal processing becomes more delicate in the case of work associated with relatively large body motions. Therefore, there are many issues that need to be tackled on the road to using this remote sensing technique in the real workplace; this technique is still in an early phase of research. However, if it becomes possible to use it in the workplace, heart rate can be monitored without large-scale equipment and without placing a heavy burden on the monitored individual. In addition, this technique of acquiring data related to cardiac activity without the need for direct contact with the body should contribute greatly to ensuring safety in the workplace since it can contribute to research in the areas of ergonomics and occupational health. Furthermore, there is a possibility of applying this technique to the simple diagnosis of disease conditions [15]. Our method appears to be promising, not only for use in ergonomics research, but also in several other fields.

References

1. Ciaccio, E.J., Hiatt, M., Hegyi, T., Drzewiecki, G.M.: Measurement and monitoring of electrocardiogram belt tension in premature infants for assessment of respiratory function. Biomed. Eng. Online 6(13), 1–11 (2007)
2. Jacobs, J., Embree, P., Glei, M., Christensen, S., Sullivan, P.: Characterization of a novel heart and respiratory rate sensor. Conf. Proc. IEEE Eng. Med. Biol. Soc. 3, 2223–2226 (2004)
3. Wang, F., Tanaka, M., Chonan, S.: Development of a wearable mental stress evaluation system using PVDF film sensor. Journal of Advanced Science 18(1&2), 170–173 (2006)
4. Matsui, T., Hagisawa, K., Ishizuka, T., et al.: A novel method to prevent secondary exposure of medical and rescue personnel to toxic materials under biochemical hazard conditions using microwave radar and infrared thermography. IEEE Trans. Biomed. Eng. 51, 2184–2188 (2004)
5. Matsui, T., Gotoh, S., Arai, I., Hattori, H., et al.: Noncontact Vital Sign Monitoring System for Isolation Unit (Casualty Care System). Military Medicine 171(7), 639–643 (2006)
6. Uenoyama, M., Matsui, T., Yamada, K., Suzuki, S., et al.: Non-contact respiratory monitoring system using a ceiling-attached microwave antenna. Med. Biol. Eng. Comput. 44, 835–840 (2006)
7. Chen, K.M., Misra, D., Wang, H., Chuang, H.R., Postow, E.: An X-band microwave life-detection system. IEEE Trans. Biomed. Eng. 33, 697–702 (1986)
8. Chen, K.M., Huang, Y., Zhang, J.: Microwave Life-Detection Systems for Searching Human Subjects Under Earthquake Rubble or Behind Barrier. IEEE Trans. Biomed. Eng. 27, 105–113 (2000)
9. Suzuki, S., Matsui, T., Imuta, H., Uenoyama, H., et al.: A novel autonomic activation measurement method for stress monitoring: non-contact measurement of heart rate variability using a compact microwave radar. Medical & Biological Engineering & Computing 46, 709–714 (2008)
10. Singh, N., Mironov, D., Armstrong, P.W., Ross, A.M., Langer, A.: Heart Rate Variability Assessment Early After Acute Myocardial Infarction-Pathophysiological and Prognostic Correlates. Circulation 93, 1388–1395 (1996)
11. Carney, R.M., Blumenthal, J.A., Stein, P.K., Watkins, L., Catellier, D., Berkman, L.F., Czajkowski, S.M., O'Connor, C., Stone, P.H., Freedland, K.E.: Depression, Heart Rate Variability, and Acute Myocardial Infarction. Circulation 104, 2024–2028 (2001)
12. Lohman, B., Boric-Lubecke, O., Lubecke, V.M., Ong, P.W., Sondhi, M.M.: A digital signal processor for Doppler radar sensing of vital signs. In: Proceedings of the 23rd annual international conference of the EMBS IEEE, pp. 3359–3362 (2001)
13. Ivashov, S.I., Razevig, V.V., Sheyko, A.P., Vasilyev, I.A.: Detection of human breathing and heartbeat by remote radar. In: Progress in Electromagnetic Research Symposium 2004, pp. 663–666 (2004)

14. Thijs, J.A.J., Muehlsteff, J., Such, O., Pinter, R., Elfring, R., Igney, C.H.: A Comparison of Continuous Wave Doppler Radar to Impedance Cardiography for Analysis of Mechanical Heart Activity. In: Proceedings of the 27th Annual International Conference of the Engineering in Medicine and Biology Society, pp. 3482–3485. IEEE, Los Alamitos (2005)
15. Matsui, T., Suzuki, S., Ujikawa, K., Usui, T., Gotoh, S., Sugamata, M., Abe, S.: The development of a non-contact screening system for rapid medical inspection at a quarantine depot using a laser Doppler blood-flow meter, microwave radar, and infrared thermography. Journal of Medical Engineering & Technology (in press)

PC-Based Rehabilitation System with Biofeedback

Chih-Fu Wu and Jeih-Jang Liou

40 Zhongshan North Road, 3rd Section Taipei 104, Taiwan(R.O.C.)
Jeih-Jang Liou,liouauto@mail.fit.edu.tw

Abstract. The purpose of this research is to emphasize on the concept of integrating computer and interactive technologies to the rehabilitation robotic with biofeedback. First, the robot is actuated with pneumatic muscle actuator which have interesting characteristics that can be exploited for upper limbed machines. The rehabilitation robotic system is using measurement which has two channels to detect and collect the rehabilitation robotic system from electromyography and the rotary encoder. Through PCI interface transferring the rehabilitation robotic system to personal computer, we can use our algorithms to attain real-time the force and/or contraction velocity of the muscle detection and other common information like the frequency of under muscle curve of user. Finally, the human-computer interface for rehabilitation system is designed. In this human computer interface consists of three main parts: detect the signal; a control scheme of robotic system combined with multimodal environment based biofeedback system; clinical database.

Keywords: rehabilitation robotic, biofeedback, human computer interface.

1 Introduction

The most of contemporary robots use DC or AC motors like the actuators. However, these implementations are often too heavy and rigid, particularly for work in contact with human. Using of these "traditional" actuators in the field of rehabilitation and force feedback devices is especially unsuitable, because rehabilitation are usually grounded on the user is can not bear while being comfortable. The DC or AC motor is relatively unfriendly in feeling. That is the reason why the researchers try to find an actuator similar to human muscles. The most promising actuator in this field of research [1] is undoubtedly McKibben pneumatic muscle actuator(PMA).

A PMA which has achieved increased popularity to provide the inherent safety and mobility assistance to humans performing tasks and another advantages such as high strength and power/weight ratio, low cost, compactness, ease of maintenance, cleanliness, readily available and cheap power source and so on [2-4]. In contrast to tradi-tional pneumatic actuators, PMA have very high power/weight and power/volume ratios [1], [2]. This is an advantage for robotic and exoskeleton applications, in which heavy actuators can add significantly to the payload.

Some scholars have already set up system modelling and performance to assess to the atmospheric pressure muscle driver [5], model analysis of the dynamic characteristic 6]. As for other application, for instance: Is it good for robot to reply [7,8], recovery

B.-T. Karsh (Ed.): Ergonomics and Health Aspects, HCII 2009, LNCS 5624, pp. 204–211, 2009.
© Springer-Verlag Berlin Heidelberg 2009

system [9], nucleon of waste material, use atmospheric pressure muscle biceps and triceps structure that driver form, simulation track, joint of angle control [10,11], applications for robotics [12,13]. Above-mentioned methods are all feedback methods. In the rehabilitation process, the user's feeling is taking most. Thus, biofeedback is considered in the rehabilitation. Originally we consider in the article the rehabilitation system include feedback and biofeedback. In addition, progress made in computer technologies has encouraged rehabilitation engineers to apply computer technologies in helping disabled people to enjoy greater degree of independence in their daily living. However, users may still rely upon special interface to communicate with a computer. Providing physically disabled persons with adequate human/computer interface may thus contribute greatly to improve their independence. The human-computer interface which operators of the rehabilitation engineer use is very important.

2 Structure in Rehabilitation System

2.1 Mechanical Structure

The PMA is a kind of principle of moving on the basis of studying the organism, change external energy but become the soft driver with similar human muscle characteristic.PMA consists of a cylindrical flexible rubber or plastic airtight tube that fits snugly inside a braided plastic sheath with helical winding. When the tube is inflated, it widens and due to the braided sheath, shortens. The axial force exerted when the PMA shortens is quite large in proportion to the PMs weight. Because of their

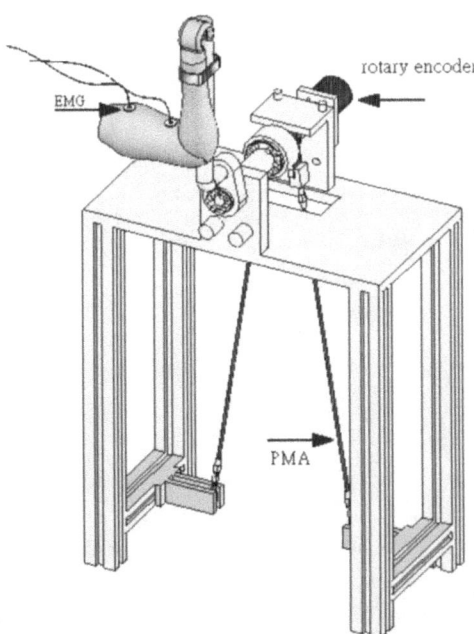

Fig. 1. The prototype of the rehabilitation robotic

construction, PMA are similar to human skeletal muscles in size and power output capability. However, PMA can only exert a single directional pulling force. In order to build a bi-directionally working revolute joint, two PMAs are coupled similarly to the antagonistic muscles of animals. Hence, the rotating torque is generated by the pressure difference between the antagonistic muscles and the external load is rotated. A joint angle is detected by rotary encoder. The prototype of the rehabilitation robotic are illustrated in Fig. 1. The operation principle of this robot, give two atmospheric pressures muscle in the regular initial pressure first, the arm is in the state of making for the first time at this moment, then mediate the pressure of both sides muscle. At this moment, the pressure expands greatly but the pressure is extended small, the arm joint will rotate the angle.

2.2 Electrical Structure

Many physiological processes can be monitored for biofeedback applications, and these processes are very useful for rehabilitation services. Biofeedback is a means for gaining control of our body processes to increase relaxation, relieve pain, and develop healthier, more comfortable life patterns. Electromyography is a seductive muse because it provides easy access to physiological processes that cause the muscle to generate force, produce movement and accomplish the countless functions which allow us to interact with the world around us [14].

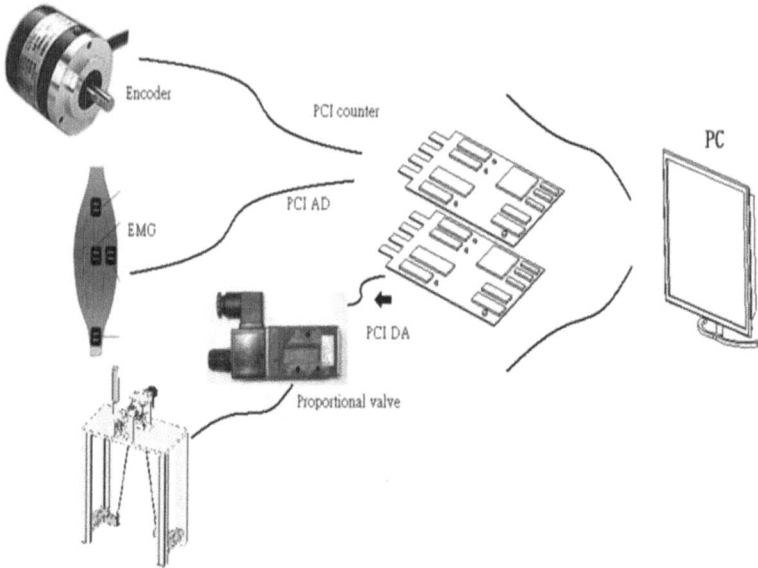

Fig. 2. Schematic diagram of the rehabilitation robotic

The experiment are carried out according to the closed-loop structure of t the rehabilitation robotic shown in Fig. 2. In the rehabilitation robotic, the joint angle, θ, is detected measured by rotary encoder and the processing of electromyography (EMG) signals from the user and feedback to PC through PCI counter board and AD board, respectively. A primary function of the robot is controlling the gas pressure sent to PMA via the processing of electromyography (EMG) signals from the user. The rehabilitation robotic system is using measurement which has two channels to detect and collect the rehabilitation robotic system from EMG and the rotary encoder. Through PCI interface transferring the rehabilitation robotic system to personal computer, we can use our algorithms to attain real-time the force and/or contraction velocity of the muscle detection and other common information like the frequency of under muscle curve of user. Besides, the personal computer calculated the control input and controlled the proportional valve through D/A board.

3 PC-Based Rehabilitation System

3.1 Software Structure

Soft Structure unit interface shown in Fig. 3. was developed for physiological monitoring of a diver using embedded digital signal process. The software is built in Visual Basic environment and runs under Windows XP. The sequence of implemented procedures follows:

- Reading of encoder via PCI counter.
- Reading of EMG signal via PCI AD card.
- Connecting the database.
- Computing of forces to be applied to control valve via PCI DA card.
- Design the man-machine interface.

The software also displays to user important data, like angle, EMG signal, desired and real pressure in muscles. User can set time, angle and force.

3.2 Human-Computer Interface

The human-computer interface which operators of the rehabilitation engineer use is very important. If there is any operation error, the consequence will cause the muscle injuring. It is necessary to verify the design of interface which operators use in advance to prevent errors for the reason of inadequate design. Then we can get the advice for improvement, and low down the chance of error. In this human computer interface consists of three main parts: detect the signal; a control scheme of robotic system combined with multimodal environment based biofeedback system; clinical database. These interfaces are shown in Fig.4-6.

3.3 Clinical Database

Users can check their medical treatment records just by entering ID numbers. Because the processing of rehabilitation, these records are very useful for long-term tracing and analyzing users' condition. In this study, the rehabilitation database system consists of three main parts: user's operating time; user's functional ability dataset and related outcome information. From the experiences of establishing the database

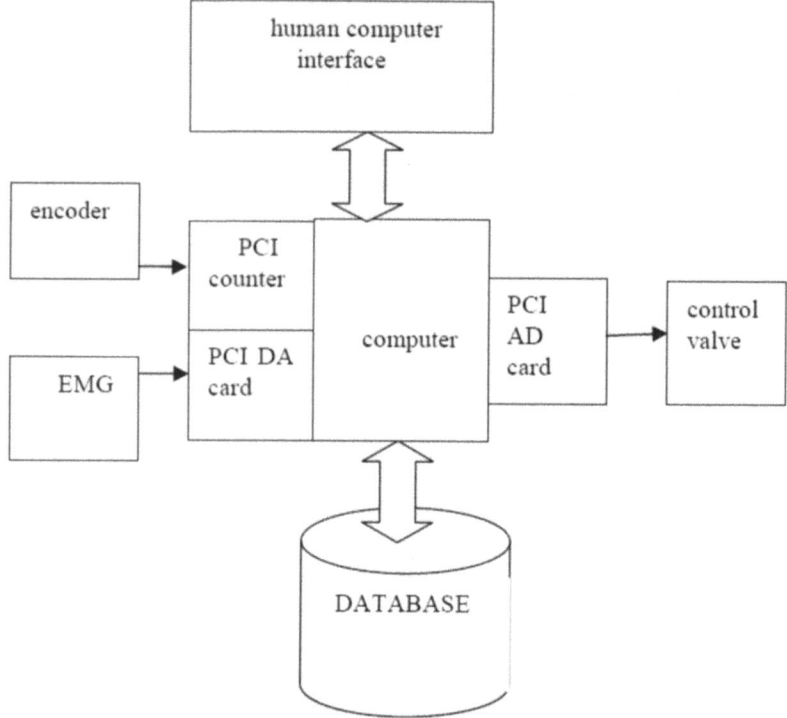

Fig. 3. Instructure of Robot Monitor

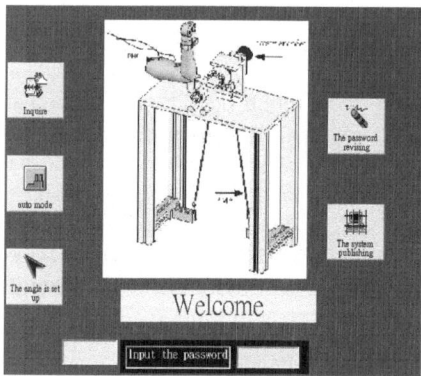

Fig. 4. Screen shot of "Multimodal environment"

as well as the clinical data collection, suggestions about the use of the database and limitations will be discussed. Moreover, the development of this project facilitates the disabled persons to use commercial pointing devices that are lowly priced and easily available. Also, with this newly developed robotic, the disabled persons can have a second choice over some specific devices that are highly priced or difficult to maintain.

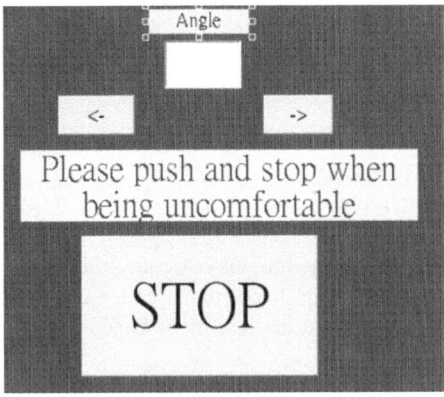

Fig. 5. Screen shot of "The joint angle testing"

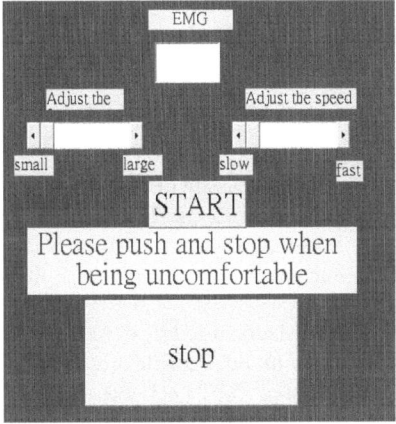

Fig. 6. Screen shot of "Force and speed adjustment"

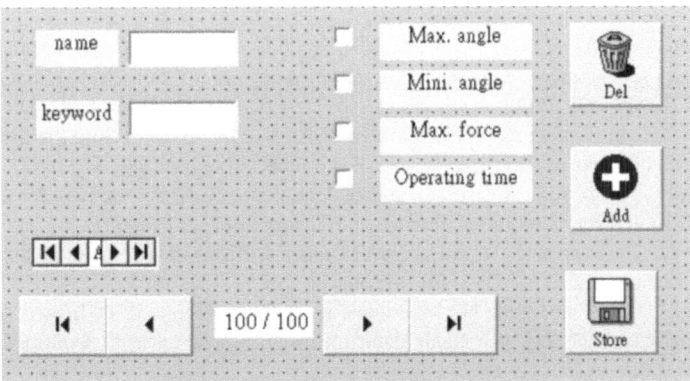

Fig. 7. Screen shot of "Clinical Database"

4 Result

The result of this paper are:

- For the purpose of rehabilitation robotic design, the concept of PMA is introduced to simplify the design procedure.
- Originally we consider in the article the rehabilitation system include feedback and biofeedback.
- For the rehabilitation system, the human-computer interface is designed. This interface consists of three main parts: detect the signal; a control scheme of robotic system combined with multimodal environment based biofeedback system; clinical database.

Acknowledgments

The work was partly supported by National Science Council, Taiwan, R.O.C., under Grant No. 97-3114-E-036-001.

References

1. Tondu, B., Lopez, P.: Modeling and Control of McKibben Artificial Muscle Robot Actuators. IEEE Control Systems Magazine, 15–38 (2000)
2. Chou, C.P., Hannaford, B.: Static and Dynamic Characteristic of McKibben Pneumatic Artificial Muscles. In: IEEE International Conference on Robotics and Automation, vol. 1, pp. 281–286 (1994)
3. Tsagarakis, N., Caldwell, D.G., Medrano-Cerda, G.A.: A 7 DOF pneumatic muscle actuator (pMA) powered exoskeleton. In: 8th IEEE International Workshop on Robot and Human Interaction RO-MAN 1999, pp. 327–333 (1999)
4. Bergamasco, M., Micheli, D.M., Parrini, G., Salsedo, F., Marchese, S.S.: Design Considerations for Glove Like Advanced Interface. In: Proceedings International Conference on Advanced Robotics, Pisa, Italy (1991)
5. Caldwell, D.G., Medrano-Cerda, G.A., Goodwin, M.: Charakteristics and Adaptive Control of Pneumatic Muscle Actuators for a Robotic Elbow (1994)
6. Caldwell, D.G., Tsagarakis, N., Medrano-CerdaS, G.A.: Bio-mimetic actuators: polymeric pseudo muscle actuators and pneumatic muscle actuators for biological emulation. Mechatronics 10, 499–530 (2000)
7. Reynolds, D.B., Repperger, D.W., Phillips, C.A., Bandry, G.: Modeling the dynamic characteristics of pneumatic muscle. Annals of Biomedical Engineering 31, 310–317 (2003)
8. Prior, S.D., White, A.S.: Measurement and simulation of a pneumatic muscle actuator for a rehabilitation robot. Simulation Practice and Theory 3, 81–117 (1995)
9. Noritsugu, T., Tanaka, T.: Application of rubber artificial muscle manipulator as a rehabilitation robot. IEEE/ASME Trans. Mechatron. 2, 259–267 (1997)
10. Caldwell, D.G., Tsagarakis, N., Medrano-Cerda, G.A., Schofield, J., Brown, S.: A pneumatic muscle actuator driven manipulator for nuclear waste retrieval. Control Engineering Practice 9, 23–36 (2001)

11. Lilly, J.H.: Adaptive tracking for pneumatic muscle actuators in bicep and tricep configurations. IEEE Transactions on Neural System and Rehabilitation Engineering 11(3), 333–339 (2003)
12. Yang, L., Lilly, J.H.: Sliding mode tracking for pneumatic muscle actuators in bicep/tricep pair configurations. In: Proceedings of the American Control Conference, Denver, Colorado, June 4-6, 2003, pp. 4669–4674 (2003)
13. No-Cheol, Hyun-Seok, Parj, H.-W., Park, Y.-P.: Position/vibration control of two-degree-of-freedom arms having one flexible link with artificial pneumatic muscle actuator. Robotics and Autonomous System 40, 239–253 (2002)
14. Inoue, K.: Rubber actuators and applications for robotics. In: Bolles, R., Roth, B. (eds.) Robotics Research: The 4th International Symposium. MIT Press, Cambridge (1988)
15. De Luca, C.J.: The use of surface electromyography in biomechanics. Journal of Applied Biomechanics 13(2), 135–163 (1997)

Part III

Interaction Devices and Environments

LED Backlight for Better Accuracy in Medical Imaging

Silvio Bonfiglio and Luigi Albani

FIMI Philips, via S. Banfi 1, 21047 Saronno, Italy
{Silvio.Bonfiglio,Luigi.Albani}@philips.com

Abstract. In clinical tasks the display is often the natural interface between the medical system and the medical professionals and in the current image-centric healthcare the accuracy of the visualized images represents a key requirement; ideally no compromise would be acceptable. In the recent past LED backlights for liquid-crystal displays have been intensively investigated for their use in displays addressed to the mainstream markets (mobile and portable displays, computer displays and TV). Accordingly adapted, they could offer new opportunities also to the displays used in healthcare by allowing better accuracy and consistency of the medical images. In this respect they could make possible a new, important advance towards a better quality of care.In this paper we will describe a novel LED backlight solution suitable for medical imaging.

Keywords: BLU, backlight, backlight unit, color gamut, display, healthcare, LCD, LED, imaging, image accuracy , medical imaging.

1 Introduction

Imaging in healthcare is opening new horizons in the continuous effort of the medical science towards a better quality of care. Images of parts of our body are used for diagnostics, to detect as earlier as possible the uprising of pathologies. Images – often in 3D format – are used for the planning of complex surgical interventions and minimally invasive, image-guided procedures are replacing traditional surgical approaches. Images are transmitted from one part to another one of the world and telemedicine and telesurgery are removing the physical distances between the patient and the physician or the surgeon. Even in therapeutic treatments the images are becoming very important: think about the virtual reality used in therapeutic programs for patients suffering from psychological stress or other mental diseases. Other new and innovative display technologies are entering into the clinical setting: large screen displays and projectors for multi-image applications, 3D displays in ultrasound and in CT or MRI, head-mounted displays for augmented reality and for immersive virtual reality experiences, portable displays for the mobile point of care, etc.

The display visualizing all these images represents the "natural interface" between the medical system and the physician. Since each detail of the image could have a "clinical relevance", the overall image chain will be effective if the display reproduces the "source image" without introducing artifacts and without reducing the quantity of "clinical information" it contains and if there is consistency over time and between same images reproduced in different displays.

B.-T. Karsh (Ed.): Ergonomics and Health Aspects, HCII 2009, LNCS 5624, pp. 215–222, 2009.
© Springer-Verlag Berlin Heidelberg 2009

Currently the display represents one of the weakest element in the medical image chain:

- spatial (dot/inch) and grayscale (number of displayed gray levels) resolutions are below the characteristics of some medical images (e.g. mammography) and below the capability of the human vision system,
- color gamut i.e. the overall range of reproduced colors is often limited and far below the overall range of available colors,
- response time, viewing angle and contrast in some displays (e.g. the liquid-crystal displays) are sub-optimal and these limitations introduce unwanted artifacts,
- brightness is often limited to avoid excessive power dissipation (e.g. in LCDs) or visual artifacts.

The backlight of the LCD monitors has been an area heavily investigated in the last decade.

In the transmissive displays such as the liquid-crystal ones the backlight represents the source of light that each LC cell - after modulating it in intensity according to the applied input video signal - will transfer outside (see fig. 1).

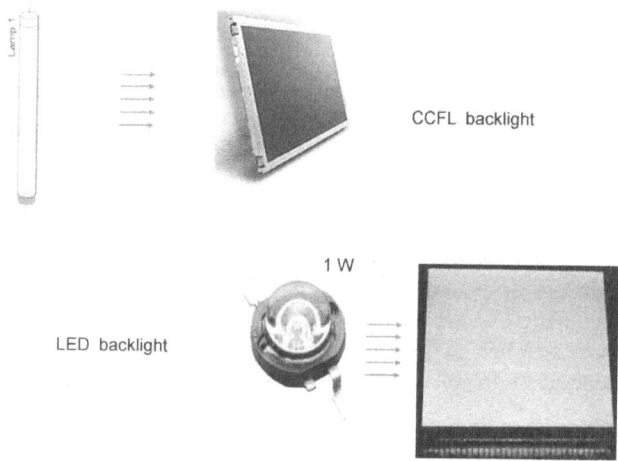

Fig. 1. CCFL and LED backlights

For long time LCD backlights have been based on the use of fluorescent lamps (cold cathode fluorescent lamps – CCFL); among the alternative technologies developed in the recent past LED backlights have been the most successful ones and are expected to replace the traditional CCFL in the coming years in all the applications (from cars and traffic lights to mobile phones, monitors and TVs) and at the same time to enter in the general lighting market.

2 LED Backlights – General Benefits

The list of benefits offered by LED backlights is quite long:

- Wider gamut: 105% of the NTSC color space compared to 65-75% of the conventional CCFL technology ; this extended color gamut allows a richer variety of colors including vivid and saturated true colors ;
- Real-Time Color Management - Instantaneously controlling of colors on a variety of data streams to enhance viewing experience;
- Fully dimmable without color variation;
- Fast response time allowing the implementation of blinking backlights for larger contrast and greater picture clarity (less blurring);
- Instant on (less than 100ns) (@ full color, 100% light);
- Higher energy efficiency;
- Very Long Operating Life (up to100k hours) and increased durability and reliability of system;
- No UV / IR in the light source (only visible wavelengths emitted) avoiding degradation of the optical system and extending product life;
- Green/Environmental : no mercury in system;
- Safe operation - low voltage.

Moreover it is important to highlight that the tuning of the white point - when using a conventional CCFL backlight - is possible only by acting on the R,G,B input video signals with the consequent drawback of a reduction of the driving levels (smaller dynamics). On the contrary in LED backlights the tuning is done by acting on the primary colors of the LEDs and the same number of reproducible colours at various colour temperatures can be achieved (see Fig. 2).

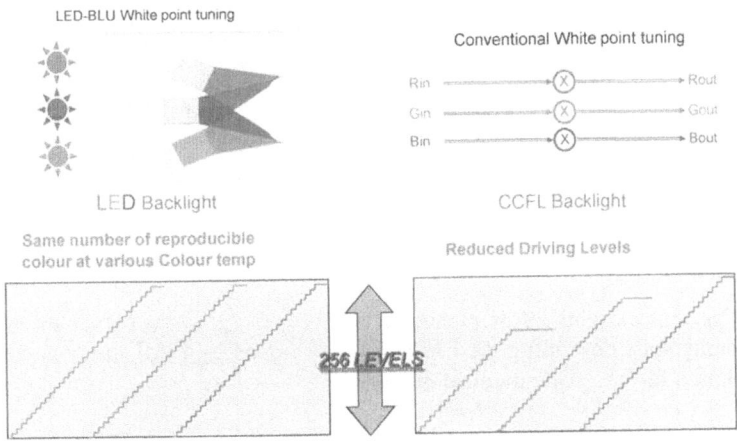

Fig. 2. White point tuning in LED and in CCFL backlights

Through the use of LED backlight the display will enrich its color gamut and enhance the effectiveness of the interfacing between the electronic equipment and the user by enriching the fidelity of the image (see Fig.3).

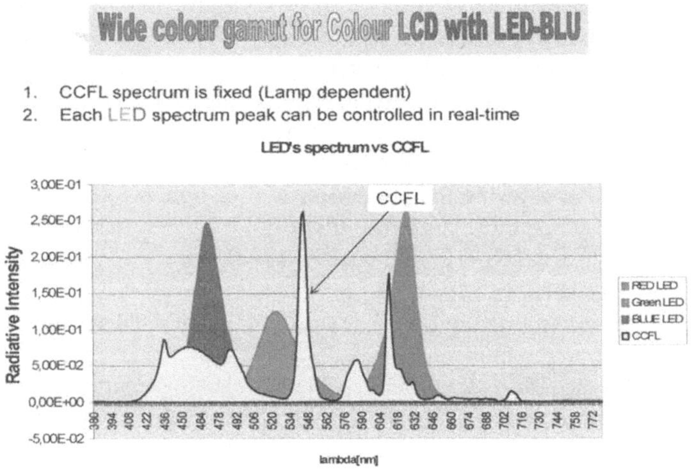
Wide colour gamut for Colour LCD with LED-BLU
1. CCFL spectrum is fixed (Lamp dependent)
2. Each LED spectrum peak can be controlled in real-time
LED's spectrum vs CCFL
CCFL
Radiative Intensity
lambda[nm]
RED LED
Green LED
BLUE LED
CCFL

Fig. 3. Wide color gamut of LED backligrhts

3 LED Backlights in LCD Displays Used for Medical Images

FIMI Philips developed a novel LED backlight specifically devoted to medical LCD displays. It includes an optical architecture and an overall design concept addressing some weaknesses currently present in the LED backlights solutions available in the market such as the limited luminous efficiency and uniformity.

Medical images visualization needs some specific requirements to be satisfied. The most important of them are:

- Luminance response compliant with the DICOM standard
- High luminance values (> 500 nit)
- Good white and color uniformity
- White point adjustability
- Accurately aligned and stabilized luminance level
- Extended lifetime

LED based backlights allow pursuing most of these goals as explained in the following paragraphs describing the LED BLU developed by FIMI in cooperation with PDS and used for grayscale medical displays.

3.1 Optical and Mechanical Architecture

The optical system was derived from a "folded mixing light guide" concept [2] where the optical function is split into two parts: one part for mixing the primary colors into white light and a second part where the light is properly distributed on the LCD glass surface (see Fig. 4). In order to get the desired output light level the system efficiency has to be maximized by reducing as much as possible the light losses along the light path.

Indeed the length of the mixing light guide has been reduced with respect to the system described in [1] and the additional mirror just in front of the LED was removed.

Since the optimal mixing light guide length is the result of a compromise between good color uniformity (achievable with a long mixing light guide) and minimal light losses (achievable with short light guide), its length was optimized considering the specific requirements of the application.

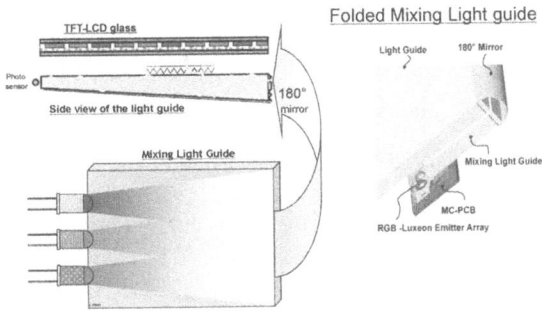

Fig. 4. The optical system of the LED Backlight developed by FIMI

A further light output improvement can be achieved by properly choosing the LED colors. LED are available in fact at several wavelength and flux. In a medical grayscale monitor very saturated colors aren't required - being the images monochromatic - so white LEDs can be included in the LED array. Doing this way some "extra light" can be added at a color temperature close to the target ones.

3.2 LED Color Mixing

Though the reasoning described in the paragraph above would let suppose that only white LED is the best solution for what concern the light output level, the color point adjustability asks for colored LED to be included in the array.

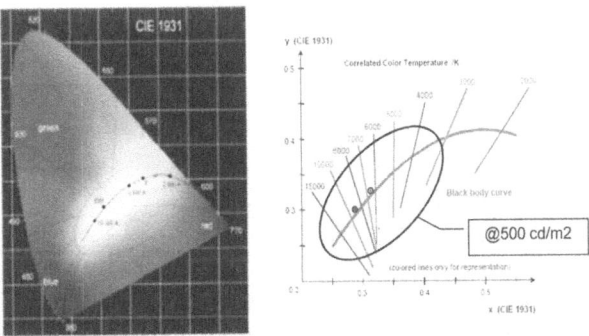

Fig. 5. LEDs enable White Point adjustability unique future in monochrome LCD monitors

The white point of the monochrome LCD Monitor can be tuned around the black body curve (see Fig. 5).

The reduced color gamut caused by the presence of white LED allows a greater accuracy in controlling each color point inside the gamut itself. Indeed, considering that the LED control is achieved through a PWM driving scheme, the same number of available PWM driving levels is spread on a smaller triangle in the x, y chromaticity diagram. This allows a more accurate adjustment and control for each point lying inside the triangle itself.

For the 18" monitor we used 40 LED's of 1 W each, binned and matched for a uniform White.

3.3 Light Loop Control

The image consistency required by the medical applications needs to keep the light performances of the monitor constant over time.

Besides that, monitors calibrated at the same color temperature must look equal when put one close to the other (e.g. in displays used in the ceiling suspensions of the operating theater)

The former goal can be achieved by keeping the driving level of LED below the maximum at the beginning of the monitor life and increasing the driving level as the LED efficiency decreases due to the aging. The latter requirement can be achieved by continuously and accurately balancing the driving level of each color.

The monitors with CCFL backlight do not allow the color temperature control therefore the display matching can only be achieved by product sorting.

In the implementation described in this paper, both goals are obtained through a closed loop control [1] implemented by a microcontroller that reads the light values supplied by a trichromatic color sensor and accordingly adapts the PWM driving levels.

The graph in the previous Fig. 5 shows the range of color temperature at 500 cd/m2 with the present implementation. The optical feedback is shown in Fig. 6.

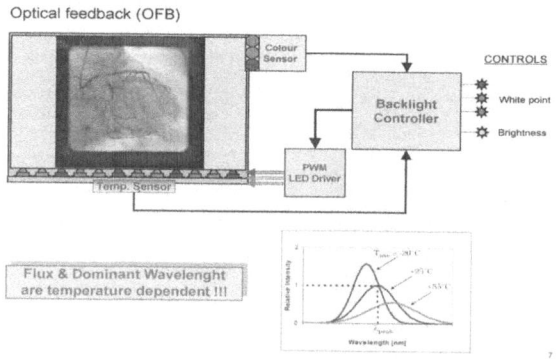

Fig. 6. The optical feedback of the LED backlight

It gives the benefits of:

- Luminance and colour consistency over time and vs. temperature changes (in fact flux and dominant wavelength are temperature dependent);
- LED aging compensation;
- Accurate white point tuning.

3.4 Thermal Management

The LED lifetime is strictly linked to the working temperature of the devices itself: lower working temperatures guarantee longer lifetimes. A good thermal management has to be implemented in order to keep the light output decay as small as possible.

In our design a set of thermal fins has been added on the back of the LED metal core PCB that efficiently spreads the heat produced by the LEDs on a wide surface keeping the devices temperature reasonably low.

Additional cooling systems with axial fans blowing on the mentioned fins could further reduce the working temperature at the expenses of an increased noise level.

4 Achieved Results

The previously mentioned techniques have been implemented in monitor samples using array of 40 high power LEDs. Some measurements were carried out in order to evaluate the system performances.

An 18" monochrome monitor was calibrated at three different color temperatures (6500K, 7600K and 9300K) and at a luminance level of 500 cd/m2. The measured power consumption of the complete set was around 49 W. The power consumption was roughly the same for a similar product provided with standard CCFL backlight and calibrated at the same luminance level was. Of course the CCFL model was not adjustable in terms of color temperature.

Further improvements in terms of efficiency are advisable in the near future since the LED performance in terms of lumen per watt is continuously improving.

The brightness and color uniformity of the complete set (including the LCD panel) was evaluated on a standard nine points pattern.

The results were:

- Brightness uniformity $\cong 85\%$
- Color uniformity ≤ 0.005 u', v' i.e. matching the typical color detectability limit of the human visual system.

5 Conclusion

The LED-based backlight offers the unique feature of controlling the white point of displayed image (fine tuning of the LCD display's white point and maintained over time); it guarantees panel-to-panel consistency in terms of white color and luminance and easier monitor replacement in multi-display installations.

The current monitors with CCFL backlights do not allow the white point control therefore the display matching can only be obtained through product sorting.

Moreover the developed solution of LED backlight overcomes the main limitations linked to the LED technology such as efficiency and uniformity of both color and brightness and offers saving in cost of ownership by achieving a longer life time

It enhances the image accuracy and stability in critical applications such as the medical imaging ones. In fact appropriate matching of the white point of two or more adjacent displays ensures consistency in the various medical images and improves the accuracy of the task of physicians and radiologists.

Acknowledgements

The authors thank Mr. Paul Aerssens of Professional Display Systems B.V. for his contribution to the design of the backlight unit.

References

1. Perduijn, A., et al.: Light Output Feedback Solution for RGB LED Backlight Applications. In: SID 2003 Symposium Digest, vol. 34, pp. 1254–1257
2. Martynov, Y.: High-efficiency Slim LED Backlight System with Mixing Light Guide. In: SID 2003 Symposium Digest, vol. 34, pp. 1259–1261

Human Factors in Lighting

Martin Braun, Oliver Stefani, Achim Pross, Matthias Bues, and Dieter Spath

Fraunhofer-Institute for Industrial Engineering (IAO) 70569 Stuttgart, Germany
martin.braun@iao.fraunhofer.de

Abstract. This paper addresses current research activities on the interaction between light and humans, including visual perception as well as cognitive, biological, and emotional factors. We focus on issues which can be deployed at office workplaces and describe how we adopt these findings at the "nLightened Workplace" at the Fraunhofer Institute for Industrial Engineering. The nLightenend Workplace integrates illumination and information displays in offices. We present our latest developments such as "Heliosity". We will give an outlook on our future research work on human factors in lighting.

Keywords: Lighting, Office Work, Human Factors, Performance and Health.

1 Introduction

Designs of ergonomic workplaces cover all elements of a working system and the relevant environmental factors. Light is an important factor for the appropriate interaction of humans, technology and information.

More than half of the people asked in a random sample in a study done by Çakir/Çakir [5] describe the lighting situation in their job with negative attributes like unpleasantly and unfriendly. Very often artificial lighting is not only considered as unpleasant, but even as health-impairing. Natural light even affects vital functions of the human organism.

Due to architectural restrictions however, healthy and productivity-enhancing natural light in offices can rarely be ensured. Missing natural light makes artificial lighting indispensable especially in winter after dusk. Sophisticated artificial lighting concepts can prevent health impairments and support motivation and performance capability of humans. To avoid tiredness during winter or noon and to prevent seasonal affective disorder or changes in mood, the employment of smart lighting concepts is essential.

The impact of light to humans can be summarized in three main topics:

- Visualization of Information
- Illumination of the environment and
- Effects on Health

In this paper we will address these topics with innovative concepts to improve the quality of life and save energy at the same time.

B.-T. Karsh (Ed.): Ergonomics and Health Aspects, HCII 2009, LNCS 5624, pp. 223–230, 2009.

2 Impacts of Light on Humans

2.1 Biological Effects of Light

The biological scope of light differs vastly from the visual effect. Light that infiltrates over the eye and skin into the body is an essential external trigger for the endogenous rhythms. It triggers the endogenous oscillator according to rhythms of days, weeks and years and therefore the function of ductless glands and cell metabolism. Hence light takes regulative effects on the complex arrangement of functions of the organism. The communication of the viscera is based on the release of the hormone melatonin into the cardiovascular system [15].

The amount of melatonin that is produced by the pineal gland is regulated by the circadian photoreceptor melanopsin in the retina of the eye. Melatonin causes tiredness and regulates the sleep-awake-rhythm and further circadian organ functions. The production of melatonin is aborted through effect of light [1].

The sensibility of melanopsin dependant on the wavelength is shown in figure 1. The maximum of the melatonin suppression and therefore the circadian activation is at 464 nanometers, which corresponds to blue light [16].

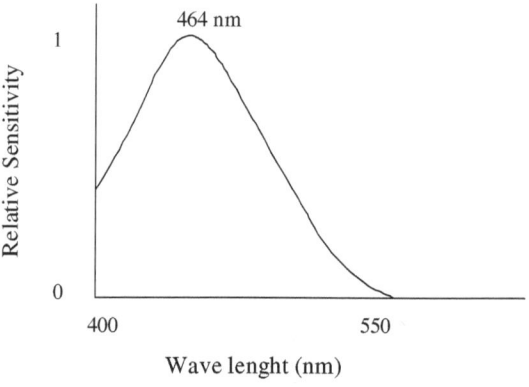

Fig. 1. Circadian sensitivity curve (Brainard et al. 2001)

2.2 Emotional Effects of Light

Balanced illumination and enjoyable colour temperatures attend the well being in the short and long term [10] [13] ascribes a relaxing effect for the raise of well being, appetite and quality of sleep to the natural sunlight. The emotional effect of light is sensed extremely individual and depends on experiences and moods. Thus light and illumination conditions that are comparably comfortable for all people do not exist. However the following effects are indentified:

Cool and white illumination with narrow spectrum lead to increased hyperactivity, exhaustion, excitability and attention deficits, whereas lamps with full spectrum contribute to an overcoming of problems with reading and learning [12].

Glaring illumination can result in an inner tension, psychological fatigue and impairment of condition. Glaring is often associated with the attributes colourless and cold (more than special colour temperatures).

2.3 Effects of Light on the Cognitive Performance

Cognitive functioning domains range from simple attention to logical reasoning, working memory, long-term memory, and complex executive functions that are usually assessed through objective, task-oriented performance measures. The main cognitive processes are shown in figure 2.

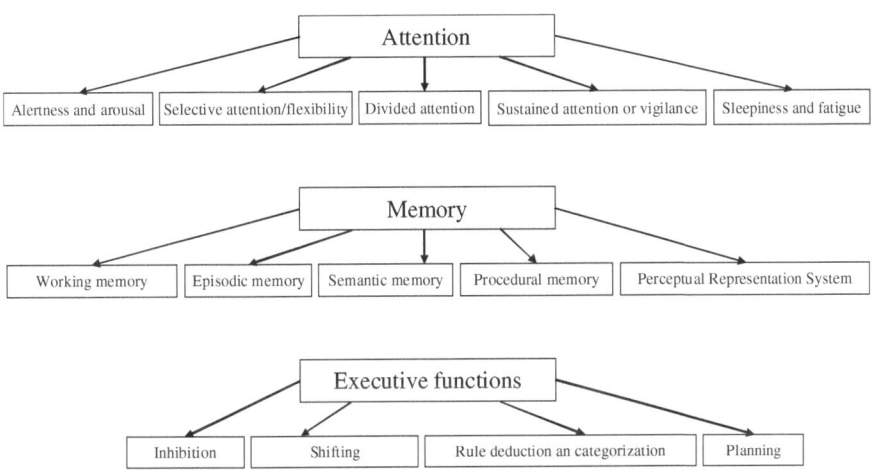

Fig. 2. Overview of the main cognitive processes

Some cognitive functions – like attention and activation – are connected to the temporary devolution of the circadian rhythm. This is revealed through the coincidence of drops in performance and a minimum of body temperature, which serves as an approved indicator for the circadian rhythm [4]. In more simple visual tasks the maxima of body temperature and performance curve occur nearly simultaneous at about 8:00 p.m.

Attention denotes a central cognitive function. It is imaginable in many degrees from casual remark to full attention, whereas the last one can be hold only a short time (Schmidt et al. 2007). *Vigilance* is related to frequency of occurrence, signal strength and other context criteria (e.g. light). [9] proved that an enhancement of illumination strength can raise vigilance. For complex tasks a precipitous ascent of vigilance in the morning, a performance maximum at early afternoon and a subsequent slow decline of performance is denoted (Folkard 1990). This difference to the devolution in simple, visual tasks arises probably from the influence of sleep regulating processes [7]. The sleep requirement increases over the period of being awake (Fig. 3). This seems to derogate the execution of more complex cognitive tasks in a bigger extent than the one of more simple visual tasks.

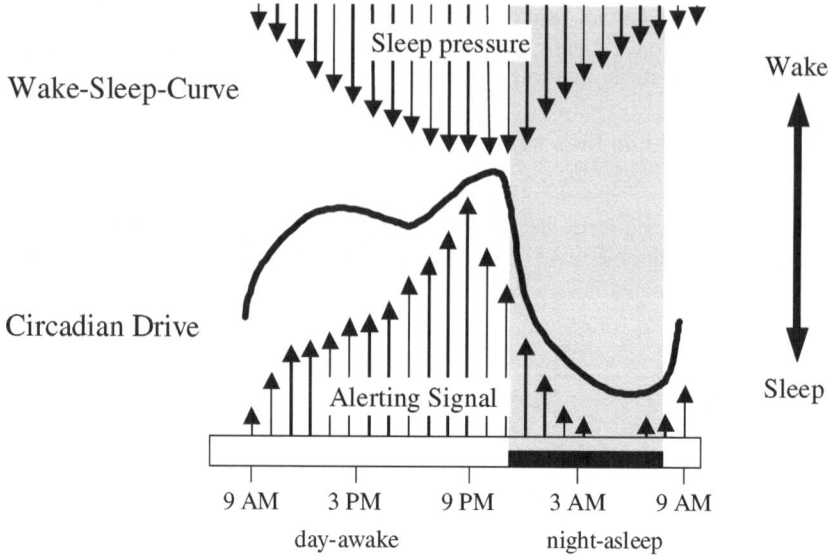

Fig. 3. Circadian und homeostatic processes as mediator of being awake and asleep (Edgar et al. 1993)

Central influence on the attention has *activation* – that is also called alertness [1]. Fluctuations of attention reflect a varying level of activation. The influence of light on the activation is obvious in the natural circadian rhythm. Corresponding to Cajochen (2007) tiredness and performance decline can be countered by short-wave blue light.

3 Impulses for the Arrangement of Light at the Workspace

Effects of light on mood, performance and health remained widely unconsidered in work design. Only since few years the interest in an integrated arrangement of light has increased. Illumination systems that are designed according to the requirements of humans establish appropriate conditions for cognitive and physiological work and contribute to maintaining health of working people. To attune the situation of illumination to human's needs the following criteria should be followed:

– Conservation of photometric quality criteria,
– with reasonable dynamic change of light,
– under inclusion of natural day light.

Emotional effects refer basically to individual subjectivity and can't be appropriately determined by means of objective criteria. For coloured lighting design the principles of harmony should be considered. Beside the principles for creation of harmony of colours mainly the avoidance of disharmonies and the comprehension of a preferably wide spectrum should be regarded.

For the human oriented light design it is recommended that illumination is not perceived as a static, consistent installation in a room and his restricting surfaces.

At present a series of prototypical installations do exist that emit blue light of high intensity with a wavelength of 464 nanometers. By suppression of the release of melatonin an activating impact of the circadian rhythm is aspired. Because the circadian effective receptor is settled in the eye, an influence over the display as primary viewing object for screen handling seems to be effective. One should keep in mind that the circadian sensitivity curve differs from the one of the blue cones. The maximum of the blue receptors is at 420 nanometers, the one of melanopsin is at 464 nanometers. The level of activation should be designed in such a manner that additional burdens or even resistances are avoided. A shift of the circadian rhythm is imaginable if strong exposure to light at the workspace occurs during the morning or in the late evening (Fig. 4). The diagram clarifies how an exhausting phase shift rises with increasing level of illumination.

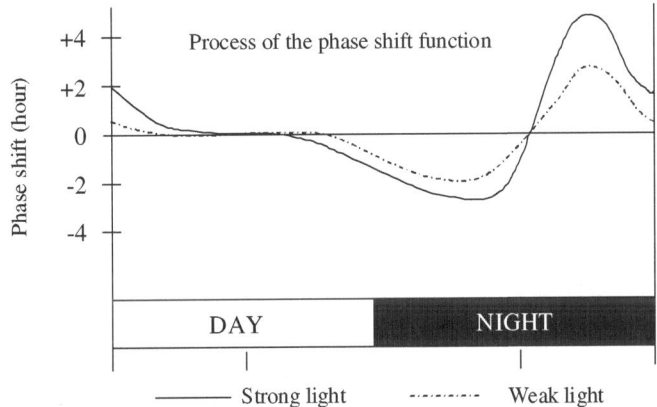

Fig. 4. Influence of the moment of exposure to light on the phase shift of body temperature for two levels of illumination (Rea 2002)

4   The nLightened Workplace at Fraunhofer IAO

Today's display workplaces have one or two screens with approximately 20 inch diagonal. These displays-centered workplaces were shaped more by technical conditions than by human requirements concerning performance and health. Apart from the ergonomic weaknesses of the limited screen surface and thereby same time representable information capacity limited the operational procedure.

The n-Lightened workplace will overcome the limits of the traditional office workplace and will replace these by the generalized concept of the digital work surface. The prototype of the n-Lightened Workplace is a 45 m² room with modular walls that can be replaced by either displays, illuminated spaces or passive spaces with additional "tracked spots" that allow for the individual highlighting of moving objects. With this modular concept we are able to integrate new display technologies as soon as they are available as prototypes. To save energy the nLightened Workplace will use natural daylight as a source of light to backlight large area, passive Displays

(LCD). A combination of a variable diffuser and a LCD panel will be used on a standard window to realise our "Smart Window". All components of the nLightened Workplace, i.e. light sources, displays, daylight elements and passive areas will be controlled by a central system which knows the geometrical distribution of all components and their physical properties such as the maximum luminance. Additionally the light emission from displayed images will be considered. The transmission of the picture information to the respective displays is network based; each display surface is a knot, visible in the network with defined parameters such as size, position, resolution and brightness. The brightness adjustment of the display surfaces is directly controlled through their sources of light.

A central control system enables the dynamic representation of an optimal light situation in space, within certain limits even selectable by the user. The n-Lightened Workplace (Fig. 5) is a research and integration platform for prototype applications, in which work and interaction concepts for concrete applications are developed and evaluated.

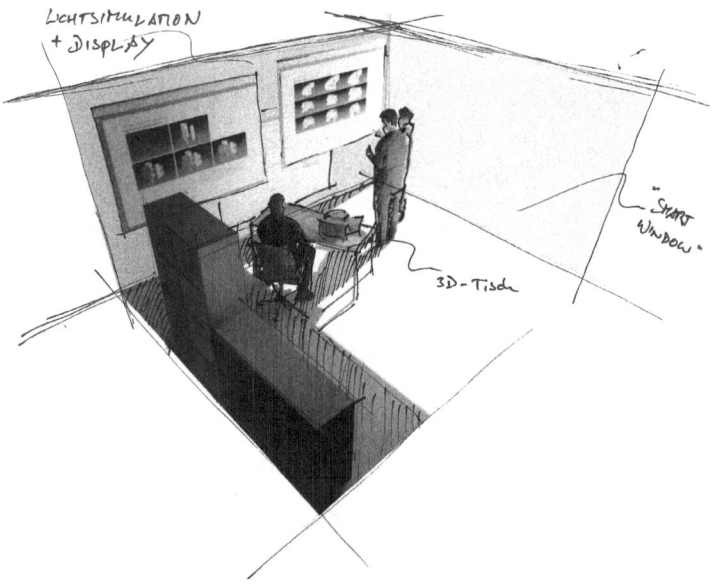

Fig. 5. Design study of the nLightenend Workplace

In nature, the colour of light changes during the day from a reddish warm white in the morning to cold, bluish tones during noon and to red during dusk. If one concludes from the evolutionary adjustment of humans to those colour changes, then it needs to be examined if artificial dynamic lighting has positive effects on humans' wellbeing and performance. Due to the coupling of human rhythms with natural light rhythms positive effects are to be expected with artificial dynamic lighting. "Heliosity" is such a light source which can be dynamically adjusted in both colour and intensity. It is based on five differently coloured LEDs plus one cold-white LED

(Fig. 6). This enables us to tune the colour of light very similar to the changes of natural daylight. If all six LEDs are turned on simultaneously, Heliosity provides a white light with a nearly continuous spectrum similar to that of daylight (Fig. 7). Therefore we expect similar advantages for health and well-being as they are known from sunlight and full spectrum lamps.

By dimming individual colours different light colours can be achieved with a discrete spectrum. The CRI (colour rendering index) with all LEDs turned on is much better than that of standard fluorescent lamps (FL) and the colour gamut is larger than that of conventional LC-displays with LED backlight. The light guide design in conjunction with the use of a *plexiglas* with specialized properties facilitates a smooth and uniform distribution of the emitted light. The *plexiglas* is a transparent, light-diffusing acrylic (PMMA) that exhibits special light-conducting and emitting properties.

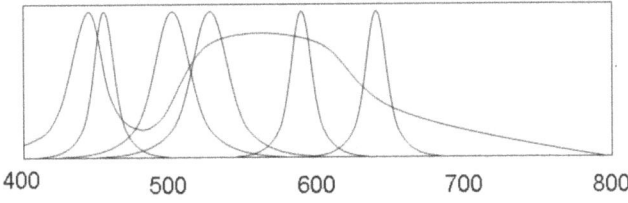

Fig. 6. Spectrum of LEDs used in Heliosity

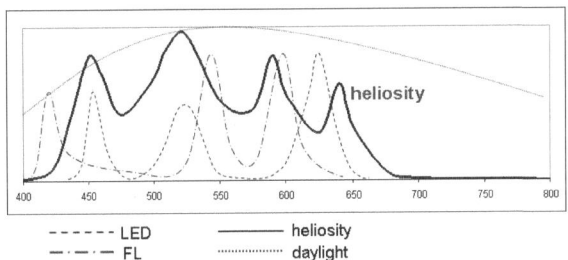

Fig. 7. Spectrum of Heliosity in comparison to daylight, LED-Backlight and fluorescent light (approximation)

5 Future Research Work

Under laboratory conditions we will examine the effects of dynamic light on humans' working performance and health. We suppose that the synchronous light will improve health and efficiency. A desynchronisation might lead to illness and incapacity to act. We need to consider that the bluish-cool white and thus the melatonin suppression during noon could suppress the afternoon low, however, the warm white tones in the evening before the end of work could promote tiredness rather than suppress it. Various colour sequences need to be investigated, compared and evaluated against their effectiveness to enhance productivity. Many cognitive functions of humans are subject to the so-called Basic Rest Activity Cycles (BRACs). Natural light changes from light to shade caused by passing clouds occur in a similar time range as BRACs. It needs to be examined whether the reproduction of the cloud play by artificial lighting can stimulate cognitive functions. To investigate our hypothesis we are currently installing a large area LED display on the ceiling which will enable us to simulate various colour and light variations.

References

1. Baumeier, D.: Der Einfluss von Licht auf die Psyche. Diss, Universität Leipzig (2000)
2. Bäumler, G.: Auf dem Weg zur operationalen Definition von Aufmerksamkeit. In: Hansen, J., Hahn, E., Strang, H. (eds.) Konzentration und Leistung, pp. 11–26. Hogrefe, Göttingen (1991)
3. Brainard, G., Hanifin, J., Greeson, J., Byrne, B., Glickman, G., Gerner, E., Rollag, M.: Action Spectrum for Melatonin Regulation in Humans: Evidence for a Novel Circadian Photorecep-tor. Journal of Neuroscience 21(16), 6405–6412 (2001)
4. Cajochen, C.: Alerting effects of light. Sleep Medicine Reviews 11, 453–464 (2007)
5. Çakir, A., Çakir, G.: Forschungsbericht des Projekts "Licht und Gesundheit". Ergonomic Institut, Berlin (1998)
6. DIN Deutsches Institut für Normung: DIN EN 12464-1; Beleuchtung von Arbeitsstätten; Teil 1: Arbeitsstätten in Innenräumen. Beuth, Berlin (2003)
7. Elmenhorst, E., Gerzer, R., Manzey, D., Samel, A., Wenzel, J.: Zirkadiane Rhythmen. In: Letzel, S., Nowak, D. (eds.) Handbuch der Arbeitsmedizin, 7, Aufl. Landsberg: ecomed, Kapitel B II-2.1 (2008)
8. Figueiro, M.: Research Recap: Light, Aging & the Circadian System – Riviving All that Jazz? Lighting Design & Application 33(6), S8–S11 (2002)
9. Fleischer, S.: Die psychologischer Wirkung veränderlicher Kunstlichtsituationen auf den Menschen. Zürich, Eidgenössische Technische Hochschule, Diss. (2001)
10. Fisch, J.: Licht und Gesundheit – Das Leben mit optischer Strahlung. Technische Universität Ilmenau (2000)
11. Folkard, S.: Circadian performance rhythms: some practical and theoretical implications. In: Broadbent, D., Baddeley, A., Reason, J. (eds.) Human Factors in Hazardous Situation. Clarendon Press, Oxford (1990)
12. Gall, D.: Die Messung circadianer Strahlungsgrößen. Tagung Licht und Gesundheit, Berlin, February 26–27 (2004)
13. Liberman, J.: Die heilende Kraft des Lichts – Der Einfluss des Lichts auf Psyche und Körper, 6th edn. München, Piper (2005)
14. Lorincz, A.: The physiological and pahtological changes in skin from sunburn and suntan. Journal of the American Medical Association 173, 1227–1240 (1960)
15. Rea, M.: Light – Much More Than Vision. In: Light and Human Health: EPRI/LRO 5th International Lighting Research Symposium, pp. 1–15. The Lighting Research Office of the Electric Power Research Institute, Palo Alto (2002)
16. Schmidt, C., Collette, F., Cajochen, C., Peigneux, P.: A time to think: Circadian rhythms in human cognition. Cognitive Human Psychology 24(7), 755–789 (2007)
17. Thapan, K.: An action Spectrum for melatonin suppression: evidence for a novel non-rod, non-cone photoreceptor system in humans. Journal of Physiology 535(1), 261–267 (2001)

Lighting as Support for Enhancing Well-Being, Health and Mental Fitness of an Ageing Population – The FP6 EU Funded ALADIN Project

Inge Gavat[1], Ovidiu Grigore[1], Marius Cotescu[1], Markus Canazei[2], Hermann Atz[3], Klaus Becker[4], Lajos Izso[5], Guido Kempter[6], Herbert Plischke[7], and Wilfried Pohl[2]

[1] "Politehnica" University of Bucharest, Splaiul Independentei 313, Ro 40063 Bucharest,
[2] Bartenbach Light Laboratory GmbH, Rinner Straße 14, A-6071 Aldrans
[3] Institute for Social Research and Opinion Polling, Dominikanerplatz 35, I- 39100 Bolzano
[4] Becker Meditec, Karl-Seckinger Straße 48 D-76229 Karlsruhe
[5] Budapest University of Technology and Economics, Egry J, u. 1. E bldg., H-1111 Budapest
[6] University of Applied Sciences Vorarlberg GmbH User Centered Technologies Research Institute Hochschulstraße 1 A-6850 Dornbirn
[7] Ludwig-Maximilians-Universität München, Generation Research Program Prof.-Max-Lange-Platz 11, D-83646 Bad Tölz
igavat@alpha.imag.pub.ro

Abstract. The paper presents the ALADIN prototype for adaptive lighting control designed to assist elderly in achieving a state of well-being, developed as a FP6 EU funded project. It uses psycho-physiological features extracted from Electro-Dermal Activity (EDA) and Pulse signals to determine the subject's mental state and adapts the lighting parameters in order to achieve a certain desired state. One of the controller implementations was done using Simulated Annealing. Field test evaluations of this implementation are discussed.

Keywords: adaptive lighting; psycho-physiological parameters; optimization algorithms.

1 Introduction

In this paper we will present the ALADIN system, built in order to enhance the well-being status of elderly by controlling light through mood dependent psycho-physiological parameters.

Due to the socio-demographic change in most developed western countries, elderly populations have been continuously increasing. Therefore, developing preventive arrangements and assistive systems that allow elderly people to live in their own homes independently as long as possible have become an economical and ethical necessity. Within the EU-funded project Ambient Lighting Assistance for an Ageing Population (ALADIN) a new adaptive lighting device that is capable to adapt to the psycho-physiological needs of an elderly person has been developed and pilot-tested. The long-term aim is to create an adaptive system capable of improving the residential

B.-T. Karsh (Ed.): Ergonomics and Health Aspects, HCII 2009, LNCS 5624, pp. 231–240, 2009.

lighting conditions of single living elderly person, so that it may support elderly individuals in the preservation of their independence. Main outcome criteria comprise wellbeing, life quality, mental and physical fitness as well as sleep quality. The system was evaluated for three months in field-tests with twelve subjects who were supported concerning technical matters by coaches during the test period. Results show a significant increase of wellbeing, life quality and mental fitness.

The project was realized by an interdisciplinary consortium of six partners, coordinated by the User Centered Technologies Research Center in the Vorarlberg University from Dornbirn, Austria. The involved partners are: APOLLIS, Institute of Social Research and Opinion Polling, Bolzano, Italy; BME- Budapest University, Department of Ergonomics and Psychologies; BLL, Bartenbach LichtLabor Innsbruck, Austria; Becker Meditec, Karlsruhe, Germany; GRP- Generation Research Program at the Ludwig Maximilian University Munich, Germany; UPB- University "Politehnica" Bucharest, Department of Applied Electronics and Information Engineering.

1.1 The ALADIN Prototype

The ALADIN prototype provides the following functions:

- An adaptive control circuit and biofeedback system which can adapt various light parameters such as intensity, light distribution or color in response to the psychophysiological data. The system therefore continuously registers physiological indicators of psychological processes on the surface of the body by wireless, smart sensors and transfers them to the adaptive feedback system. For this adaptive algorithms are used to compute the lighting conditions best suited to the individual or to a particular situation.
- A manual control system that can be adjusted via graphical user interfaces (GUI). This system does not only permit to override the computationally derived lighting parameters by the algorithms, but also allows the resetting of all light parameters to their default values. Moreover, supervisors may also change the individual configuration of the adaptive algorithms by defining individually suitable values of the light parameters. These adjustments can in turn be used by the system for further refining and optimizing the adaptive algorithms.
- An advice and support application based on the most recent findings on the factors that influence people's sense of well-being, their mental alertness and physical fitness to assist older people in becoming aware of their own affective-cognitive states including their circadian rhythms. This is achieved by visualizing the psycho-physiological data received from the individual in a clear and accessible way.

The structure of the system is represented in Fig. 1. The system user activates in an enlightened environment and has sensors that measure the interesting psycho-physiological parameters. If they do not correspond to the desired person's status, they could be changed by the adaptive light control circuit; it will modify the lighting conditions (intensity and spectral competence of the light) in order to bring the psycho-physiological parameters to the desired situation's target values. The change of the light parameters can be done also manually by the user. The system can advise the user regarding the mental state enhancement.

Users can control the ALADIN system by a standard remote control. The chosen parameters and settings are displayed on a standard TV screen. From the main menu they can select individual applications of the ALADIN system, like for example adaptive lighting or exercises. During adaptive lighting and biofeedback exercises psychophysiological data of the user are monitored and are either used to calculate and apply new lighting situations (adaptive lighting), or visualized on the TV screen (biofeedback) for giving the user feedback of his current state. In both cases a feedback loop is created. In addition to adaptive lighting, users can also switch to a manual lighting mode at any time. Furthermore, activation exercises are supplied to help users get mentally activated. After finishing the exercises their results are then visualized in an accessible manner, where users can see how they improved over time. Based on these results also well-being advices are provided by the system to support the users.

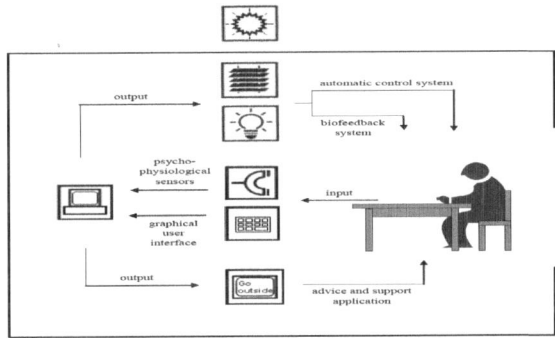

Fig. 1. Structure of the ALADIN system

1.2 Realization Steps of the System

The system was realized, tested and refined in less than two years, in a collaborative work between partners.

The prototype of the ALADIN system was developed in the first year of the project based on the results of the requirements analysis. However, elderly people were involved in the development of the software as well as invited to provide feedback used in the prototype at all stages. The system was tested from January until August 2008 and evaluated in twelve households in Germany (Bad Tolz), Austria (Innsbruck, Dornbirn) and Italy (Bolzano) under field conditions.

Essential to build the prototype was to establish the light sensible psychophysiological parameters of users. This was the major responsibility for the team of Budapest, Prof. Lajos Izsó with his Ph.D. students Lazsló Laufer and Ádám Horváth. They established by experiments done on elder people that especially the skin conductance and the heart rate could be light controlled and that they have variation trends which can be associated with a state of relaxation or activation.

Also very important was to have adequate sensors to measure these parameters and transmit the results wireless to the processing part of the prototype. Each user has to keep on him these sensors during the experiment, and put them easy up and down. That was the task of Becker Meditec, directed by Klaus Becker.

In order to use this signals, a signal processing chain was devised, with contribution of all partners, after long discussions, in order to fulfill best possible the requirements for the developed algorithms.

Two teams were responsible to develop algorithms: the team Andreas Künz, Philipp von Hellberg and Karl-Heinz Emich directed by prof. Guido Kempter from the Applied Sciences University of Vorarlberg (FHV) and the team prof. Inge Gavat, prof. Ovidiu Grigore and Marius Cotescu from the University "Politehnica" Bucharest (UPB). FHV developed the manual control, the advice program and a genetic algorithm to automatic light control. The basic soft installation and the supervision of the platform programs was also their responsibility. UPB developed three light control algorithms in form of stochastic optimization algorithms: the global random search, the local random search and the simulated annealing.

The controllable lighting system was realized by Bartenbach LichtLabor (BLL) team, Markus Canazei, and Siegfried Mayr directed by Wilfried Pohl. They also provided an interesting evaluation of the light controlling algorithms, the genetic one and the simulated annealing.

The field tests, during from January 2008 until august 2008 were conducted in 12 households: in Italy by the Apollis team, Ulrich Becker and Elena Vanzo directed by Hermann Atz, in Germany by the GRP team, Astrid Schuelke, Astrid Plankensteiner, and Guido Haase directed by Herbert Plischke and in Austria by the FHV team Edith Maier and Guido Kempter. The tests were very laborious but successful and proved for the test subjects' enhancements in mental fitness and quality of life.

The results determined long discussions in the project team continued during the congress "Light and the Ageing Society" held in October 2008 in Bad Tolz. At the end of the congress we could conclude that the ALADIN project is a first, but important step on the way to help elderly to live independently in their own homes as long as possible with light based assistive technology.

2   Signals and Control Algorithm

The Adaptive Lighting System is composed of two main modules: the Signal Processing Module, and the Light Control Module. The Signal Processing Module records and analyses the data collected from the subject in order to extract three features, while the Light Control Module uses the information provided by the features to determine the new lighting parameters.

2.1 The Signal Processing Module

The information of the subject's psycho-physiological state is extracted from two sources: Electro-Dermal Activity (EDA) and Pulse signals [1]. The EDA signal is collected using two electrodes placed on the subject's hand and The Pulse signal is measured using a pulse-oximeter. From these two signals, three features are extracted: Skin Conductance Level (SCL), Skin Conductance Response (SCR), and Inter Beat

Interval (IBI). The SCL and SCR features are extracted from the EDA signal and offer important information of the subject's psycho-physiological state, while IBI is extracted from the Pulse signal, offering complementary information on the subject's activation or relaxation state.

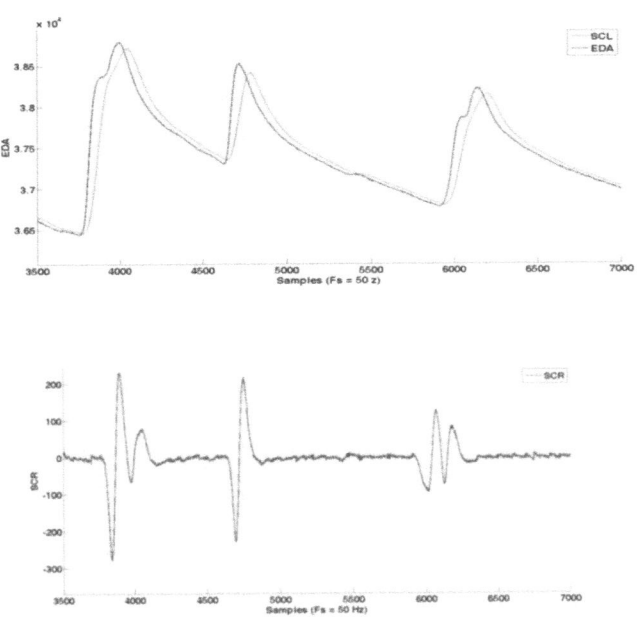

Fig. 2. EDA processing for extracting SCL (top) and SCR (bottom) features

$$SCL(t_1) = \frac{1}{2 \cdot K} \sum_{j=-K}^{K} EDA(t_1 + j \cdot T) \tag{1}$$

$$SCR(t_1) = StDev(EDA(t_1) - SCL(t_1)) \tag{2}$$

SCL and SCR are the continuous and, respectively, alternative components of EDA. The SCL is computed as the moving average of the skin conductance calculated using a certain time window, while the SCR feature is obtained by subtracting the SCL feature from the raw EDA data. In our measurements the time window was 2 seconds long, but slightly shorter or longer windows are also applicable. It is worth trying to experiment with different window sizes in order to maximize the algorithms' light adaptation capability.

Both features show a strong response to the light stimulus. The subject reacts to a light stimulus by a sudden rise of the EDA signal, followed by a slow decrease of the signal's value. Tests performed by our partners from the University of Budapest [2], show that a relaxed subject should have small values both for the SCL, and SCR features. But because of the EDA's reaction to light, the SCL feature might not fall quick enough after the reaction to the light stimulus, thus building up in value even though the SCR feature shows that the subject is relaxed.

The Electro-Dermal Activity (EDA) is measured in micro-Siemens; the value of an average adult is between 10 – 20 micro-Siemens. According to our and BLL's experiments elderly sometimes does not have almost any skin conductance, sometimes have only up to 4 micro-Siemens. This means that if we are developing algorithms for elderly, in the software development period we have to use elderly as test person, otherwise the algorithms might not be applicable for them.

IBI (Inter-Beat Interval) is the time interval elapsed between two heart beats. It is measured as the distance in time between two maximums of the pulse signal. As we said earlier, the Pulse signal is measured using an oximeter. This technique is frequently subject to artefacts caused by the patient's movements that are propagated into the IBI signal as high frequency spikes. These can be easily removed from the signal through integration.

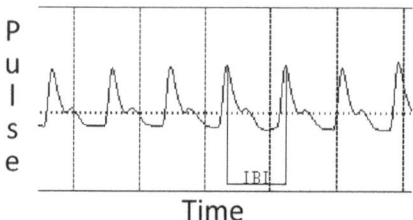

Fig. 3. Pulse signal processing

After each change in the lighting conditions, the SCR, SCL and IBI features are monitored for 20 seconds in order to extract the mean SCL, the standard deviation of the SCR feature and the mean IBI over the analysis window. Further on, by SCL, SCR and IBI we will be referring to the values computed from the 20 second analysis window. The three features are integrated in an objective function through the following equation:

$$E = 0.7 \cdot SCR + 0.2 \cdot SCL + 0.1 \cdot IBI \qquad (3)$$

2.2 Simulated Annealing

Simulated annealing is a generalization of a Monte Carlo method for examining the equations of state and frozen states of n-body systems [3]. The concept is based on the manner in which liquids freeze or metals re-crystallize in the process of annealing. In an annealing process a melt, initially at high temperature and disordered, is slowly cooled so that the system at any time is approximately in thermodynamic equilibrium. As cooling proceeds, the system becomes more ordered and approaches a "frozen" ground state at $T=0$. Hence the process can be thought of as an adiabatic approach to the lowest energy state. If the initial temperature of the system is too low or cooling is done insufficiently slowly the system may become quenched forming defects or freezing out in meta-stable states (i.e. trapped in a local minimum energy state).

The original Metropolis scheme was that an initial state of a thermodynamic system was chosen at energy E and temperature T, holding T constant the initial configuration is perturbed and the change in energy dE is computed. If the change in energy is negative the new configuration is accepted. If the change in energy is positive it is accepted with a probability given by the Boltzmann distribution $\exp(-dE/T)$. This processes is then repeated sufficient times to give good sampling statistics for the current temperature, and then the temperature is decremented and the entire process repeated until a frozen state is achieved at $T=0$.

The most commonly used annealing schedule is the *exponential cooling*. Exponential cooling begins at some initial temperature T_0, and decreases the temperature in steps according to $T_{k+1}=\alpha \, T_k$ where $0<\alpha<1$. Typically, a fixed number of moves must be accepted at each temperature before proceeding to the next. The algorithm terminates either when the temperature reaches some final value T_f, or when some other stopping criterion has been met.

The choice of suitable values for α, T_0 and T_f is highly problem-dependent. However, empirical evidence suggests that a good value for α is 0.95 and that T_0 should be chosen so that the initial acceptance probability is 0.8. The search is terminated typically after some fixed, total number of solutions has been considered. A more detailed description of the algorithm and parameter optimization can be found in [2] and [4].

3 Algorithm Evaluation in Field Tests

The field tests were performed at three locations: one in Austria at Innsbruck, one in Germany at Bad Tolz, and one in Italy at Bolzano. At each location, four volunteers were chosen, age 65 or older, who received an Adaptive Lighting System for their personal use. The tests lasted for four weeks. During this period they were asked to do at least one test lasting 30-60 minutes every day. The data was recorded and later analyzed at Bartenbach LichtLabor.

The lighting system is shown in Fig. 4, and it consists of four ambient and one local light systems. Each light system has two independent light sources, one with a Colour Temperature of 2700K, and one with 8000K. Each light source is dimmable, covering a spectrum from 2700K to 8000K. The ratio between local and ambient light is adjustable.

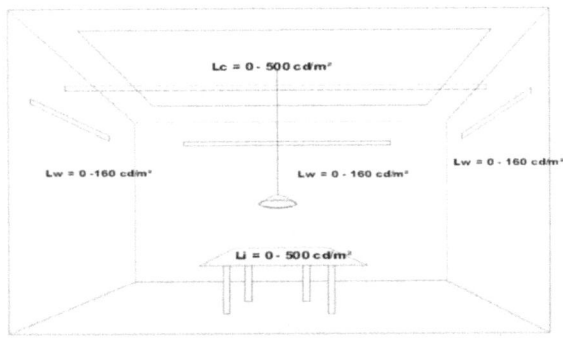

Fig. 4. Lighting system components

The main goal of the analysis was to determine whether the system functioned correctly and succeeded in inducing the subject a state of relaxation. We have analyzed the variation of lighting parameters and psycho-physiological features during the tests. The mean and standard deviation was computed for the psycho-physiological and lighting parameters at the beginning and end of every test. The biological features' evolution is shown in Fig. 5. The SCR feature clearly shows a descending trend, indicating that the system succeeds in relaxing the subjects. The SCL shows a small variation towards lower values, but it is too small to be considered significant. The IBI feature remains relatively constant. These results are in accordance with the study performed by our partners at the University of Budapest.

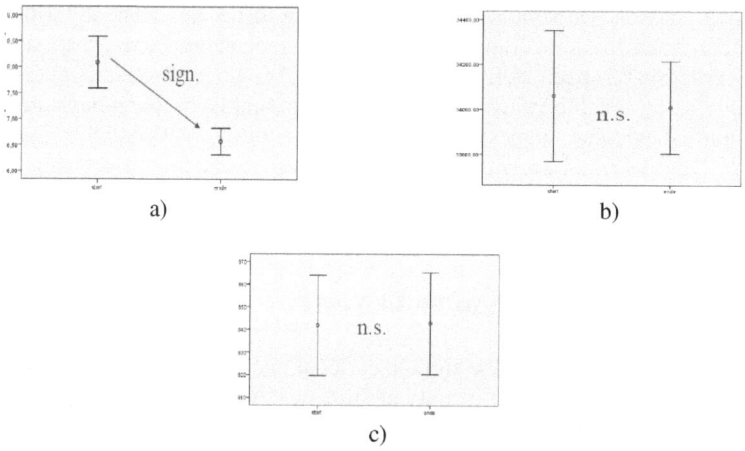

Fig. 5. Psycho-physiological features variation: a) SCR, b) SCL, c) IBI

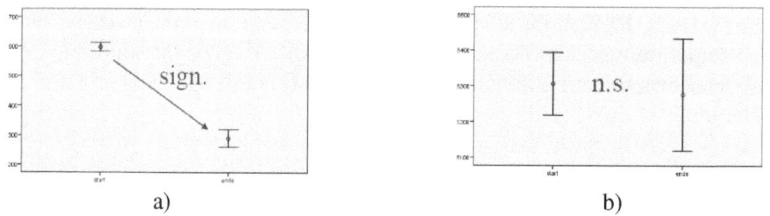

Fig. 6. Lighting parameters variation during tests. a) Intensity, b) Color Temperature.

Fig. 6 shows the variation of the lighting parameters during the tests. The light's Intensity clearly moves toward lower values, which seem to induce the relaxation state. The light's Color Temperature, on the other hand doesn't show the same kind of variation, indicating that its influence on the subject's state is much lower.

Fig. 7 depicts the SCR map over the Lighting Parameters space for one of the subjects. The surface is similar with the one that we have obtained during laboratory tests, and shows a global optimum towards lower Intensity and Color Temperature, but also the same local optimum in the middle of the map.

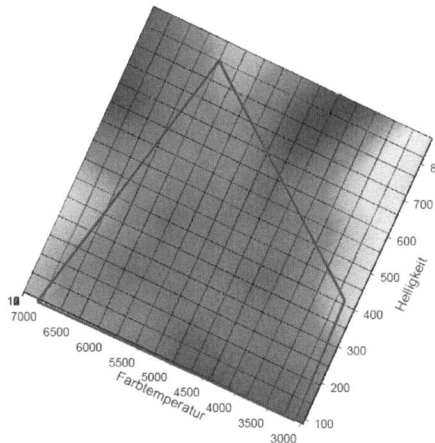

Fig. 7. SCR feature map for one of the volunteers

4   Conclusion

We have developed and adaptive lighting system intended to enhance the elderly population's state of well-being by assisting them in achieving the desired mental state – either relaxed or activated. The system relies on 10 independent channels of light – half providing a 2700 K white light, and half 8000 K – to deliver a large palette of light intensity and color temperature. The lighting parameters can be controlled either by manual input, or by automatic control provided by the Adaptive Lighting Controller which was implemented using the Simulated Annealing algorithm.

The system was tested on 12 volunteers, older than 65 years, in three different European locations. The field tests showed that the SCR feature was more dependent of the lighting situations than the other two psycho-physiological features. It also showed that the light intensity played a more dominant role in determining the subjects' psycho-physiological state over the color temperature.

We consider the system to be an important step towards commonly using adaptive lighting in households to improve the inhabitants' well-being by providing assistance in achieving a desired mental state.

Acknowledgments. The work and results presented in this paper are part of the FP6-2005-IST-6 framework, for the "ALADIN - Ambient Lighting Assistance for an Ageing Population" project.

References

1. Grigore, O., Inge, G., Grigore, C., Cotescu, M.: Psycho-Physiological Signal Processing and Algorithm for Adaptive Lighting Control. In: 2nd International Symposium on Electrical and Electronics Engineering, pp. 13–18. Galati University Press, Galati (2008)

2. Grigore, O., Inge, G., Grigore, C., Cotescu, M.: Stochastic Methods Used in Adaptive Lighting Control. In: International Multi-Conference on Engineering and Technical Inovetion 2008, Orlando (2008)
3. Metropolis, N., Rosenbluth, A.W., Rosenbluth, M.N., Teller, A.H.E., Teller, E.: Equation of state calculations by fast computing machines. The Journal of Chemical Physics 21, 1087–1092 (1953)
4. Grigore, O., Inge, G., Grigore, C., Cotescu, M.: An adaptive lighting system using the simulated annealing algorithm. In: 8th conference on Simulation, modelling and optimization, pp. 142–147. World Scientific and Engineering Academy and Society (WSEAS), Stevens Point (2008)

The Evaluation of Operating Posture in Typing the QWERTY Keyboard on PDA

Han-Chi Hsiao, Fong-Gong Wu, Ronald Hsi, Chih-I Ho, Wen-Zhou Shi,
and Chien-Hsu Chen

Department of Industrial Design, National Cheng Kung University, 1,
Ta-Hsueh Road, Tainan, Taiwan 70101, Taiwan
hedyhanchi@yahoo.com.tw

Abstract. In this research, we observed the user's posture while using PDA. 30 participants typed the keys with standard QWERTY keyboard on the PDA. At the end of the experiments the participants who have professional background in design were asked to complete an open-ended questionnaire, which is in order to evaluate the usability of the PDA. In the final, we presented the suggestion of design criterion for keyboard, as to provide the references for future PDA design. The statistical result of the posture while using the PDA revealed that the most users held PDA with both hands and pressed keys with both thumbs. The findings in this research suggest that when we design small input devices such as PDA in the future, the stability of the keyboard usage should be taken into considerations to enhance its input performance and improve user experience.

Keywords: Letters Key Design, PDA Typing Posture.

1 Introduction

The use of digital mobile devices is becoming popular with the fast growing economy, many business workers have grown used to working with a PDA to do computer related work. The most common work done on a PDA is text input, which includes the input of electronic mails or SMS text messages. Many past researches had focused on the muscle and bone injury caused during text input using a keyboard: Serina and others [1] found that incorrect wrist and forearm posture during text input is a risk to indisposed upper limb muscle and bone; Straker and others[2]did research on the comparison of text input posture between the use of desk top computers and laptop computers back in 1997, along with the effect on typing posture change under different types of working environment; Kotani and others[3] brought forward the effect different horizontal positions of keyboards have on forearm and wrist posture during typing; the further the keyboard is from the user the smaller the ulnar deviation angle and the larger the back bending angle, a supporting mattress could help with the back bending problem. As for posture analyzing, Baker and others [4] brought forward the study of kinematics of fingers and hands during computer operation.

Colle et al . [5]studied the features of the keys, focusing on the experiments on the different sets of key sizes (10, 15, 20, 25mm) and gaps (1.3mm) between virtual number

B.-T. Karsh (Ed.): Ergonomics and Health Aspects, HCII 2009, LNCS 5624, pp. 241–249, 2009.
© Springer-Verlag Berlin Heidelberg 2009

keys. The best size was found to be between 15~20mm, and no obvious effect was found in the gap differences. Gong and Tarasewich[6]designed a new alphabetical distributed input pattern to be used on mobile phone keypads. Sears et al. [7]studied the effects of different key sizes and user operation on virtual key data input on mobile devices. Many others studied different types of keys [8][9][10][11], including varies virtual and concrete keypads and small-sized concrete keypads designed for mobile devices. Li et al.[12]studied single-handed input keypad design. Kim et al.[13]studied the use of small QWERTY keypads on portable electronic devices. Wobbrock et al.[14]studied the integration of joystick control and touch screen as an input pattern on small devices. As for key operation efficiency, Silfverberg el al.[15] established a formula predicting text input speed on mobile phones. Mizobuchi et al.[16]focused on the connection between walking speed and the level of mobile phone text input difficulty.

From earlier researches, many human-engineering related problems on standard computer keyboard input operation have already been discovered, especially problems with diseases caused by long-term incorrect posture. However, these standard keypad arrangements are still very common in the market today. With increased functions and decreased sizes on mobile devices, small-sized standard keypads are being used, especially on personal digital assisting devices. Using a large number of keys in a limited space with a repetition of incorrect posture often causes injury around hand areas (fingers, wrists, forearms etc.). For fingers, past studies focused on thumb posture during mobile phone operation [17], thumb adduction/abduction and palm flexion/extension problems were found. Since no literature has fully covered the study of PDA keypad operation posture, our research will focus on the observation of vertical QWERTY keypad operation on text input, with further advice on key designs.

2 Method

The NOKIA E71 model has been chosen for our experimental observations. There are two major stages to the research. The first stage covers the observation of PDA operation posture of users and the later stage focuses on the connection between PDA operation posture and the pain caused. Our goal is to conclude suitable operation posture for PDA and recommend better PDA key designs.

2.1 Experiment A: PDA Operation Posture Observation

Experiment A observes the different types of PDA operation posture. That is, observing vertical PDA users typing English on QWERTY keypads, focusing on the operation posture while standing and sitting. The independent variable being the operation style (standing, sitting), the dependent variable being hand posture types, the controlled variable being gender, distance between screen and participant, and experimental environment. Data obtained from the experiment is handed to four human-engineering specialists for further classification according to posture.

2.1.1 Subjects
Thirty subjects were obtained from National Cheng-Kung University. They were asked to be right-handed with no RSI or other hand injuries, to frequently input text,

and to have normal eye-sight with or without lenses. All subjects need to sign an agreement prior to the experiment. The 30 subjects participating in the experiment all came from a design background, between the ages of 21-37 with an average age of 24.7±3.2, and an average palm width of 78.42 mm(SD: 6.55). Subjects include 15 male, with an average age of 26 (SD: 1.08) and average palm width of 84.07 mm (SD: 0.80); 15 females with an average age of 24 (SD: 0.47) and an average palm width of 72.77mm (SD: 0.85).

2.1.2 Experimental Procedure and Measurements

Describe the goal and task of the experiment to subjects in advance and ask for basic information and measure palm width. Then ask subjects to operate on the PDA models in the two operation styles of standing and sitting. The subjects are asked to input English text once for the two operation styles, with the text given to them on a Microsoft Power Point 2003 file 460 cm in front of them. The operation style order and one of the two English text is given in random. 15 subjects are asked to stand first and 15 to sit. The distance between standing and sitting subjects is 91.7cm.

Prior to the experiment, researchers describe experiment procedures to the subjects and do test runs. Photographs are taken to keep a record of posture before and after operation. Subjects are asked to input an English text with a model of the NOKIA E71 mobile phone and are asked to read each letter as they type to record the input speed. For example, when inputting the sentence "Do not laugh", subjects will need to read "D" after typing it, read "o" after typing "o" and say "space" after entering a space and so on. During the standing operation experiment, subjects are asked to operate in a natural and comfortable manner. During the sitting operation experiment, a table of 73cm in height, 69cm in width and 59.5cm in depth is placed in front of the subjects. The subjects are asked to operate in a natural and comfortable manner with or without hands on the table. During the experiment, researchers record the sitting experiment with a CANON IXU 600 digital camera and the standing experiment with a CANON IXU 800 digital camera, focusing on hand movement operation posture. Another Panasonic digital camera is used to record hand posture before and after operation of both styles; shooting a hand-held posture photograph from each of the front angle, upper angle, right angle, and left angle. Lastly, the subjects are asked to fill out a questionnaire concerning PDA keypad operation analysis and related questions.

2.2 Experiment B: Observation of the Connection between Various Posture and Pain

Experiment B focuses on the connection between various posture and pain. According to the hand-held and thumb typing posture concluded from experiment A, study the connection between different PDA typing posture and pain(including index finger support, little finger support, ring finger support, and four finger support). The independent variables include index finger support posture, little finger support posture, ring finger support posture, and four finger support posture; the dependent variables include the level of pain in the thumb, wrist, elbow, forearm, shoulder and neck; the control variables include the distance between drawing board and subjects, and experimental environment. Lastly, data is analyzed using repeated measures.

2.2.1 Subjects

Thirty subjects participated in the experiment, with 14 male and 16 female. They are all right-handed with no RSI or other hand injuries. They are familiar with text input and all have normal eyesight. The average height for male subjects is 174±6.98 cm, average left hand length being 186.21±17.78 mm and right hand length being 183.25±17.41 mm; average left palm width being 80.32±5.01mm, right palm width being 82.21±4.61 mm. The average height for female subjects is 162.5±5.39 cm, average left hand length being 172.19±8.83 mm and right hand length being 171.53±9.70 mm; average left palm width being 73.5±3.55mm, right palm width being 74.86±3.61 mm.

2.2.2 Experimental Procedure and Measurements

First explain the goal and tasks of the experiment to the subjects and ask them to fill out basic information and sign an experiment agreement. Then, subjects must support the PDA in certain posture to input an English text, one specific posture for each text message. Specific supporting posture includes index finger support, little finger support, ring finger support, and four finger support. Subjects draw out the posture order before typing, each subject is required to type four different texts with a different posture for each. The texts are four short descriptive articles chosen from the website: http://health.discovery.com, each contain about 179-184 words without punctuations. The procedure for each posture has a time limit of six minutes. Since PDA is a mobile device that is mostly used standing, hence subjects are asked to stand for the experiment. During the input process, subjects are allowed to move their bodies but not their hand posture. Researchers will record the standing posture by taking a photograph every 2 minutes with a digital camera on the front-right and the front side of the subject. When one text is done, researchers make a record of the number of words, and the subject is asked to complete a questionnaire about the pain caused by the posture. Analysis is done on five parts of the body (thumb, wrist, elbow, forearm, shoulder and neck), rating from 0~10, where 0 stands for no pain and 10 stands for the most pain. After completing the analysis for each of the four posture, researchers will measure the palm width and hand length of the subject.

3 Results and Discussion

3.1 Experiment A: Observation Results of PDA Operation Posture Types

In this subject we have differentiated PDA operation posture into standing and sitting, hand-held posture into left hand support, right hand support and two hands support. With a standing posture, 90% (27 subjects) supported the PDA with two hands, 6.7% (2 people) supported with left hand, and 3.3% (1 person) with right hand; with a sitting posture, 83.3% (25 people) supported with two hands, 6.7% (2 people) supported with left hand, 3.3% (1 person) with right hand, and 6.7% (2 people) set it on the desk for operation.

There are four posture for pressing the keypad (Fig. 1): right thumb pressing, right index finger pressing, two hands thumb pressing and two hands finger pressing. With a standing posture, 13.3% (4 people) pressed the keypad with right thumb, 3.3% (1 person) pressed with right index finger, 73.5% (25 people) pressed with two

Table 1. Handheld posture

	Standing	Sitting
Two hands support	27	25
Left hand support	2	2
Right hand support	1	1
Lying on desk	0	2
Total	30	30

Table 2. The Pressing and support posture

Pressing posture on keypads.	Standing	Sitting
Right hand thumb pressing	4	3
Right hand index finger pressing	1	2
Two hands thumb pressing	25	24
Two hands all fingers pressing	0	1
Total	30	30
Upper edge support posture.	Standing	Sitting
Two hands index fingers	8	6
Single hand index finger supporting upper edge of PDA	5	3
No upper edge suppor	17	21
Total	30	30
Lower edge support posture.	Standing	Sitting
Middle finger support lower edge	3	2
Ring finger	9	12
No lower edge support	6	9
total	12	7
Total	30	30

thumbs in turn; with a sitting posture, 8.8% (3 people) pressed the keypad with right thumb, 5.9% (2 people) pressed with right index finger, 70.6% (24 people) pressed with two thumbs in turn, and 2.9% (1 person) pressed with two index fingers in turn.

During PDA operation, users often use finger support to gain stability, we will look at upper edge support and lower edge support: With a standing posture, 16.7% (5 people) uses an index finger to support the upper edge of the PDA, 26.7% (8 people) use two index finger, 56.7% (17 people) did not support the upper edge; With a sitting position, 10% (3 people) used a middle finger to support the lower edge, 30% (9 people) used a ring finger, 60% (9 people) used a little finger, and 13.3% (7 people) did not support the lower edge.

To sum up, we have concluded 4 types of holding posture from the observation in experiment A (Fig. 2). They are two hand holding posture, thumb pressing, upper edge support, and lower edge support. The results show that the two hand holding posture and two thumb typing in the main stream for PDA operation. During the sitting and standing posture, subjects used two index fingers to support the upper edge of PDA or simply no upper edge support; With a standing posture, subjects either support the lower edge of PDA by using ring fingers or simply did not support the lower edge; with a sitting posture, many support the lower edge with ring finger and little finger to gain stability.

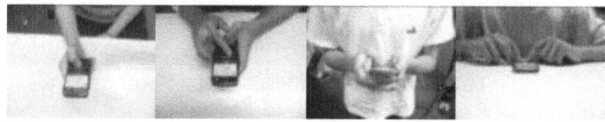

Fig. 1. Key pressing posture

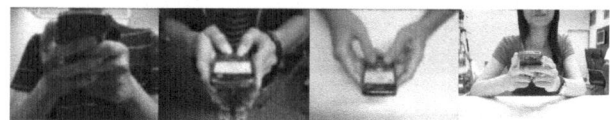

Fig. 2. Grip and stability posture

We looked at the connection between the various posture using χ^2 , and found a positive connection between handheld posture and fingers used for typing with both standing and sitting posture, a connection between upper edge support and lower edge support, a connection between handheld posture and whether forearm is leaning against table in a sitting posture, a connection between elbow support and hand support in a sitting posture, and a connection between elbow support and forearm learning against desk in a sitting position.

As for the keys, subjects generally commented on PDA keys being too small, causing a high error rate, and the large number of characters causes confusion in recognition. The clarity and choice of icons and the convenience of symbol and input language switching both need to be worked on, feedback sounds should be considered too; distance between keys needs to be clear for recognition and the keypad curving angle needs to avoid reflection. As for key arrangements, subjects declared that although the arrangement is similar to a computer keyboard, keys may be hard to find for non-computer users, hence training may be needed. If chord corresponding keys are used then comfort needs to be considered, an alphabetical order arrangement may be more appropriate than a computer keyboard arrangement. After learning and training, chord corresponding keys should be able to reach the same average speed as the standard keyboard arrangement, the key size problem could also be solved. As for the PDA width size, subjects suggested a width that is comfortable to be held single-handed, so it is comfortable to operate with one or two hands. This could be shown on the LCD screen by a horizontal displacement mechanism.

3.2 Experiment B: Observation Results of the Connection between Posture and Pain During PDA Operation

From experiment A, we found that most people take the posture of two hand holding and two thumb pressing, and users take different posture to support PDA to gain stability. Since mobile devices require a fast-speed data transfer, stability in hands is a must. According to the stability supporting posture in experiment A, Experiment B focuses on the connection between supporting posture and pain during speed input operation.

When supporting the lower edge of PDA with the index finger, the pain level caused from severe to mild goes from shoulder and neck(51.57), thumb(49.07), wrist(39.70), forearm(39.37), to elbow(37.47). When supporting the lower edge of PDA with the little finger, the pain level caused goes from shoulder and neck(47.23), thumb(42.73), forearm(37.37), wrist(35.83), to elbow(33.80). When supporting the back of PDA with four fingers, the pain level caused goes from shoulder and neck(53.23), thumb(40.70), forearm(40.43), elbow(33.63), to wrist(29.80). When supporting the lower edge of PDA with the ring finger, the pain level caused goes from shoulder and neck(53.30), forearm(40.73), thumb(39.53), wrist(38.60), to elbow(34.67).

We can see that with either of the four posture, should and neck pain level were the most severe, followed by forearm, wrist, and elbow. After observing the full-body photographs, we found that subjects often make changes with standing posture, the shoulder and neck pain is caused by the long-term standing posture and the head movement due to the need of viewing the screen and external information. However, whether the connection exists between viewing the screen to input data and the shoulder and neck pain, is yet to be verified. The thumb pain caused by speed input with a fixed posture is rated second in the pain level. From this we can see that most people input with their thumbs, this creates speed, but causes excess burden on the thumbs even only for a short period of input time. Forearm and wrist pain were rated third. This could be caused by the wrist and forearm turning inwards, causing discomfort during speed data input. Elbow caused the least pain, and this could be due to the support given by chest and waist when placing elbows on the two sides of the body.

Table 3. The consistency of pain analysis in the five areas. (LSD comparison afterwards)

Area	Thumb	Wrist	Elbow	Forearm	Shoulder and Neck
Thumb		◎△	◎		
Wrist	◎ △			△	◎ △ ●
Elbow	◎				◎ △ ●
Forearm		△			◎ △ ●
Shoulder and Neck	◎ △ ●	◎ △ ●	◎ △ ●		

◎: when supporting PDA with index finger support, $p<0.05$

△: when supporting PDA with four finger support, $p<0.05$

●: when supporting PDA with ring finger support, $p<0.05$

The repeated measures result shows no significant difference in the connection be-tween thumb pain, wrist pain, elbow pain, forearm pain, shoulder and neck pain and the four supporting posture. Hence, the four posture do not cause significant pain in the five body areas. However, when testing the consistency of pain analysis in the five areas (Table 3), it shows a higher level of shoulder and neck and thumb pain in all except for the little finger support posture. Including when supporting PDA with in-dex finger, thumb pain was more severe than the wrist and elbow pain, and shoulder and neck pain was more severe than the elbow, forearm, and wrist; when supporting PDA with four fingers, the thumb pain was more severe than wrist pain, shoulder and neck pain was more severe than elbow, forearm, and wrist pain, and the forearm pain more severe than wrist pain; when supporting with the ring finger, shoulder and neck pain was more severe than wrist, elbow, and arm pain. The reason why it shows no connection between supporting posture and pain, could be due to the length of opera-tion, or the disturbance on analysis standards caused by analyzing five body areas for each posture. This means that subjects could forget the standard used for analyzing one posture from another. However, regardless of the supporting posture, thumb and shoulder and neck pain is easily seen during short-term fixed input posture compared to other body parts.

4   Conclusion

To make PDA portable, they are made small in size and light in weight. Due to its small-sized keys and limited space between the keys, users tend to use a single finger such as thumbs to press the keys. The size of PDA and its keys has a profound effect on the way people use them. We recommend designers to thoroughly consider the connection between key designs and operation posture.

It has become a trend for PDA to be small in size. Hence the only change we could make to avoid physical burden during operation is to improve key designs and input styles. We found that most users hold PDA with both hands and type with both thumbs. Supporting the PDA with the index finger, little finger, ring finger, and four finger postures do not cause obvious pain in thumb, wrist, elbow, forearm, and shoul-der and neck. There is a higher level of shoulder and neck and thumb pain compared to the other parts with all supporting posture except for the little finger support. There is no connection between the pain level caused and supporting posture, it has more to do with operation time period. Disregard the supporting posture used, when operating for a short time period with fixed posture, thumb and shoulder and neck feels a higher level of pain than the other body areas. Hence, designs should try to avoid the excess use of thumbs. Designers could improve on key arrangement designs to change the operation style of PDA input, in order to avoid users pressing the keys with only their thumbs; also improve on the shape of PDA to increase stability, in order to avoid the pain caused due to excess pressing motion.

Acknowledgments

The authors would like to thank the National Science Council of the Republic of China for financially supporting this research under Contract No. NSC 97-2221-E-006 -169 -MY3.

References

1. Serina, E., Tal, R., Rempel, D.: Wrist and forearm postures and motions during typing. Ergonomics 42, 938–951 (1999)
2. Straker, L., Jones, K.J., Miller, J.: A comparison of the postures assumed when using laptop computers and desktop computers. Applied Ergonomics 28, 263–268 (1997)
3. Kotani, K., Barrero, L.H., Lee, D.L., Dennerlein, J.T.: Effect of horizontal position of the computer keyboard on upper extremity posture and muscular load during computer work. Ergonomics 50, 1419–1432 (2007)
4. Baker, N., Cham, R., Cidboy, E.H., Cook, J., Redfern, M.S.: Kinematics of the fingers and hands during computer keyboard use. Clinical Biomechanics 22, 34–43 (2007)
5. Colle, H.A., Hiszem, K.J.: Standing at a kiosk: Effects of key size and spacing on touch screen numeric keypad performance and user preference. Ergonomics 47, 1406–1423 (2004)
6. Gong, J., Tarasewich, P.: Alphabetically Constrained Keypad Designs for Text Entry on Mobile Devices. In: CHI 2005, pp. 211–220. ACM Press, Portland (2005)
7. Sears, A., Zha, Y.: Data Entry for Mobile Devices Using Soft Keyboards: Understanding the Effects of Keyboard Size and User Tasks. International Journal of Human-Computer Interaction 16, 163–184 (2003)
8. MacKenzie, I.S., Zhang, S.X., Soukoreff, R.W.: Text entry using soft keyboards. Behaviour & Information Technology 18, 235–244 (1999)
9. Zhai, S., Hunter, M., Smith, B.A.: The Metropolis keyboard—an exploration of quantitative techniques for virtual keyboard design. In: UIST 2000 Proceedings of the ACM Symposium on User Interface Software and Technology, pp. 119–128. ACM Press, San Diego (2000)
10. Goldstein, M., Book, R., Alsiö, G., Tessa, S.: Non-keyboard QWERTY touch typing: a portable input interface for the mobile user. In: CHI 1999, pp. 32–39. ACM Press, Pittsburgh (1999)
11. Sears, A., Jacko, J.A., Chu, J., Moro, F.: The role of visual search in the design of effective soft keyboards. Behaviour and Information Technology 20, 159–166 (2001)
12. Li, Y., Chen, L., Goonetilleke, R.S.: A heuristic-based approach to optimize keyboard design for single-finger keying applications. International Journal of Industrial Ergonomics 36, 695–704 (2006)
13. Kim, S., Sohn, M., Pak, J., Lee, W.: One-key keyboard: a very small QWERTY keyboard supporting text entry for wearable computing. In: 18th Australia conference on Computer-Human Interaction: Design: Activities, Artefacts and Environments, pp. 305–308. ACM Press, Sydney (2006)
14. Wobbrock, J.O., Myers, B.A., Aung, H.H., LoPresti, E.F.: Text entry from power wheelchairs: edgewrite for joysticks and touchpads. In: 6th international ACM SIGACCESS conference on Computers and accessibility, pp. 110–117. ACM Press, Atlanta (2004)
15. Silfverberg, M., MacKenzie, I.S., Korhonen, P.: Predicting text entry speed on mobile phones. In: CHI 2000, pp. 9–16. ACM Press, Hague (2000)
16. Mizobuchi, S., Chignell, M., Newton, D.: Mobile text entry: relationship between walking speed and text input task difficulty. In: 7th international conference on Human computer interaction with mobile devices & services, pp. 122–128. ACM Press, Salzburg (2005)
17. Jonsson, P., Johnson, P.W., Hagberg, M.: Accuracy and feasibility of using an electrogoniometer for measuring simple thumb movements. Ergonomics 50, 647–659 (2007)

Vector Keyboard for Touch Screen Devices

Martin Klima and Vaclav Slovacek

Czech Technical University in Prague, Czech Republic
{xklima,slovav1}@fel.cvut.cz

Abstract. Paper introduces a vector keyboard for touch screen devices. Characters are typed by drawing a vector starting from a dedicated area. The typing area is divided into three clusters, each containing 9 characters. Measurement of typing speed and of number of typos reveals that the keyboard is comparable to ABCDEF virtual keyboard.

Keywords: vector keyboard, virtual keyboard, touch screen, PDA, QWERT.

1 Motivation

The motivation of this work is to introduce a new, user friendly method for inserting text input on handheld devices. The widely spread insert methods are either using a limited hardware keyboard, graffiti, or a virtual QWERTY keyboard. Despite the fact that experienced users, who are well trained to use any of the named input methods, can be very efficient in typing text, each of the methods suffers with some limitations. The limited hardware keyboards are usually very small and difficult to press, graffiti is not intuitive and difficult to learn and finally the virtual QWERTY keyboard is, similarly to the hardware keyboard, small and often requires usage of stylus. The virtual QWERTY keyboard occupies a significant portion of the display that should be used for the application. We propose a method that was meant to solve most of the named weaknesses.

2 State of the Art

The current trend in mobile devices is to maximize the display area and to minimize the hardware buttons necessary to control the system. This aim leads to large touch screens with either virtual clickable keyboards or to vector, respectively gesture based text input. Palm Computing 5 introduced graffiti in Palm OS, a touch screen gesture input method, Microsoft implemented a similar system on its Pocket PC platform called Block Recognizer. The advantage of these methods is that the shapes to be drawn on the touch screen are similar to regular Greek alphabet. Nevertheless the shapes are quite complicated and the usage is not possible without an initial training.

Other approaches like 1, 2 use gestures either on a virtual keyboard or within a dedicated area for writing letters. In each case, the gesture made on the touch screen is a complicated shape, typically a polyline. An interesting approach is introduced in 3 where the virtual keyboard is split into several regions, each containing up to five

B.-T. Karsh (Ed.): Ergonomics and Health Aspects, HCII 2009, LNCS 5624, pp. 250–256, 2009.

characters. The user can draw a curve which will select one character. The above mentioned methods suffer with one or more significant drawbacks. Either the user has to learn a completely new set of gestures or the typing is extremely difficult on the handheld due to a reduced screen space. The first is true in case of 2 and the graffiti system. These (and similar) writing systems try to introduce gestures that are somewhat similar to the Latin alphabet nevertheless they are significantly different in many cases. The second is true in case of 6 or 7 where the individual letters are not typed directly but are passed over by a pen stroke. This method is vulnerable to errors on mobile devices when the user is in movement.

3 Our Approach

In our approach we introduce a method that enables for one stroke, simple non curved line character typing on a touch screen. The primary idea was to introduce an input method that would make it possible to use both hands simultaneously for typing on a touch screen devices. When holding a mobile device, typically a PDA (Personal Digital Assistant) or a Smart Phone in both hands, only the thumbs are available for typing on the touch screen, see Fig.1. In such a case, considering a small dimensions of the touch screen and relatively big dimension of the thumbs, it is difficult to use a standard QWERTY keyboard. The regular way of touching the keyboard becomes difficult in a mobile environment, users tend to mistype the proper area touch screen or touch them accidentally multiple times. Our approach uses typing gestures on the touch screen instead of typing. The gestures are extremely simple so that the users do not need to learn them or use some mnemonics. In our case the screen is divided into virtual keyboard area and the application area. The virtual keyboard requires less space than a QWERTY virtual keyboard.

The keyboard is divided into three major clusters, each containing an array of nine characters. There are four additional functional buttons that switch beween upper/lowercase letters, numbers and special characters, backspace key and enter key. See Fig. 4 for details.

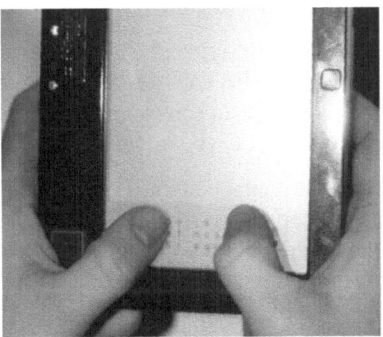

Fig. 1. Typing letter

The usage of the keyboard is the following: The eight characters on the edge of each cluster are typed by drawing a vector starting wherever in the given area and pointing in parallel with a straight line from the middle of the box to the character typed. The method is displayed in Fig. 2.

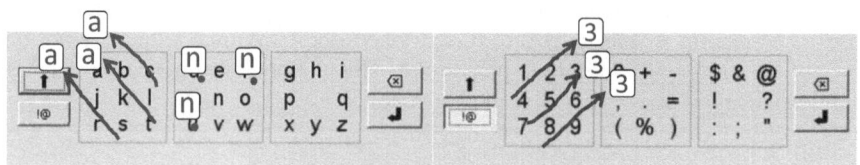

Fig. 2. Typing the character a, n, and 3

The character in middle of each cluster is typed by single tapping anywhere on the cluster area. For the user convenience the typing algorithm was enriched so that two spaces in a sequence are transformed into comma and a space followed by a capital letter.

For the sake of simplicity this keyboard is currently not enriched by special national characters, only the basic set of characters conforming the US QWERTY keyboard is present.

4 Evaluation and Testing

The evaluation of the usability of the vector keyboard was based on a combination of a subjective evaluation of the evaluators and an objective performance measurement. The test conditions were following:

4.1 Test Setup

Each tests consisted of an introduction of the device, several types of keyboards, pre-test interview, test of different keyboards and a post-test interview.

Number of users: 9

Device used: Mivvy UM-400 with stylus

Input methods: external QWERTY keyboard, internal sliding keyboard, QWERTY touch screen, ABCDEF touch screen and vector keyboard touch screen.

Each user was to use five different keyboards for typing texts. The keyboards were:

1. Regular 105 keys PC keyboard attached via USB. Typing on such a keyboard reveals the experience of the user with work on a PC.
2. Sliding keyboard of the ultra mobile PC Mivvy UM-400. This keyboard has a limited size and 65 keys, see Fig. 4. This keyboard has principally a QWERTY layout but should be operated by thumbs only. Typing on this keyboard reveals the user's capability to use thumbs only on a quasi normal keyboard.
3. QWERTY keyboard on the touch screen operated by stylus. The dimension of the keyboard does not allow for using fingers (thumbs). Similar to the previous case, this keyboard reveals the user's capability to use stylus.

Table 1. User overview

Nr.	Age	Gender	PC Exp.	Handheld Exp.	Touchscreen Exp.	Type Style	Layout
1	24	Male	Yes	Occasional	Occasional	8	QWERTY
2	31	Female	Yes	No	No	10	QWERTZ
3	12	Female	Yes	No	No	8	QWERTY
4	47	Male	Yes	No	No	2	QWERTZ
5	27	Male	Yes	Yes	Yes	8	QWERTY
6	33	Female	Yes	No	No	2	QWERTZ
7	44	Female	No	None	No	2	none
8	63	Male	Yes	No	No	2	QWERTZ
9	35	Male	Yes	Yes	Yes	10	QWERTY

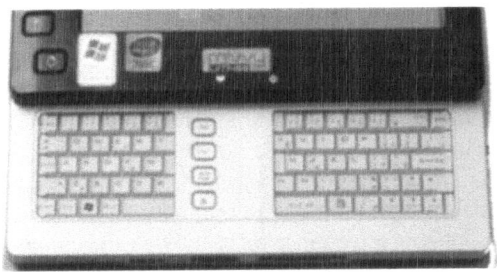

Fig. 3. Mivvy UM-400 sliding keyboard

4. ABCDEF keyboard on the touch screen operated by stylus. This keyboard has physically the same geometrical layout of keys but the keys are ordered in an alphabetical order. Typing on this keyboard shows the contrast between the layout the user is used to from the PC and a new layout which is easy to understand but not fully adopted by the user.

5. Vector keyboard, which is the primary subject of testing. Due to the sensitivity of the touch screen used, stylus was used for operating it.

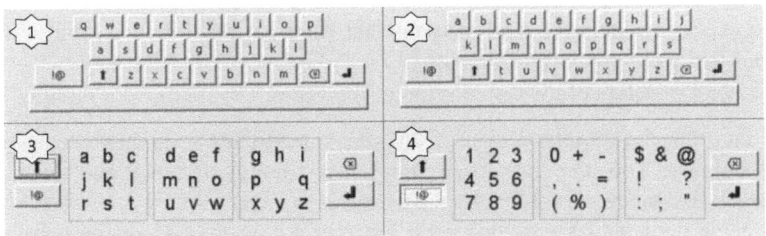

Fig. 4. 1- QWERTY touch screen keyboard, 2 – ABCDEF touch screen keyboard, 3 – vector keyboard, 4- vector keyboard numeric set

Texts: We used texts of equal complexity, thematic and size that were dictated to the user so that the attention was not disrupted. Each text was approximately 100 words in length. All eventual foreign words or grammatical structures were dictated phonetically in order to minimize the cognitive load dedicated to text structure.

Recording: Every letter typed was automatically logged with exact time and order. The evaluation was done by measuring various aspects of typing.

4.2 Evaluation

The evaluation has taken into account two aspects. The first one was the actual performance of each user. The collected typing data were filtered so that all pauses between two characters longer than 3 seconds were removed. The reason for this was that such long pauses were always caused by influences different from typing difficulties, for example by not understanding the dictated text or by interruption by external sources.

By our observations the pauses between individual words were significantly longer than pauses between individual characters. Therefore we measured only times between characters within a single word, not between words. Number of typos was measured and number of deletes was measured. A multiple delete in a row was suggested as a single delete operation due to the fact that some users deleted a series of characters after recognizing a typo instead of moving the cursor to the typo first.

5 Results

Experienced users showed very good performance in typing with QWERTY layout both hardware and virtual keyboard, see Fig. 5. This is an expected result since the layout is well memorized from previous experience.

The most relevant comparison can be made between the ABCDEF keyboard and the vector keyboard, since the ABCDEF partly eliminates the user's experience.

The typing speed was comparable to the ABCDEF, see Fig. 5, which is considered a good result considering a new way of interaction (draw instead of tap). The drawing itself takes longer.

Writing on vector keyboard caused significantly higher number of typos for most users (6 of 9). Fig. 6 shows sum of typos that were corrected by user during the test and typos that were not corrected at all.

As a major problem of the tested setup of the vector keyboard were reported:

1. The fact that the current design of the vector keyboard combines vector gestures with tapping. The tapping caused significant amount of typos and was also reported as a subjective problem by the users.
2. The angle dedicated for writing each letter in a cluster is 45 degrees that caused accidental write of a neighboring letter.
3. The quality of the touch screen of the Mivvy UM-400 made it sometimes difficult to draw the vector in a satisfactory level.

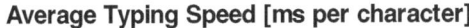
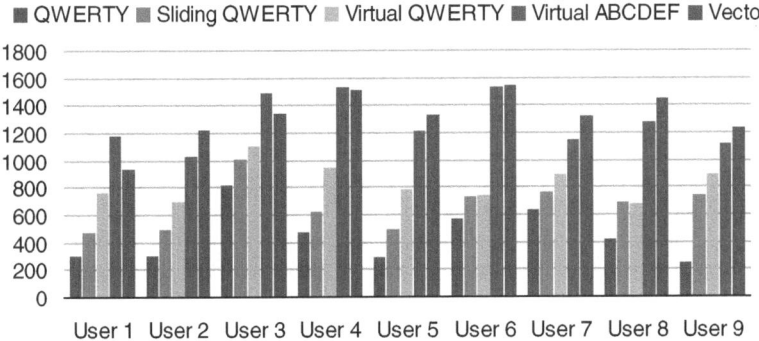

Fig. 5. Average typing speed of one character on various keyboards

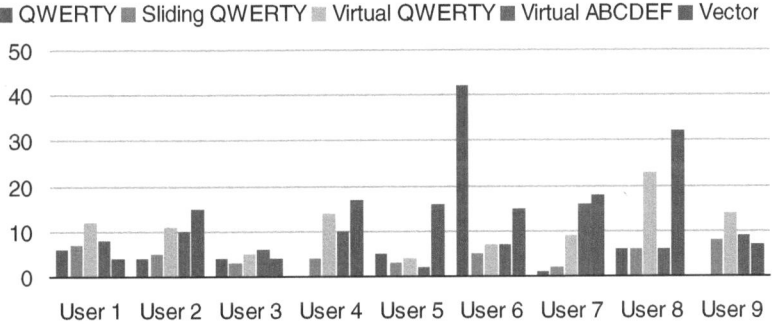

Fig. 6. Number of typos on various keyboards

As a future improvement we recommend to introduce a layout with one more cluster, each having eight characters only (with no letter in the middle) and thus omitting the tapping at all.

Implementing an error correction based on a dictionary may also lead to reducing number of typos. The correction of typo of two neighboring characters can be done in case the direction of a stroke is close to a threshold between the two characters.

We recommend developing and testing of a new prototype for capacitive touch screen device. Capacitive touch screen enables higher level of precision when recognizing strokes and also makes it possible to control the vector keyboard by thumbs that may lead to different results.

As a result we state that the vector keyboard as it was implemented does not compete to the virtual QWERTY keyboard due to the generic experience with this keyboard. On the other hand, the vector keyboard was performing almost equally to the ABCDEF keyboard which shows that the method itself is as good as the tapping. We believe that further development of the vector keyboard, as it is suggested above, will lead to significant improvement of typing performance.

References

1. Kristensson, P.O., Zhai, S.: Command Strokes with and without Preview: Using Pen Gestures on Keyboard for Command Selection. In: Proc. CHI 2007: ACM Conference on Human Factors in Computing Systems, San Jose, California (2007)
2. Wobbrock, J.O., Myers, B.A., Kembel, J.A.: EdgeWrite: A stylus-based text entry method designed for high accuracy and stability of motion. In: Proceedings of the ACM Symposium on User Interface Software and Technology (UIST 2003), Vancouver, British Columbia, pp. 61–70. ACM Press, New York (2003)
3. Perlin, K.: Quikwriting: continuous stylus-based text entry. In: UIST 1998: Proceedings of the 11th annual ACM symposium on User interface software and technology, pp. 215–216 (1998)
4. Yatani, K., Truong, K.N.: An Evaluation of Stylus-Based Text Entry Methods on Handheld Devices in Stationary & Mobile Settings. In: The Proceedings of MobileHCI 2007: The 9th International Conference on Human-Computer Interaction with Mobile Devices and Services, Singapore, September 11-14, pp. 145–152 (2007)
5. Shoemaker, P.B.: Designing interfaces for handheld computers. In: Conference on Human Factors in Computing Systems, pp. 127–127. ACM, New York (1999)
6. Kristensson, P.O., Zhai, S.: Command Strokes with and without Preview: Using Pen Gestures on Keyboard for Command Selection. In: Proc. ACM CHI 2007, New York, NY, USA, pp. 1137–1146 (2007)
7. Kristensson, P.-O., Zhai, S.: SHARK2: a large vocabulary shorthand writing system for pen-based computers. In: Proc. the 17th annual ACM Symposium on User Interface Software and Technology, pp. 43–52 (2004)

Evaluation of a Functional Film Attached on Top of a Tablet PC

Yugo Kobayashi, Tatsuya Terada, Toshiyuki Kondo, and Masaki Nakagawa

Tokyo University of Agriculture and Technology,
2-24-16, Naka-cho, Koganei, Tokyo, Japan
{50008646117}@st.tuat.ac.jp

Abstract. This paper presents usability evaluation of a functional film named PenFit attached on top of a tablet PC. We compared a tablet PC with PenFit and that without PenFit from the viewpoint of the ease of writing. We considered several measures to evaluate the ease of writing. We propose "how people can write letters neatly (neatness)", "how people can write quickly (speed)" and "how people can write without fatigue (fatigue)" as the measures to evaluate the ease of writing. As a result, it is suggested that the functional film provides the ease of writing.

Keywords: pen interface, functional film, ease of writing, electromyogram.

1 Introduction

A Tablet PC is gradually getting common. The price-down is promoting its wider use in many scenes. However, the surface of LCD integrated tablets has been very hard so that a pen is slippery, people feel hard reaction from the surface, and they feel tired after writing. Although a tablet PC is promising for school children, this strange feeling of writing is not favored by them.

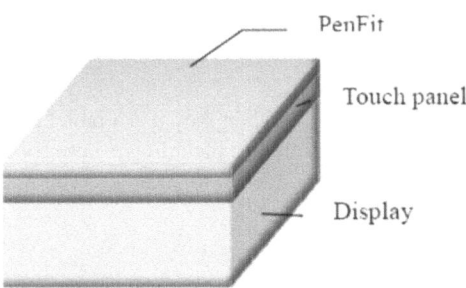

Fig. 1. PenFit on top of writing surface

A functional film is proposed to enhance the ease of writing and provide smooth feeling of writing on a tablet PC. We select the product named PenFit, which has the largest sale, to evaluate whether it realizes the aimed effect.

B.-T. Karsh (Ed.): Ergonomics and Health Aspects, HCII 2009, LNCS 5624, pp. 257–263, 2009.

2 Evaluation Measures

We considered several measures to evaluate the ease of writing. We asked people to write on a tablet PC with PenFit and that without PenFit (naked tablet PC) and evaluated the ease of writing according to these measures.

We propose "how people can write letters neatly (neatness)", "how people can write quickly (speed)" and "how people can write without fatigue (fatigue)" as the measures to evaluate the ease of writing.

Moreover, for pen interfaces, such as menu selection, pen tap, dragging, and so on, pen operability is also important. On top of that, writing pressure is available from a pen so that we also measure it.

We should measure these factors for people who are familiar with a tablet PC and people who have no experience of using it.

2.1 Neatness

The measure "neatness" is still broad so that we decompose it into 6 factors as follows:

- Control: being able to control a pen just as we want.
- Smoothness: feeling smooth when we write.
- Continuation: being able to move a pen as we write.
- Feedback: feeling proper reaction from the surface.
- Naturalness: feeling natural as if writing on a paper
- Tiredness: feeling tired (distinguished from physical fatigue).

We let subjects to write text at three writing conditions, i.e., "Write it slowly", "Write it as usual", and "Write it as fast as possible" on a tablet PC with PenFit and on a naked tablet PC. We don't tell the subject of using PenFit or not. After the experiment, we let them evaluate the ease of writing.

2.2 Speed

We measure writing speed when the above subjects write text at three writing conditions of "slowly", "as usual", and "as fast as possible" on a tablet PC with PenFit and without it.

2.3 Fatigue

We measure the fatigue of the subjects when they use a tablet PC with PenFit and without it. The subjects write text for 60 minutes including 5 minutes break after 30 minutes. We measure electromyogram after 10, 20, 30,45,55 and,65 minutes from the start.

2.4 Pressure

We measure the pressure of a pen to writing surface when the subjects write a tablet PC with PenFit or not.

2.5 Operation

We perform an experiment on pen operations on Windows GUI with a pen using PenFit or not. The operations are "Double tap", "Pen hold "and "Drag & Drop".

- Double tap: attaching a pen to the same screen position twice quickly.
- Hold: fixing a pen at the same screen position for some predefined period.
- Drag & Drop: choose an object by putting down a pen, moving (dragging) the pen, and lifting the pen off at a destination.

We count how many times subjects succeed to make each operation.

3   Result

3.1   Neatness

We asked subjects to express their subjective evaluation on control, smoothness, continuation, feedback, naturalness and tiredness into 6 ranks (0 as worst to 5 as best). Fig. 2 to Fig. 4 shows the average at 3 kinds of writing speed.

We performed t-test on the questionnaire result for the 6 measures. Table 1 shows either of writing on PenFit or without it is superior to the other significantly. The mark "-" denotes no significant difference between the two.

Generally speaking, PenFit provides better control, continuation, and feedback but posed drawback in tiredness. This is probably because people feel friction when they write on PenFit while they can run a pen almost without friction on a naked tablet PC. We should recognize that the hard surface of LCD-integrated tablet is different from

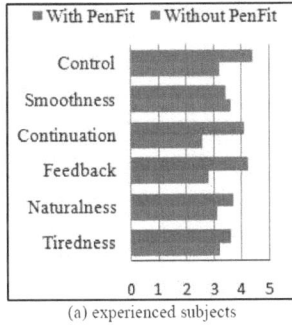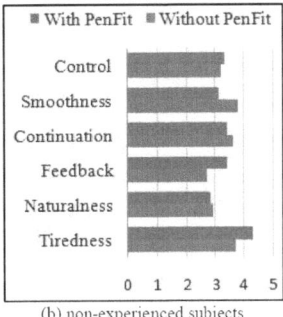

Fig. 2. Neatness when writing slowly

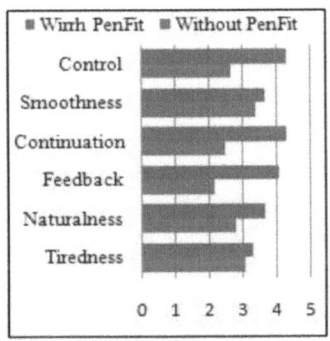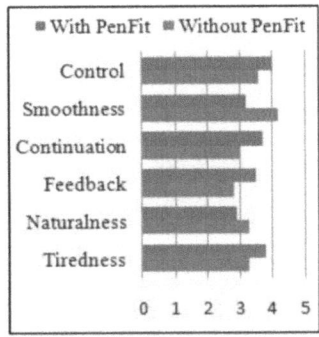

Fig. 3. Neatness when writing as usual

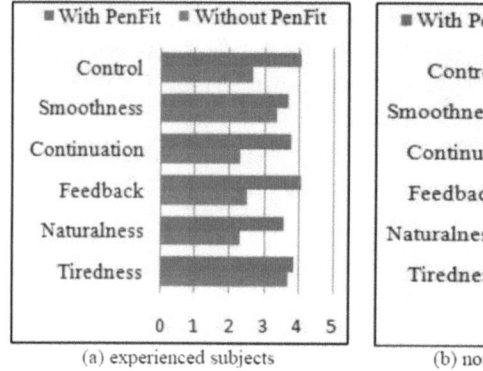

Fig. 4. Neatness when writing as fast as possible

Table 1. Superiority of writing on PenFit or without it

(a) experienced subjects

measure. / writing speed.	Control.	Smooth ness.	Continua- tion.	Feedback.	Nutural ness.	Tired ness.
slowly.	-	-	-	PenFit	-	Without PenFit
as usual.	PenFit	-	-	-		Without PenFit
as fast as possible	PenFit	-	-	-		Without PenFit

(b) non- experienced subjects

measure. / writing speed.	Control.	Smooth ness.	Continua- tion.	Feedback.	Nutural ness.	Tired ness.
slowly.	-	-	-	PenFit	-	Without PenFit
as usual.	PenFit	-	-	-		Without PenFit
as fast as possible	PenFit	-	-	-		Without PenFit

real paper and a new writing condition. There remains comparison between PenFit and real paper. If PenFit provides equivalent evaluation in other measures as real paper, we consider the PenFit's superiority in control, continuation and feedback is important, although it has the drawback in tiredness in comparison to a naked tablet PC.

3.2 Speed

We measured writing speed when the subjects wrote text at three writing speeds on a tablet PC with PenFit and without it. Fig. 5 shows the time spent for writing a certain

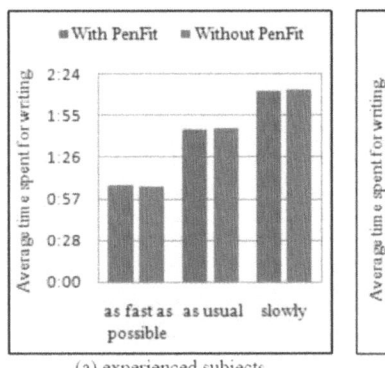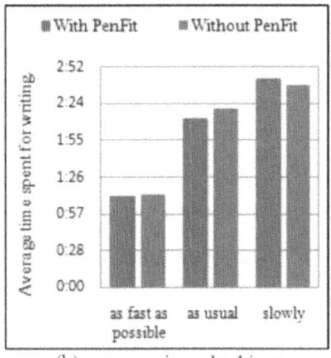

(a) experienced subjects   (b) non-experienced subjects

Fig. 5. Average time spent for writing

amount of text (100 characters). Significant difference was observed between experienced and non-experienced subjects and among the three writing speeds but not between writing on PenFit and without it.

3.3 Fatigue

We measured electromyogram of 8 experienced subjects and 8 non-experienced subjects at 10 minute later and 60 minute later after starting writing.

As for the fatigue measure, t-test did not show significant difference between writing on PenFit or not regardless of experience.

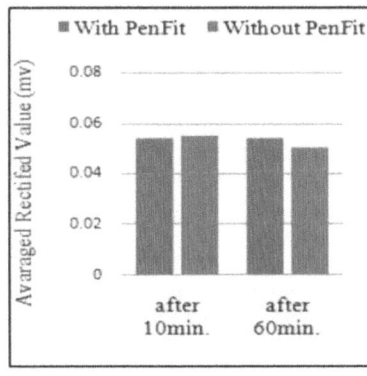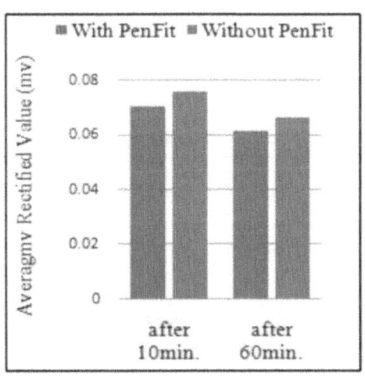

(a) experienced subjects   (b) non-experienced subjects

Fig. 6. Averaged Rectified Value

3.4 Pressure

We measured the pressure of a pen to writing surface from 8 experienced subjects and 8 non-experienced subjects when they wrote a tablet PC with PenFit or not. Table 3 shows the average score of the pressure. Pressure score has a 0 ~255 grade.

Table 2. Pressure of a pen to writing surface

(a) experienced subjects.

	PenFit	Without PenFit
experience1	198.02	197.75
experience2	197.24	187.67
experience3	157.49	155.14
experience4	152.55	177.44
experience5	162.20	174.13
experience6	140.43	154.97
experience7	182.96	201.89
experience8	201.54	177.25
Average	174.05	178.28

(b) non-experienced subjects.

	PenFit	Without PenFit
no-experience1	163.73	170.67
no-experience 2	145.76	160.67
no-experience 3	118.20	129.84
no-experience 4	191.15	188.82
no-experience 5	115.20	106.79
no-experience 6	170.38	170.37
no-experience 7	205.57	211.25
no-experience 8	178.29	183.64
Average	161.04	165.26

T-test did not show significant difference between writing on PenFit or not regardless of experience.

3.5 Operation

We performed an experiment on pen operations on Windows GUI with a pen using PenFit or not. We measured success rate of 8 experienced subjects and 8 non-experienced subjects to make each operation. Table 3 shows the rate.

As for the operation of "Double tap", "Hold", the average success rates of PenFit are better than without PenFit regardless of experience. However, t-test did not show significant difference between writing on PenFit or not regardless of experience.

As for "Drag & Drop", the success rates is about 100% regardless of experience.

Table 3. Averaged of success rate of each operation

(a) experienced subjects.

	PenFit	Without PenFit
Double tap	90%	89%
Hold	100%	90%
Drag & Drop	98%	98%

(b) non-experienced subjects.

	PenFit	Without PenFit
Double tap	94%	83%
Hold	97%	91%
Drag & Drop	100%	98%

4 Conclusion

This paper has presented to what extent a functional film named PenFit solves problems of writing on a tablet PC and enhance ease of writing. We have proposed neatness, speed and fatigue as the measures to evaluate the ease of writing. As for the neatness, we have decomposed it into control, smoothness, continuation, feedback, naturalness and tiredness.

Experiments have suggested that PenFit provides better control, continuation, and feedback. As for the tiredness, however, it posed drawback to a naked tablet PC. This is probably because PenFit provide friction. There remains comparison between PenFit and real paper.

As for pen operations, PenFit provides superiority in "Hold" and "Double tap" while no significant difference in "Drag&Drop" in comparison to a naked tablet PC. Moderate friction provides by PenFit makes careful operations easy and provides better control of a pen.

On the other hand, PenFit provides no significant difference from a naked tablet PC in writing speed, fatigue and pressure.

Acknowledgement. The work is being supported by the Special Coordination Funds for Promoting Science and Technology, Ministry of Education, Culture, Sports, Science and Technology Japan.

References

1. Hara, Y., Yoshida, M., Matumura, M., Ichihashi, N.: The Quantitative Evaluation of the Muscle Activity by Integrated Electromyogram (in Japanese). IEEE J. Trans. EIS 124(2), 431–435 (2004)
2. Osamu, N.: The Relationship between the EMG Signal and Force Output 21(4), 641–645 (2004) (in Japanese)

Interaction between Dynamic LED-Light
and Color Surfaces

Ralf Michel

Vice Head Institute of Design & Technology/Managing Team Color-Light Center
Zurich University of the Arts
Hafnerstrasse 29, CH-8005 Zuerich, Switzerland
ralf.michel@zhdk.ch
www.colourlight-center.ch
http://idt.zhdk.ch

Abstract. The many different interactions between light and colours represent a
very important research topic at the Zurich University of the Arts. This is why
the Zurich ColourLight-Center was set up at the Institute for Design und Technology, idt. For more than 15 years, we have been investigating the potential of
interactions of light and colour and asking fundamental questions about the
relevance of the subject to the development of design education and practice. In
the ColourLight-Lab, the research project, which we present from the Zurich
ColourLight-Center, products and methods of presentation were created, which
describe the sensory perception of light and colour as a phenomenon of seeing.
The LED-ColourLab research project specially takes as its theme, the interaction of dynamic LED light and colour surfaces.

1 ColourLightLab

The ColourLightLab is a research project of the Zurich University of the Arts and
DORE (Swiss National Fund). At the meeting point of art, science and the communication of art and design, methods of presentation and products were developed in
2005/2006, which take as their theme the sensory perception of colour and light as a
phenomenon of seeing.

Central problems:

- How are the effects of colours influenced by different light as a result of their
  arrangement / positioning in the room?
- How do different combinations of various light sources and materials affect the
  perception of colours?
- How can the findings regarding the questions of visual perception be implemented
  topically and by the senses in the development of theory?

1.1 Research Project

Discovering colours in the field of tension between light and darkness and experi-
menting with their effects, is the central concern of our research publication, "Colours

B.-T. Karsh (Ed.): Ergonomics and Health Aspects, HCII 2009, LNCS 5624, pp. 264–267, 2009.
© Springer-Verlag Berlin Heidelberg 2009

between light and darkness"(1). Phenomena of the sensory perception of colour and light are visualised by pictures and videos. Different media, such as colour charts for the new colour painting system, interactive tools and software for setting up installations, invite playful handling of colour and light. The documented projects of students at the Zurich University of Art and Design provide varied suggestions for design practice. Theoretical knowledge can be deepened using our compendium. Our work is directed at teachers, students and others interested in colour. The colour-light installations (e.g. pigment carpet) are recorded as videos and some can be reconstructed using the software contained on the CD ROM and the instructions.

Using interactive tools on the CD ROM (e.g. Bezzold spreading effect) questions of the perception of colour can be reconstructed and tried out by way of a virtual demonstration room. The theoretical aspects of colour and light are presented in a richly illustrated compendium in a way that is understandable to all. All 70 illustrated compendium terms (e.g. binding agents) can be printed out as PDF files. The documented teaching projects (e.g. "Light staging") are sources of inspiration for students and teachers, for example in Project Weeks / seminars / workshops or at interdisciplinary events at the interface of arts, science and artistic topics. All documented teaching projects contain series of pictures/videos or animations and can likewise be printed as PDF files.

2   Research in the LED-ColourLab

LED-ColourLab is our second research project and co-financed by KTI (Committee for Technology and Innovation, Swiss Research Promotion). The research partners are: Philips AG Lighting Switzerland; IGP Pulvertechnik Switzerland; kt.color Switzerland.

LED is a light technology is forecast to have great economic potential (justified by low electricity consumption whilst simultaneously producing high luminosity). The successful implementation of this potential gives rise to the development of concrete, design-driven applications for diverse user groups, as well as the development and prototype implementation of innovative representative processes and products. Experiments in the field of interactions between dynamic LED technology with surface colours / coatings and space are the main subject matter of research of the LED-ColourLab project. The author will give an insight into the methods of the research and the results concerning the interaction between dynamic LED-light and coloured surfaces as well into the results concerning the hue shift.

2.1   The Scientific and Technical Aims of the Research Project

In the area of dynamic LED interaction with surface colours, there are hardly any systematised investigations, which are useful in terms of design, into the specific influence of the relevant factors of light / colour / space / surface.

The scientific aim of LED-ColourLab is to gain knowledge that can at least be roughly generalised, and which will result in a method of efficient and realistic simulation of the interactions of light, colour, space and surface. The principles for a planning and design tool based on such knowledge, can be used by architects, interior designers, designers, scenographers etc.

The knowledge mentioned above is to be obtained by answering the following questions:

- How is the perception of colours with different LED illumination on surfaces, materials and spatial areas influenced by their material composition?
- How is the perception of colours on surfaces and in spatial areas influenced by LED illumination?
- How is the perception of colours on surfaces and in spatial areas influenced by LED illumination in the spatial arrangement of the illuminated surfaces?
- How do subtractive and additive mixtures of colour and light behave as a result of illumination by and radiation of LED light?

2.2 Method(s)

The above aim is achieved by simulation and evaluation in experimental facilities (referred to as laboratories for the sake of simplicity). The method follows the idea of research through design, which was expressed by Bruce Archer in 1995 as research through practice: "Action Research: Systematic investigation through practical action calculated to devise or test new information, ideas, forms or procedures and to produce communicable knowledge." The design driven experiments were based on specific light and colour measurements and combined with evaluation methods.

In other words, our procedure is a systematic examination of the interaction of design-relevant parameters (light [concentrating here on LED lighting technology], colour, space and surface).

2.2.1 Prototypes and Pilot Methods
The experimental investigations form the basis for the development of pilot methods for visualising dynamic LED technology in interaction with surface colours and coatings and spaces, using the following equipment

- LED-ColourBox: modular system model
- LED-ColourCase: Test room
- LED-ColourInstallations and Laboratory Exhibition: 3-D design

2.3 Transfers to Design Studies

The experimental investigations are evaluated with respect to teaching applications in design studies. Educational concepts have been designed and put into practice, based on development to date, for one module each in the Department of Design / Consolidation of scenographical design and in the BA/MA, teaching art and design.

2.4 Results

We are currently examining the initial results of the series of tests and evaluation for their relevance with respect to the design support tools that are to be developed. Furthermore, we are working on the didactic and scenographic implementation of the results. The exhibition which is at the same time our 3rd research laboatory "Staging LED – colour. Light and colour surfaces in 3D" will be shown from 9 November 2008 – 03 May 2009 at the Gewerbemuseum in Winterthur, Switzerland.

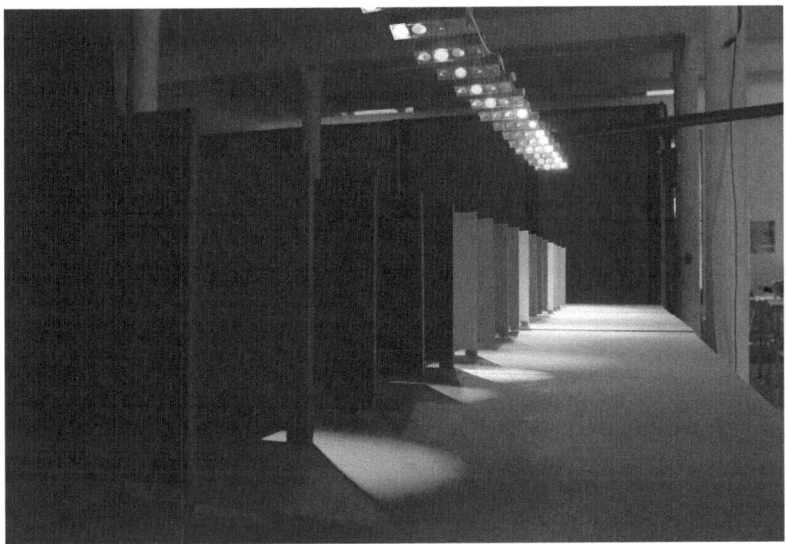

Fig. 1.

The installation "LED colour keyboards" (see model, Fig.1) is one of the exhibits at the "Staging LED – light. Light and coloured surfaces in 3D" exhibition. Dimensions: 2500 x 250 x 260 cm; 15 coloured wall panels; 14x4 RGB- Philips LED Lines; Dynamic Colourlight Score.

References

1. Archer, B.: A view of the nature of design research. In: Jacques, R., Powell, J. (eds.) Design:Science:Method. Westbury House, Guildford (1981)
2. Bachmann, U.: Farben zwischen Licht und Dunkelheit / Colours between light and darkness. Verlag Niggli AG, Sulgen/ Zurich (2006)
3. Bachmann, U., Michel, R.: Hochparterre: Light and Colour Research. Special Ediion Hochparterre Magazine (November 2008)
4. Jonas, W.: Research through DESIGN through research - a problem statement and a conceptual sketch. In: Proceedings of wonderground, DRS international conference, Lisbon (November 2006)
5. Michel, R. (ed.): Design Research Now – Essays and Selected Projects. Birkhäuser, Basel Boston Berlin (2007)
6. Michel, R. (ed.): Forschungslandschaften um Umfeld des Designs. Museum für Gestaltung, Zürich (2005)
7. Michel, R., Léchot, L.: Drawing New Territories - 3rd Design Research Symposium of the Swiss Design Network. Zürich (2006)
8. Schön, D.A.: The Reflective Practitioner. How Professionals Think in Action. Basic Books (1983)
9. Rittel, Horst, W.J.: Second-generation Design Methods. In: Cross, N. (ed.) Developments in Design Methodology. John Wiley, Chichester (1984) (Original 1972)

Color Model for Human Visual Environment and Physical Interaction

Tsutomu Mutoh and Kazuo Ohno

International Media Research Foundation,
Kagurazaka1-1, Shinjuku, 162-0825, Tokyo, Japan
{mutoh,ohno}@imrf.or.jp

Abstract. The authors explored a method to control dynamic RGB light source in accordance with human visual environment and possibilities of physical interaction with light source of full color capabilities. We developed a color model composed of hue, grayscale, brightness components and an algorithm to transform RGB values into the color space of the model. We implemented the color model using full color light emitting diode (LED) in a light source device designed for people to interact with color physically. We set up an experimental environment for human color perception to prove visual and physical interaction effect of dynamic light source and object with color composition governed by the color model and the device.

Keywords: color model, visual interaction, physical interaction, full color LED.

1 Introduction

As one of the color output peripherals of computer, we have light emitting diode (LED) as a light source with comparable range of colors as digital RGB monitor to display information in characters, images, motion pictures. Cost of LED device unit has been reduced and its usability including the lifetime improved, and we occasionally see a modern architecture being illuminated by huge numbers of them.

In the history of illustration, art and craft, human being started expression by scratching cave walls with stone or charcoal, then invented lampblack, pigment from ground minerals or dye and methods to deposit them with oil or glue on such media as paper (papyrus), animal skins (parchment or vellum), clay boards or wood walls, textiles, glasses. In modern age of communication, product and industrial design, colors are obtained by elaborative process of mixture of chemical ink and paint to be fixed on paper, metal or plastic. They are selected and designed to show colors under sunlight or a light environment of expecting space for the object to be used or placed. Those reflecting object colors are analyzed by the three pure colors of cyan, magenta, yellow, called subtractive primary and synthesized by their subtractive mixture. Color solid based on such as Munsell color appearance system (1912) [1], for example, organizes object colors by three dimension values of hue, value (lightness), chroma.

Contrary to the long history of color of object, candles, beautiful stained glass of churches from medieval era or gas street lamp as precedents, color control of light source or lighting design has been only ventured on the latter years of 20th century

B.-T. Karsh (Ed.): Ergonomics and Health Aspects, HCII 2009, LNCS 5624, pp. 268–275, 2009.
© Springer-Verlag Berlin Heidelberg 2009

along the development of new type of light systems such as halogen lamp, high intensity discharge lamps such as mercury, high pressure sodium and metal halide lamp including recent laser or fiber optical technology and their combination or arrangement technique.

The color of light source consists of three pure stimuli of red (R), green (G) and blue (B) called additive primary and are synthesized by their additive mixture. CIE standard colorimetric reference system (1932) is the standard system to organize and specify color of light by three dimension components derived by RGB values.

But in actual world of lighting design, hue of light source color is decided by selection of type of light bulbs and their mixture which are measured by color temperature or described by the term of color rendition. Vivid hue of light has been obtained by tinted bulbs as ornament, by neon sign as advertisement in a dark environment, or by color screen filters in theater, but their numbers and sequence of color hue change are limited in several patterns. Only continuous changes in brightness and saturation are obtained simultaneously by control of power supply.

Computer displays are limited in size for human visual field but are able to control one million pixels independently in ten million different colors, each of them more than ten times in a second. Full color LED's consist of RGB luminous elements invented late 20th century are catching up those displays in speed and color varieties, and they are improving in brightness to replace lighting bulbs as light source in public space or living environment.

It is not difficult to light a LED device on and off by setting RGB value. If you develop a program to choose a series of color, set the corresponding RGB values and send them sequentially or randomly to LED output from computer, you can obtain a dynamic color source. A couple of commercial products implemented such function are already found on market. But if you plan to design a continuous change of color hue from one to the other responded to dynamic input data, or design subtle color changes such as expression of the sky at sunrise or sunset, we have few design principles other than prescribed cell animation technique.

Although we have systems to organize and describe colors of static object or static light source, we do not have much knowledge about:

– Color system for visual interactive environment to harmonize dynamic light source and object
– Interface to control dynamic light source color

In this paper, we explore these problems in a color model to control RGB light source and design an interactive device based on current computer and LED technology.

2 Optical Tone Color Model

Human being perceives color in lightness, hue and chroma. On the other hand, color outputs from device such as computer monitor or full color LED are light which consist of red, green and blue by additive mixture color method. To adjust RGB values for computers to control colors visually for human being, we must be sensitive the difference and find a practical way to manipulate colors by numbers.

If you imagine you are in a living room and able to select one color for the room light and to change hues continuously, it will be preferable their brightness to be constant for smoothness in the eye. Current sequences of color hue change, typically observed at popular live music spaces, ignore brightness control and the light stimuli will be perceived uneven to eyes time to time. To remove this discomfort, we explore a color model focused on constant brightness as the first principle.

The brightness value b is defined by RGB values using the luminous coefficients (α, β, γ) unique to the device and defined by CIE standard.

$$b = \alpha R + \beta G + \gamma B \qquad (1)$$

Then we collect constant brightness colors on a flat plane and arrange their pure colors around a hue circle. Hue is defined by the ratio of RGB value and pure colors are a set of hues that have the largest difference in RGB values. Our color model is intended to use in a visual environment coexisting of dynamic source color and object colors, we selected a color system to arrange hues based on psychological four primary colors of red(R), green(G) , blue(B) and yellow(Y) harmonizing additive primary for light source and subtractive primary for static objects. Practical Color Coordinate System (PCCS) defined by Japan Color Research Institute [2] is one of the widely accepted system in designing color tone of objects in Japan. We interpolate and extend 24 hue values of the PCCS color system to 256 of hue values h, and allocate pure colors around the hue circle for each brightness value plane (2).

Fig. 1 illustrates the difference of RGB value distribution for a hue circle in HSB (hue, saturation, value for brightness) color model [4] and for a hue circle of a constant brightness value in PCCS color model.

If you keep brightness value constant and increase the maximum value from RGB, and decrease the minimum value to the intermediate one, you reach a gray (no color) of the brightness. The grays should be located on the center of color circles for each brightness value. Mixed colors of the same brightness will be distributed on a circle from the center for gray and to circumference for pure colors according to its grayness. The value in radial dimension defines the grayscale g of colors (3).

Thus we obtain a color model named "Optical Tone color model" defined by hue, grayscale and brightness (h, g, b) components. A color represented by RGB values will be transformed to hgb and allocated in a cylindrical space defined by color circle of constant brightness stacked by its gray value from black to white in height. Grayish colors are located near the center axis, and pure colors on circumference of the cylindrical space.

Color circles from three types of color model are illustrated in Fig. 2. The lowest ones are Johannes Itten's 12-hue color circles in which yellow, red and blue are specified as primary colors and arranged complement colors in opposite diagonals [3]. The uppermost ones are HSB hue color circles consist of RGB additive primary colors and obtained by linear mixture of the RGB values (Fig. 1). The middle ones are of the Optical Tone color model which maintain complementary characteristics with diagonal colors and their brightness in a circle as constant. On HSB model, hues are defined by proportional RGB ratios, but we observe in the diagram the brightness is not constant on a circle. Johannes Itten's model is visually proportional but numerical continuity is broken in a circle and hard to manipulate by computers. The Optical Tone color model is designed in visually proportional still computational to control hues.

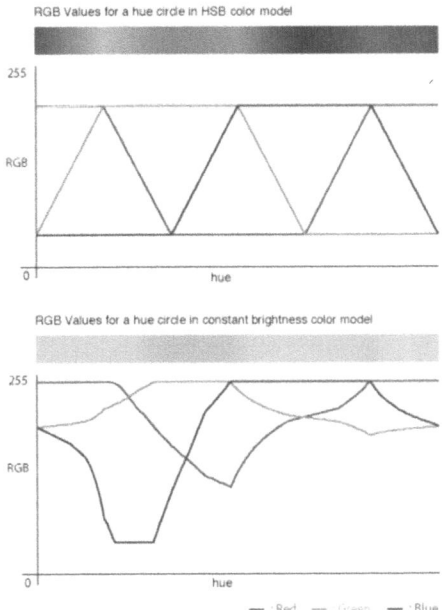

Fig. 1. RGB value distribution for HSB and constant brightness hue circle

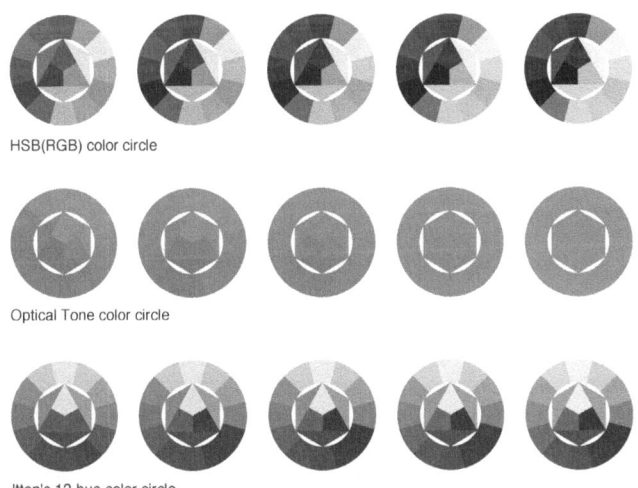

Fig. 2. Color circles based on HSB, Optical Tone and Itten's color model

If you transform RGB values to *hgb* by the algorithm with process (1)(2)(3) described above, you are able to manipulate a color of light independently along hue (*h*), grayscale (*g*) and brightness (*b*) in the Optical Tone color model space. If you specify one color in the Optical Tone color space (a point in *hgb* space) and inversely transform the *hgb* values to RGB, you are able to obtain the adjusted color emission of the hue, grayscale, brightness from RGB device. If a point moves around in the Optical Tone color space (*h(t), g(t), b(t)*), the LED will perform dynamic color emission accordingly. Fig. 3 shows the RGB-*hgb* transformation diagram.

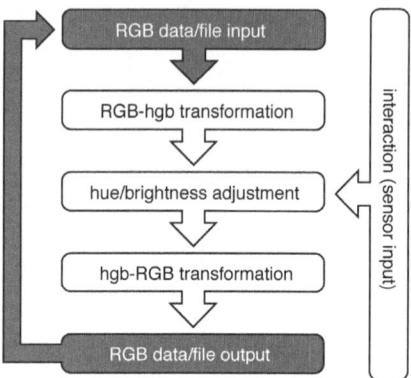

Fig. 3. RGB-*hgb* transformation diagram

Typical lighting controller of today for a single color light bulb regulates power supply by slider or rotator to control intensity of illumination. If the Optical Tone color model is applied to a RGB light source such as LED device and RGB-*hgb* transform algorithm is implemented, you are able to control the hue, brightness, grayscale of the light independently. If you follow the cylindrical space and dimension of Optical Tone color model, you may able to assign your arm motion of rotating action to change of hue, of vertical action to brightness and of horizontal action to gray scale, for example, to control light source color of a RGB output device.

3 Physical Interaction with Optical Tone Color Model

To prove perceptional and psychological smoothness of the Optical Tone color model for dynamic color environment, we designed and manufactured a light source object (Optical Tone light source device) that allows us to control hue and brightness of light intuitively by physical interaction.

The basic concept of the Optical Tone light source device is a tumbler (Fig. 4). The top globe implemented LED light is designed as same shape and same size as the bottom part (250 mm in diameter). The twos are connected by a metal rod (1150 mm in height). The shape has an effect for people to draw their visual attention to the top part and give them an impression of a globe emitting color light floating in the dark. The weight in the bottom (approximately 11kg) is carefully adjusted to balance and to provide a comfortable response when people touch and push the top to swing at a moderate period. In the bottom, a three-axes acceleration sensor is embedded and detects swinging motion to control color output of LED's (6 units, 3W for each). The *hgb*-RGB algorithm transfers round motion of the device to hue control and swing

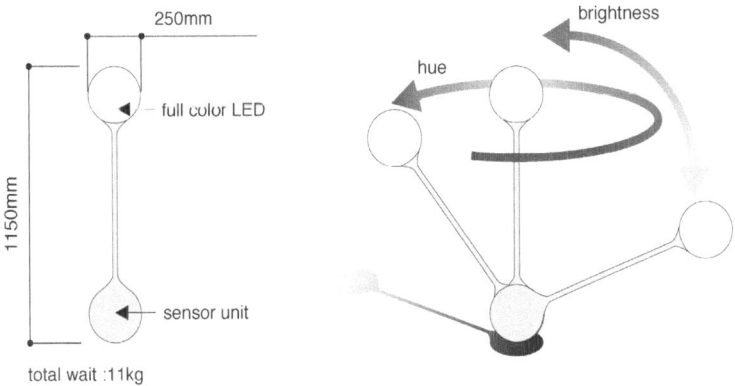

Fig. 4. Optical Tone dynamic light source device

motion to brightness control in accordance with the Optical Tone color model. Fig. 4 shows dimension and color control of the Optical Tone device. The device allows people to interact physically with color dynamism in the Optical Tone color space.

4   Visual Interaction Experiment of Optical Tone Color Model

As Optical Tone color model is based on hue circle of PCCS color system composed from psychological four primary colors, and the model provide a method to control light source color with constant brightness, it is applicable in designing visual environment to harmonize light source of full color capability and color of objects (products or printing materials) in a space.

As an experiment of visual interaction, we set up in a closed dark space several Optical Tone devices which function as dynamic light source based on the Optical Tone color model with graphically composed walls which function as a static reflecting object governed by the same Optical Tone color model (Fig. 5).

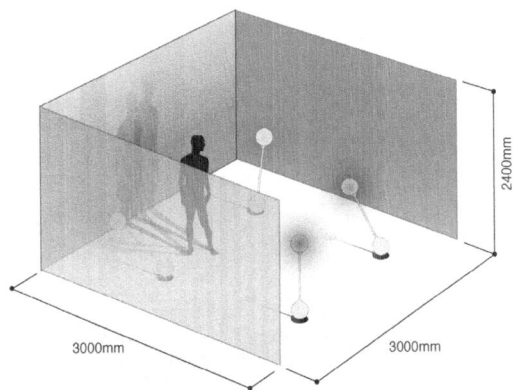

Fig. 5. Experimental space for visual interaction based on Optical Tone color model

The wall graphic pattern consists of vertical stripes to be visually effective with Optical Tone light source which swings horizontally (Fig. 6). To disturb human color perception of foreground and background of the pattern, we designed stripes of same width and in a complicated color combination for each side, and the height of them to be tall enough to cover the viewer's perspective. To maximize the visual effect of reflection of dynamic light source, we kept the lightness of each stripe color as a constant. The chromas of them are adjusted to arouse a sense of visual resistiveness and sense of depth in dimension. 3 side walls covered by stripes with large dynamic hue range are intended to produce a spectacles of color interaction with dynamic lights from several swinging devices at a time. The graphic patterns are printed on a large size paper by a printer in our office and pasted on the walls.

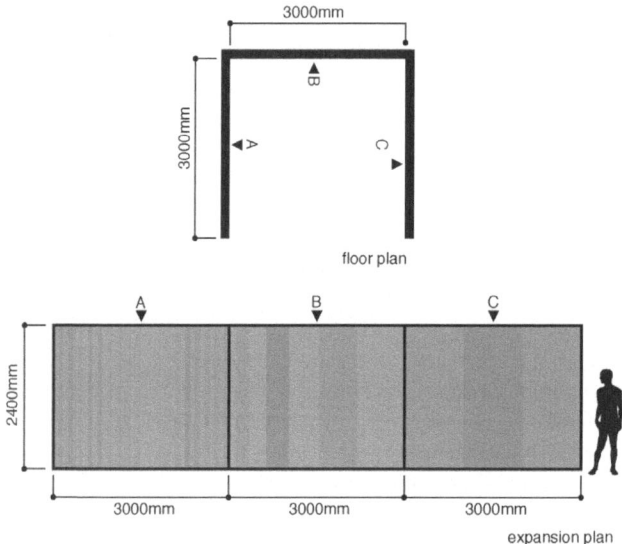

Fig. 6. Wall graphic for visual interaction experiment

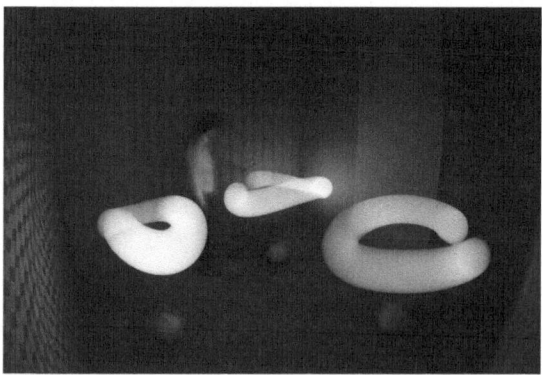

Fig. 7. Visual interaction of dynamic light source and static object

The experiments for visual interaction are carried out as art installation style in several places [5] (Fig. 7) but not under a strict scientific control.
The observations at the experimental spaces are:

- comfortable motion and dynamism of color by intuitive physical interaction with Optical Tone device draws not a least interests of people.
- illusions of colors by visual interaction between the dynamic color of light and wall graphics are perceived spectacularly.

Some people refer to playfulness, healing effect, communication inviting characteristics of the device. Others check the relation between globe position of the device and hue and brightness of the light by rotating or swinging. Some of them confirmed such visual perception phenomena as complementary characteristics or color consistency in the experimental space.

5 Conclusion

Expecting visual environment of dynamic full color light with static object coexistence in a living space of near future, the authors developed a color model based on color circle harmonized for light and material and focused on smoothness of brightness. The color model is implemented in a light source device controllable along hue and brightness by intuitive physical interaction. The experiments are carried out in a space surrounded by graphic walls composed by the same color model. Comfortable responsibility of physical interaction to control color by the device and optical illusion caused by visual interaction between the dynamic light source and the wall object are observed at a considerable level. The methodology is to be explored in further application to lighting product or visual communication.

References

1. Munsell Color Company: Book of Color. Munsell Color Company. Baltimore MD (1976)
2. Japan Color Research Institute: Digital Color Manual. Creo. Tokyo (2004)
3. Itten, J.: The Elements of Color: A Treatise on the Color System of Johannes Itten. Van Nostrand Reinhold, New York (1971)
4. Smith, A.R.: Color Gamut Transform Pairs. In: SIGGRAPH 1978, pp. 12–19 (1978)
5. Mutoh, T.: Optical Trajectory 2. NTT Inter Communication Center. Tokyo (2007); Mutoh, T.: Optical Tone. In: Ars Electronica Festival, CyberArts 2008. Linz (2008); Mutoh, T.: Optical Tone: Dynamic Color Composition. In: SIGGRAPH 2008, New Tech Demo, Los Angeles (2008)

Improvement of the Design Quality of 3D-Input Devices Using Motion Analyses and Biomechanical Comparisons

Tobias Nowack[2], Stefan Lutherdt[1], Manuel Möller[1], Peter Kurtz[2], and Hartmut Witte[1]

[1] Ilmenau University of Technology, Dept. of Biomechatronics, Ilmenau
[2] Ilmenau University of Technology, Dept. of Working Sciences, Ilmenau
PF 10 05 65, 98684 Ilmenau, Germany
tobias.nowack@tu-ilmenau.de, stefan.lutherdt@tu-ilmenau.de,
peter.kurtz@tu-ilmenau.de, hartmut.witte@tu-ilmenau.de

Abstract. Due to the lack of investigations and standards describing the design of real 3D input devices a real 3D input device was develop. To compare several devices a test task was created and performed with combination of a motion capturing system. During the experiment 19 attendees with different levels of experience performed the test with this setup. Several intra-individual motion patterns and using strategies belonging to different input devices could be observed.

Keywords: User-centred design, 3D-input, evaluation software, reachable space of motion, ergonomically motivated equipment, motion analyses of input tasks.

1 Introduction and Motivation

International standard DIN ISO 9241-400 (last version 2007) describes principles and requirements for physical input devices. One of these principles is to minimize biomechanical strains, but there is no explanation how to reach this goal. Typically input devices (and in our case 3D-input devices as well) are evaluated during the stage of development by different usability test methods, like questionnaire-based test tasks. These predominately subjective evaluations indicate physical strain of the hand–arm–shoulder-system to be very high. But no simple relation to the objective parameters describing usability (course accuracy and handling time) could be identified [1]

Our hand is a tool adapted to "manipulation", a multitude of functions, most of which yet are even unknown, but not optimized for "indirect" manipulation of computer devices. But in a lot of industrial applications it is necessary to use indirect manipulations due to "wrong" size (too big or too small), dangerous environmental conditions or security aspects which provokes a few diverse discrepancies. Thus for industrially used machines it is necessary to have a control by human computer interfaces, does mean brain-hand-computer interfaces, where functions of brain and hand are coupled in mostly (yet) unknown manner. Present input devices for such interfaces restrict movements of the hand in comparison with direct manipulation, and in contrast to common 3D-use of hands. These restrictions force to develop attitudes of usage which never are comfortable or ergonomically.

B.-T. Karsh (Ed.): Ergonomics and Health Aspects, HCII 2009, LNCS 5624, pp. 276–285, 2009.

In 2007 the International Standard on "Ergonomics of human-machine-interaction – Part 400: Principles and requirements for physical input devices" (ISO 9241-400) had been published as well as "Part 410: Design criteria for physical input devices" (ISO 9241-410). In these documents only generic ergonomic principles are given without any kind of data or evaluation criteria [3]. For 1D and 2D input devices literature gives good advices how the device should be constructed (see [4]). Krauss in 2003 [5] published an evaluation concept for 2D pointing devices.

During the last years several tests have been created to measure usability aspects of input devices with more than 2 input dimensions. One of these tests used at Ilmenau University of Technology is a migration of Krauss' tests tasks from 2D to 3D environments [6]. This test has been developed on the basic usability criteria "effectiveness, efficiency and satisfaction".

Within these experiments applied to the as well in Ilmenau developed 3D input device "*Haptor*" [7] several tests were performed. The results of these first studies are based on questionnaires and subjective impressions. Only time to solve the tasks (duration) could be objectified. After first tests it becomes obvious that it is necessary to measure more parameters than demanded by the basic test tasks. Therefore we extended the setup to measure motions and current positions of input devices, to allow to compare them kinematically.

2   Description of Experiments

2.1   Test Equipment and Setup

All experiments were executed in a laboratory protected against physical and psychological disturbances by other people, noise, machines or mechanical systems. The only confounder besides the presence of measuring systems was the laboratory temperature, because during winter time we were not able to securely assure living room temperature.

The measuring system used was a passive infrared motion capturing system called *ProReflex* from Swedish company *Qualisys® AB*. This system consists of 6 IR-cameras, IR-reflecting (passive) spherical markers and a laptop with the measuring software necessary to record and analyze motion data. The software used for recording was *Qualisys Track Manager* (QTM version 1.9.254). Analyzes also were made with *QTM*, with *Microsoft® Excel2007*, with *SPSS v.14* and *Matlab® R2007b*.

Fig. 1. shows the whole setup with the used hardware components, without experimentees and test executives.

The above-mentioned test setup was prepared and tested for this special task within a pre-test stage over several months before the experiments started. During this time all influences of the system by the laboratory were minimized; the setup was adjusted, tested and finally recorded to ensure the reproducibility of the setup in later stages of (re-)experiments.

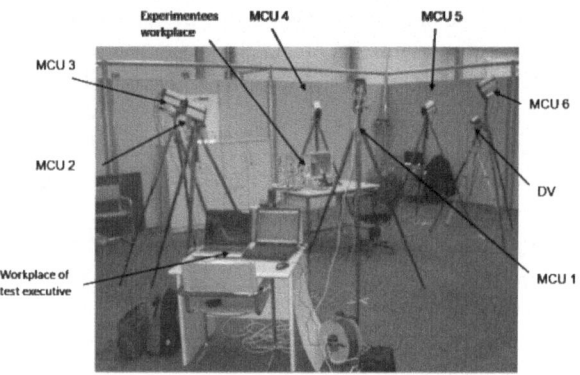

Fig. 1. Test setup for motion analyses with *Qualisys*® *ProReflex*

2.2 Objects of Investigation

During the tests the motions and motion ranges used by the utilization of three different input devices for the same standardized input task was investigated. These input devices were two market available pseudo 3D input devices: a gamepad from *Hama* and a joystick from *Saitek* (see fig. 2a and 2b). They are called "pseudo-3D" because only two axes are controllable at the same by one hand and one input action; the third axis had to be controlled by the other hand via an additional input element (a second mini-joystick and a throttle). Normally the gamepad is able to control 6 DOF (joystick 5 DOF), but ever only two dimensions at the same time. Both devices are angle based, but the test software generates a test task in which only the dead stop in each direction and the central position is necessary to be used. Therefore both devices can be compared with the *Haptor* as (discretely) "translation based" input devices.

In the gamepad input device, x- and y-axes can be simultaneously controlled by the right mini joystick; z-axis has to be controlled by left mini joystick. Both joysticks are self-resetting to their initial central position by small springs. These springs impresses a light force which is not perceivable during use. The design of this gamepad (and others) is so that the user has only one way to hold and use it: with both hands and the thumbs forming input elements. The kind of use (hands-free, partially or totally propped) was not dictated and could be changed during the test too.

In *Saitek's* joystick the big shaft was used to control x- and y-axes and the throttle for z-axis. The small knob at the top is also a mini joystick but was not used in tests. The shaft is self-resetting to the initial center position by a spring, and this center position is well perceivable. The throttle has no perceivable position and is not self-resetting. The attendees could not use the joystick with their preferred hand because the necessity of controlling the throttle with the left hand (thumb or two fingers). The position on the table was not fixed; therewith the attendees could adjust the distance between them and the device to their physical needs.

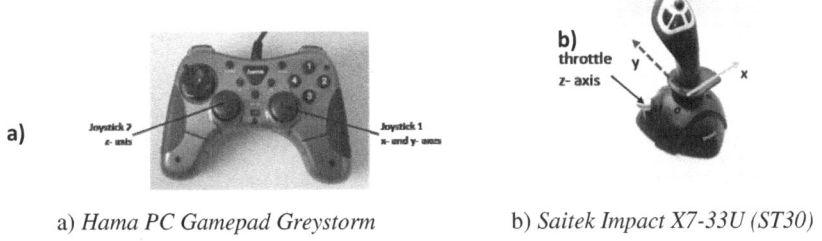

a) *Hama PC Gamepad Greystorm*   b) *Saitek Impact X7-33U (ST30)*

Fig. 2. Input devices tested

The third input device investigated was a prototype of the self-developed real 3D input device called *Haptor*, from the Dept. of Working Sciences of the Ilmenau University of Technology (see fig. 3). All axes at this device can be controlled by one hand at the same time. The additional throttle function (for speed acceleration) of arm rest was not used during these tests. The grip (and therewith the coupling point between human and machine) is represented by a ball. All three axes are not self-resetting and have no perceivable center position. Irrespective to the handiness, all the attendees had to use their left hand for input actions.

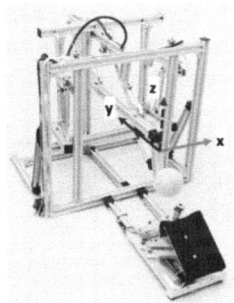

Fig. 3. Self-developed *Haptor* (Dept. of Working Sciences, TU Ilmenau) [7]

2.3 Test Software and Test Tasks Performed

To allow a standardization of the tests and to make the results comparable the experimentees had to perform a software given test task (see fig. 4). During this test they had to approach several goals marked by red dots. The current position was marked by green dots, and the whole test space was a cube with an edge length of 1024 pixel. The test consists of nine subtasks formed by translations from start via eight defined points to stop (which was equal to start position, for the whole test task see Tab. 1). The time to solve the test task was not restricted, but measured as "duration". The test software writes a log file with a timestamp (in milliseconds), the position in x-, y- and z-coordinates (increments) and a marker "ze" for "goal reached". These data have been written to file whenever new data were available at the USB interface.

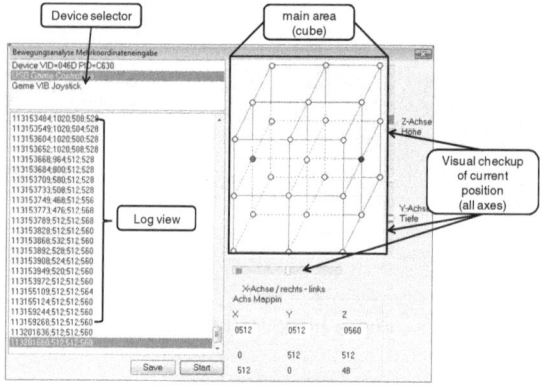

Fig. 4. Test Software

To support the experimentees during the tests, esp. to use the *Haptor* without other possibilities to control the spatial position, additional visual checkups were added on the right and bottom side of the main area.

Table 1. Description of subtasks

	No. of subtask	Starting point (x;y;z)	Goal (x;y;z)
	0	Undef.	P1
		Undef.	(512;0;512)
	1	P1	P2
		(512;0;512)	(512;1024;512)
	2	P2	P3
		(512;1024;512)	(1024;512;512)
	3	P3	P4
		(1024;512;512)	(0;512;512)
	4	P4	P5
		(0;512;512)	(0;1024;1024)
	5	P5	P6
		(0;1024;1024)	(1024;0;0)
	6	P6	P7
		(1024;0;0)	(0;0;0)
	7	P7	P8
		(0;0;0)	(1024;1024;1024)
	8	P8	P9
		(1024;1024;1024)	(512;512;512)

Fig. 5

Due to hard- and software specificities not all input devices could reach the maximum of 1024 increments as well as the minimum of zero increments, according to the pixels of the cube shown. It was necessary to create an area of about 60 increments (depending on the type of input device) as a trapping area around the goal, which was accepted as "goal reached".

2.4 Characterization of Experimentees (Test Subjects)

The tests were performed with 19 attendees (14 male, 5 female) with a mean age of 23.5 years (range 19 from to 30 years). Two of the attendees are left-handed (but this was not considered as a co-factor). All of them stated that they were in good physical condition without any discomfort or diseases of neck-shoulder-arm-hand system. The anthropometric data of the attendees were measured three times each, as well before and after the tests. The anthropometric data measured were tested for normal distribution and statistical deviations to the control data of DIN [8] and [9].

Because the attendees were a highly selected group (students) they could not match the means of the German overall population. Standard t-test confirmed significant differences ($p < 0.05$).

2.5 Experimental Chain

Each test started with an explanation of the whole experiment to the attendees, and a short training period with each input device, if necessary. Afterwards the first two measurements of anthropometric data were conducted. After this 22 IR-reflecting spherical markers were fixed at shoulder and arms like described in [10]. Additional five markers were fixed at each hand (shown in fig. 5), and three markers at the head (both temples and chin, see fig. 6). The points to fix the markers were palpated, but the markers could not be applied at bare bodies of attendees because of the low temperature.

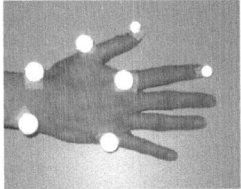

Fig. 5. Position of the hand markers

The investigator started the test software and the motion capturing system for the first run, the order of devices was: joystick, gamepad, *Haptor*. After this run the test person had to perform some physical actions (static: hold a weight of 2.5 kg in each hand; dynamic: squeeze a spring dumb-ball with a compression force of 100 N by each hand). Then the whole test was repeated. The second test additionally has been videotaped.

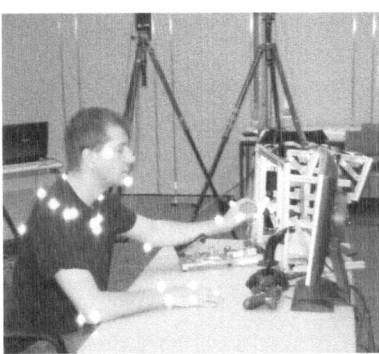

Fig. 6. An experimentee performing the test (with *Haptor*)

2.6 Aims, Hypotheses and Methods

With the experiment described at first we simply but necessarily tried to test whether a motion capturing system with passive IR-markers is appropriate to investigate motions occurring during the use of 3D input devices. A second aim was to investigate the usefulness of different input devices for 3D input tasks by the use of standardized tests.

The hypotheses for the first experimental stage were:

1. For each input device different patterns are detectable and characterizable.
2. Due to the different design of the devices investigated the duration and the time to execute discrete parts of the tests differ.
3. Individuals have different motion patterns, but remodeled by the device used.
4. These patterns also depend on the grade of experience with such devices.
5. The patterns change after a provoked fatigue.

To test the hypotheses motion capturing system (*QTM*) data were collected and conditioned. Synchronously log-file data were recorded and also conditioned, especially adequately scaled to *QTM* data. Afterwards relevant *QTM* data (data of markers at the elbow, wrist, fingers, acromium and vertebra C7) were filtered and their specific velocities and accelerations were calculated (by *MATLAB* routines with algorithms taken from [11]). All data chosen were tested with statistic standard methods.(by *SPSS*).

3 Results

3.1 Analyses of Hardware Log-Files

Haptor shows up to be the slowest input device (as well what concerns point-to-point as overall duration of task) shown in fig. 7, but on the other hand deviations between demanded and realized trajectories are lower than in the two other devices, as long as real 3D-movements (including a z-component like in subtasks four to seven like shown in fig. 8) are on demand.

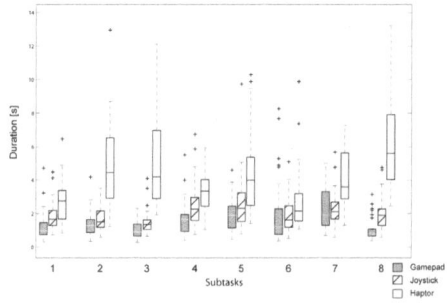

Fig. 7. Comparison of subtask duration of all input devices

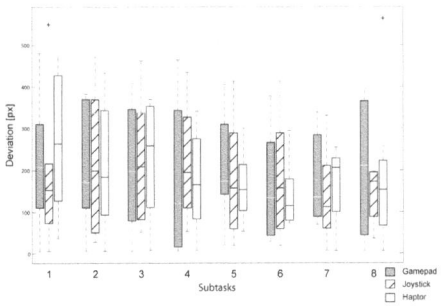

Fig. 8. Comparison of subtask deviations of all investigated devices

3.2 Analyses of QTM®-Data

In all trials, no significant motion of the upper body (represented by marker C7) could be observed. Observable kinematics were restricted to hand-arm-system.

Vice versa mobility was realized by giving up fixation of wrist, in extreme visible in case of *Haptor*, where the lift of the arm from the hand rest is represented by lift of elbow and extension of wrist joint (cf. fig. 9). All attendees used hand rest had also negative values of lifting but a smaller range of wrist joint angle than attendees which are had not used the rest. The extension of wrist joint were significantly lower at attendees which are had not used the rest.

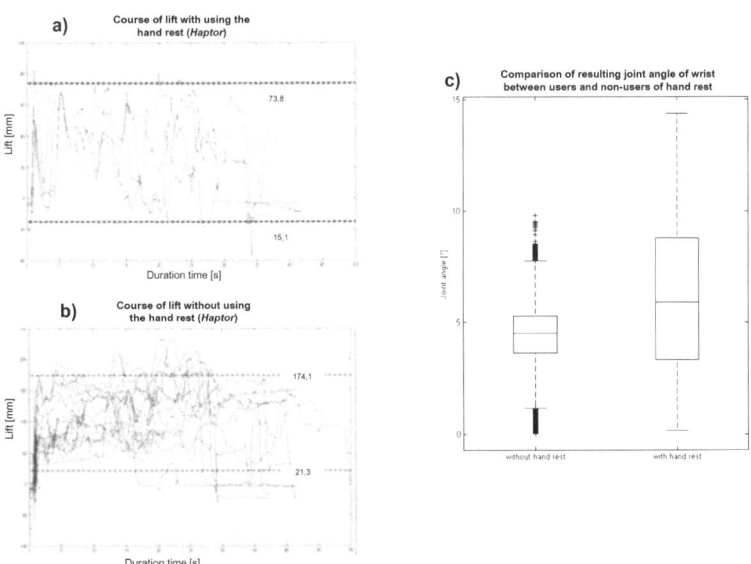

Fig. 9. (a) Lift of attendees using the hand rest, (b) Lift of attendees not using the hand rest, (c) Comparison of resulting wrist joint angle of both

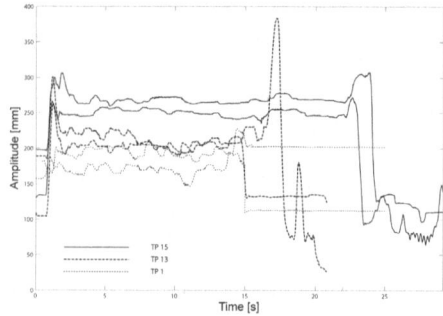

Fig. 10. Intra-individual patterns of three experimentees at a gamepad (right thumb, x-component *QTM* data)

Intra-individual patterns of kinematics did not occur systematically, but were observable in a subset of experimentees (fig. 10).

Another pattern could be abstracted: In case of gamepad, experienced users ("gamers") keep contact to the mini-joysticks only during "action", as long as a position is intended to be kept thumbs are lifted (fig. 11). This is represented by peaks which are correlated with reversal points of the logged input action.

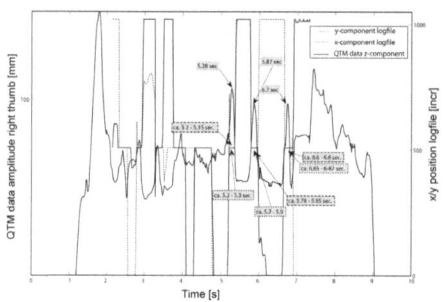

Fig. 11. Effect of thumb lifting at an experienced gamepad user

No effects of fatigue could be shown.

4 Discussion

The missing observation of fatigue effects indicates that our "loading" of experimentees was too low – obviously today usage of computer mice provokes a general training effect on endurance of hand-arm-system.

None of the devices analyzed provided observable inter-individual patterns. The occurrence of intra-individual patterns in subsets of the experiments indicates the adaptivity of users to devices – primary goal of ergonomics is the adaptation of devices to the physiology (and thus needs) of users.

From our bionic synthesis of manipulative robots we know, that human grasping (and as well pointing) at minimum is composed of two atavistic factors:

1. reaching, performed by long elements (lower arm, upper arm, scapula),
2. grasping *sensu strictu*, performed by the hand

Both functions in the multifunctional human hand-arm-systems are adapted to a variety of yet not completely identifiable, partly diverging tasks, leading to compromises in structure and control. To mirror that nature given boundaries into human-machine-interfaces in future more intensely has to be based on function-morphological knowledge on reaching and grasping. Thus in our experiments in the next steps we shall focus on human and primate biology incl. handiness more than on technical devices.

References

1. Nowack, T., Kurtz, P., Lutherdt, S.: Ergonomische Gestaltung eines 3D-Eingabegerätes und Evaluation des Bedienkomforts. (Ergonomic design of a 3D-input device and evaluation of operational comfort. Only in German) In: Technische Universität (Hg.): Arbeitsgestaltung für KMU. Ilmenau: ISLE (Herbstkonferenz der Gesellschaft für Arbeitswissenschaft e.V.), pp. S.249–S.256 (2008)
2. DIN ISO 9241-410: Ergonomie der Mensch-System-Interaktion - Teil 410: Gestaltungskriterien für physikalische Eingabegeräte. DIN e. V. Berlin, Beuth (2008)
3. Keller Chandra, S., Hoehne-Hückstädt, U., Ellegast, R.: BGIA- Report 3/2008. Ergonomische Anforderungen an Eingabemittel für Geräte der Informationstechnik. BGIA- Institut für Arbeitsschutz der Deutschen Gesetzlichen Unfallversicherungen, Sankt Augustin (2008)
4. Krauss, L.: Entwicklung und Evaluation einer Methodik zur Untersuchung von Interaktionsgeräten für Maschinen- und Prozessbediensysteme mit grafischen Benutzungsoberflächen. Universität Kaiserslautern, Diss. (2003)
5. Nowack, T., Lutherdt, S., Gramsch, T., Kurtz, P.: An Evaluation Study for a 3D Input Device Based on Ergonomic Design Criteria. In: Dainoff, M.J. (ed.) HCII 2007 and EHAWC 2007. LNCS, vol. 4566, pp. 257–266. Springer, Heidelberg (2007)
6. Nowack, T., Kurtz, P., Lutherdt, S., Gramsch, T., et al.: Design of an Evaluation Study for 3D Input Devices. In: Proc. of the 9th ERCIM Workshop User Interfaces For All (UI4All), Königswinter (2006)
7. Nowack, T.F., Kurtz, P., Gramsch, T., Lutherdt, S., Schäfer, S.: Ergonomisch motiviertes 3D-Eingabegerät - "Haptor". In: Restorff, W.v. (ed.) Forum Arbeitsphysiologie 10. Symposium Arbeitsphysiologie für Nachwuchswissenschaftler, München, p. S20 (2006)
8. DIN 33402-2: Ergonomie – Körpermaße des Menschen - Teil 2: Werte. Deutsches Institut für Normung e. V.Berlin, Beuth Verlag GmbH (2005)
9. Flügel, B., Greil, H., Sommer, K.: Anthropolog. Atlas. Frankfurt/M. Edition Wötzel (1986)
10. Wu, G., van der Helm, F.C., Veeger, H.E., Makhsous, M., Van Roy, P., Anglin, C., Nagels, J., Karduna, A.R., McQuade, K., Wang, X., Werner, F.W., Buchholz, B.: ISB recommendation on definitions of joint coordinate systems of various joints for the reporting of human joint motion–Part II: shoulder, elbow, wrist and hand. J. Biomech. 38, Seite, 981–992 (2005)
11. Andrada, E.: A new model of the human trunk mechanics in walking. In: Berichte aus der Biomechatronik. Witte, H. (Hs.) Fachgebiet Biomechatronik an der TU Ilmenau Band 1, Ilmenau, Universitätsverlag (2008)

Author Index